Surgical Principles in Inguinal Hernia Repair

Melissa Phillips LaPinska
Jeffrey A. Blatnik
Editors

Surgical Principles in Inguinal Hernia Repair

A Comprehensive Guide to Anatomy and Operative Techniques

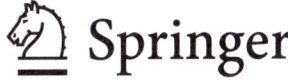 Springer

Editors
Melissa Phillips LaPinska
Department of Surgery
University of Tennessee Health Science
Center
Knoxville
TN, USA

Jeffrey A. Blatnik
Department of Surgery
Washington University Medical Center
Department of Surgery
St Louis
MO, USA

ISBN 978-3-030-06540-9   ISBN 978-3-319-92892-0   (eBook)
https://doi.org/10.1007/978-3-319-92892-0

This Springer imprint is published by the registered company Springer Nature Switzerland AG
The registered company address is: Gewerbestrasse 11, 6330 Cham, Switzerland

To our surgical mentors for helping us stand on the shoulders of giants – especially Dr. Bruce Schirmer, Dr. Jeff Ponsky, and Dr. Jeff Marks – and to our family for loving us as we share our time with teaching others.

Preface

Inguinal hernia repair remains one of the most commonly performed operation in the United States and internationally. The multiple surgical procedures that have been described to address this show the challenge that surgeons face on a daily basis – that is, there is not a single "best" operation to suit a wide variety of patients with significantly different clinical scenarios. Currently, texts have addressed the ventral and incisional hernias, but there has not been a comprehensive guide to the management of the inguinal hernia, which represents a large number of surgical procedures performed. *Surgical Principles in Inguinal Hernia Repair* has been written by many of the key leaders in hernia surgery with the hopes of being able to share not only the latest literature but also the "tricks and tips" that really make up the details of these surgical procedures. It presents a curriculum for basic and common general surgery procedures while detailing the complex scenarios in which one can encounter an inguinal hernia such as in the setting of bowel injury or contamination or in a patient needing prostatectomy. The technical details including online access to surgical videos are discussed for many different scenarios. It is our hope that this text will guide the reader to consider and learn to apply each of these surgical techniques to optimize their individual patient as the center of the surgical choice in management of the inguinal hernia. The text also addresses important topics for the community and academic surgeon, such as the training of residents in inguinal hernia and the importance in surgeon kept outcome data. This book would not be possible without the help of each author who has contributed his or her time and effort in the submission of the individual chapters and the publishing team at Springer for their guidance and direction in this project. *Surgical Principles in Inguinal Hernia Repair* will be an invaluable resource to the practicing general and trauma surgeon including residents and fellows in these areas. On behalf of my coeditor and I, we hope you enjoy *Surgical Principles in Inguinal Hernia Repair.*

Knoxville, TN, USA Melissa Phillips LaPinska
St Louis, MO, USA Jeffrey A. Blatnik

Contents

Contributors

Gina L. Adrales Department of Surgery, Johns Hopkins Hospital, Johns Hopkins University School of Medicine, Baltimore, MD, USA

Vamsi V. Alli Division of Minimally Invasive and Bariatric Surgery, Department of Surgery, Penn State Hershey Medical Center, Hershey, PA, USA

Mariah Alexander Beasley University of Tennessee School of Medicine, Department of Surgery, Knoxville, TN, USA

David J. Berler Resident in General Surgery, Icahn School of Medicine at Mount Sinai, New York, NY, USA

Jeffrey A. Blatnik Section of Minimally Invasive Surgery, Department of Surgery, Washington University School of Medicine, St. Louis, MO, USA

Vandana Botta University of Tennessee School of Medicine, Memphis, TN, USA

Michael Bottros Department of Anesthesiology, Washington University School of Medicine, St. Louis, MO, USA

Benjamin Carr Department of Surgery, University of Michigan, Ann Arbor, MI, USA

Nicholas H. Carter Department of Surgery, Vanderbilt University Medical Center, Nashville, TN, USA

David C. Chen Lichtenstein Amid Hernia Clinic, David Geffen School of Medicine at UCLA, Los Angeles, CA, USA

Sherard Chiu Department of Surgery, University of Tennessee Graduate school of Medicine, Knoxville, TN, USA

Domenic R. Craner Akron Children's Hospital, Department of Pediatric Surgery, Akron, OH, USA

Ian C. Glenn Akron Children's Hospital, Department of Pediatric Surgery, Akron, OH, USA

Matthew I. Goldblatt Medical College of Wisconsin, Milwaukee, WI, USA

Brian P. Jacob Icahn School of Medicine at Mount Sinai, New York, NY, USA

Garth R. Jacobsen University of California San Diego, San Diego, CA, USA

David M. Krpata Cleveland Clinic Comprehensive Hernia Center, Digestive Disease and Surgery Institute, Cleveland Clinic Foundation, Cleveland, OH, USA

Sepehr Lalezari Johns Hopkins University Bayview Medical Center, Baltimore, MD, USA

Melissa Phillips LaPinska Department of Surgery, University of Tennessee Medical Center, Knoxville, TN, USA

Nicole Kissane Lee Indiana University School of Medicine, Department of Surgery, Indianapolis, IN, USA

Gregory J. Mancini Department of Surgery, University of Tennessee, Knoxville, TN, USA

Matthew L. Mancini Department of Surgery, University of Tennessee Medical Center, Knoxville, TN, USA

Luis A. Martin-del-Campo Columbia University Medical Center, New York, NY, USA

Stephen Masnyj Medical College of Wisconsin, Milwaukee, WI, USA

Jared McAllister Section of Minimally Invasive Surgery, Department of Surgery, Washington University School of Medicine, St. Louis, MO, USA

John Mark McLain Department of Surgery, University of Tennessee Medical Center, Knoxville, TN, USA

L. Michael Brunt Department of Surgery and Section of Minimally Invasive Surgery, Washington University School of Medicine, St. Louis, MO, USA

Yuri W. Novitsky Columbia University Medical Center, New York, NY, USA

Sean B. Orenstein Oregon Health & Science University, Portland, OR, USA

Eric M. Pauli Division of Minimally Invasive and Bariatric Surgery, Department of Surgery, Penn State Hershey Medical Center, Hershey, PA, USA

Arielle J. Perez Cleveland Clinic Comprehensive Hernia Center, Digestive Disease and Surgery Institute, Cleveland Clinic Foundation, Cleveland, OH, USA

Richard A. Pierce Department of Surgery, Vanderbilt University Medical Center, Nashville, TN, USA

Todd A. Ponsky Akron Children's Hospital, Department of Pediatric Surgery, Akron, OH, USA

Bruce Ramshaw Department of Surgery, University of Tennessee Medical center and Graduate school of Medicine, Knoxville, TN, USA

Janavi Rao Department of Anesthesiology, Washington University School of Medicine, St. Louis, MO, USA

Jessica L. Reynolds University of California San Diego, San Diego, CA, USA

Michael W. Robinson Lichtenstein Amid Hernia Clinic, David Geffen School of Medicine at UCLA, Los Angeles, CA, USA

Arghavan Salles Department of Surgery and Section of Minimally Invasive Surgery, Washington University School of Medicine, St. Louis, MO, USA

Amber Shada Department of Surgery, University of Wisconsin School of Medicine and Public Health, Madison, WI, USA

Steve R. Siegal Department of Surgery, Oregon Health & Science University, Portland, OR, USA

Nathaniel Stoikes Division of Minimally Invasive Surgery, University of Tennessee Health Science Center, Memphis, TN, USA

Wen Hui Tan Section of Minimally Invasive Surgery, Department of Surgery, Washington University School of Medicine in St. Louis, St. Louis, MO, USA

Dana Telem Department of Surgery, University of Michigan, Ann Arbor, MI, USA

Dennis R. Van Dorp Department of Surgery, University of Tennessee, Knoxville, TN, USA

Guy Voeller Division of Minimally Invasive Surgery, University of Tennessee Health Science Center, Memphis, TN, USA

David Webb Division of Minimally Invasive Surgery, University of Tennessee Health Science Center, Memphis, TN, USA

Part I

Preoperative Evaluation

Preoperative Considerations and Patient Optimization

Amber Shada

Current Trends

About 700,000 inguinal hernias are repaired annually in the USA, making this one of the most commonly performed operations [1]. While some inguinal hernias must be repaired urgently if incarcerated or strangulated, the majority of repairs in the USA are done in an elective setting. Current controversies in repair include timing of repair (versus watchful waiting or nonoperative management) and surgical approach. Additionally, modifiable patient factors are an important consideration in any elective surgery, and inguinal hernia repair is no exception.

To Repair or Not to Repair

Randomized studies have suggested that watchful waiting of minimally symptomatic hernias can be appropriate [2]. There are, however, predictable reasons that patients will be more likely to proceed to repair if they initially elect not to have their hernia repaired. Those with chronic constipation, with prostate problems necessitating straining to urinate, who are married, and in good health were more likely to proceed to repair

A. Shada
Department of Surgery, University of Wisconsin School of Medicine and Public Health, Madison, WI, USA
e-mail: shada@surgery.wisc.edu

rather than successfully manage their groin hernia with long-term watchful waiting [3]. For minimally symptomatic hernias, the risk of postoperative groin pain can outweigh the benefit of early repair in many patients. Factors like age, activity level, comorbidities, and prior or future surgeries must be taken into account when deciding on optimum time for repair. Additionally, patients over 70, those with a femoral or recurrent hernia, or obese patients are more likely to need emergent hernia repair and thus should be considered higher risk for nonoperative management of inguinal hernia [4]. For these reasons, I counsel my patients about the risks and benefits of both repair and no surgery, but I encourage those at higher risk of needing an emergent repair to consider surgery in an elective setting. Female patients, as well as those with femoral hernias, should not be offered watchful waiting as an option for their hernia, due to a paucity of data supporting observation of this group and a higher risk of complications with an untreated femoral hernia than inguinal hernia.

Preoperative Risk Factors

To maximize success, it is important to do a high-quality repair using proper materials. Surgical details are outlined in Chaps. 5–12 of this text. Patient preoperative risk factors should be evaluated, and any modifiable preoperative risk factors

© Springer International Publishing AG, part of Springer Nature 2018
M. P. LaPinska, J. A. Blatnik (eds.), *Surgical Principles in Inguinal Hernia Repair*,
https://doi.org/10.1007/978-3-319-92892-0_1

be identified and minimized prior to surgery. Examples include tobacco use, obesity, diabetes and diabetic control, nutritional status, and identification and decontamination of resistant organisms prior to surgery. There are also a host of risk factors that are less modifiable. Use of patient immunosuppression, presence of prior inguinal hernia repair, history of prior wound or skin infections, and presence of underlying liver disease can negatively impact the success of repair, but there is less ability to directly impact these prior to surgery.

Tobacco Use

Tobacco use is arguably one of the most important modifiable risk factors to consider for patients undergoing hernia repair. Smoking creates a decrease in end-tissue oxygenation as well as aerobic metabolism. This leads to impairment of healing of tissues after surgery, both by reducing the inflammatory healing response and impairing the proliferative response [5]. A single cigarette has been shown to decrease cutaneous blood flow in both smokers (38% reduction) and nonsmokers (28% reduction). This takes up to 5 min to be restored to levels prior to active cigarette smoking [6]. Conversely, quitting smoking can create a relatively rapid improvement in tissue oxygenation, down to the cellular level with restoration of inflammatory cell response within 4 weeks after smoking cessation. The proliferative response does not rebound quite as well [5]. Studies have shown lower perioperative complication rates after 4 weeks of preoperative smoking cessation as compared to patients who continued to smoke prior to surgery [7]. Smoking has also been directly linked to increased rates of recurrence of inguinal hernia [8, 9]. While I do not demand smoking cessation prior to primary/nonrecurrent hernia repair, I certainly suggest it. For any patients with a non-incarcerated, minimally symptomatic but recurrent hernia, I do ask them to stop smoking for 4 weeks prior to repair.

Obesity

Obesity is becoming more and more prevalent, with 66% of American adults falling into the category of obese (BMI $\geq$ 30). This creates complexity for virtually all types of surgery, and inguinal hernia is no exception. Overall, there is a paucity of published outcomes of inguinal hernia repair in obese patients. Technically these cases can be more challenging as compared to patients with a normal body habitus. Certainly, we have seen an increase in incidence of abdominal wall hernias in the obese [10]. Interestingly, there may be a lower incidence of inguinal hernias in those with a BMI over 30 [11]. However, obese patients have a higher risk of recurrence of inguinal hernia after repair [12]. There have been studies in inguinal hernia as well as abdominal wall hernia as a whole that found an increased rate of surgical site infections in obese patients [13, 14]. Several studies have shown a decreased rate of complications such as surgical site infection in laparoscopic inguinal hernia repair as compared to open repair [13, 15]. Thus, it may be prudent to consider laparoscopic inguinal hernia repair for the obese patient.

A recent NSQIP evaluation of open versus laparoscopic inguinal hernia in the obese found similar short-term outcomes with open and laparoscopic repair [15]. However, this fails to evaluate recurrence rate. Another study found higher morbidity in open inguinal hernia repair as compared to laparoscopic [13]. However, this did not exclude emergency cases or cases including a bowel resection, which may have skewed the results in favor of laparoscopic repair. Rates of obesity continue to rise, and as such inguinal hernia repair techniques will have to accommodate this. Whether that means an increase in use of laparoscopy remains to be seen, but I suspect the trend will be increased use of laparoscopy for inguinal hernia repairs and particularly so in the morbidly obese patient. I do not currently employ a BMI cutoff in my decision-making for repairing inguinal hernias, but I do counsel patients that their recurrence rate is likely higher if they are obese.

Nutrition

Like many types of surgery, there appears to be an association with lower perioperative morbidity in patients with better nutrition. While there are no studies evaluating the role nutrition plays in inguinal hernia repair, there are studies of abdominal wall hernias suggesting that a lower preoperative albumin level is predictive of increased length of stay [16]. Additionally, there are studies demonstrating that those who are underweight (BMI < 18.5 kg/m^2) have a higher risk of postoperative complications after inguinal hernia repair [12]. In a minimally symptomatic patient, it may be prudent to determine the underlying reason for a lower than normal BMI and attempt to remedy all pathologic etiologies if possible prior to surgery.

Diabetes

Patients with diabetes are well-known to have impaired wound healing and, as a result, higher perioperative morbidity for a variety of operations. This has been best studied in cardiothoracic surgery, where wound complications increased in those without well-controlled blood sugar perioperatively [17]. Furthermore, those with poorly controlled diabetes at baseline (hemoglobin A1C >8) had double the rate of superficial site infections [17]. Diabetic patients also have an elevated risk of recurrence of abdominal wall hernias. While there is no literature stratifying operative risks based on preoperative glycemic control, we can extrapolate the existing literature in other disciplines to assume that diabetics with better glycemic control will likely do better and are unlikely to do worse than patients with poorer glycemic control. Short-term complications after inguinal hernia repair, including bleeding, wound infection, and superficial wound dehiscence, are higher in patients with diabetes [18]. I do not repair inguinal hernias in an elective setting unless hemoglobin A1C is less than 8.0%.

MRSA

Though infection after inguinal hernia repair is relatively rare, it can be devastating. The incidence of drug-resistant bacteria, such as methicillin-resistant *Staphylococcus aureus* (MRSA), continues to rise, and MRSA colonization can put patients at increased risk of perioperative infection. The literature in surgical patients supports decolonization with nasal mupirocin and topical chlorhexidine in those colonized with MRSA [19]. Despite a paucity of evidence to suggest this improves outcomes in inguinal hernia repair, I feel as though the benefit of decontamination outweighs risk, and I employ this for all of my patients with a history of MRSA infection or any history of prior hernia repair complicated by mesh infection.

Conclusion

Surgery is the only definitive way to treat inguinal hernias. Patients with minimally symptomatic hernias consider watchful waiting rather than repair, but those with symptomatic hernias or those at high risk of developing symptoms should consider elective repair. Modifiable patient risk factors, including tobacco use, obesity, nutritional status, diabetes, and presence of MRSA colonization, should be optimized prior to inguinal hernia repair.

References

1. Schumpelick V, Treutner KH, Arlt G. Inguinal hernia repair in adults. Lancet. 1994;344(8919):375–9.
2. Fitzgibbons RJ Jr, Giobbie-Harder A, Gibbs JO, Dunlop DD, Reda DJ, McCarthy M Jr, et al. Watchful waiting vs repair of inguinal hernia in minimally symptomatic men: a randomized clinical trial. JAMA. 2006;295(3):285–92.
3. Sarosi GA, Wei Y, Gibbs JO, Reda DJ, McCarthy M, Fitzgibbons RJ, et al. A clinician's guide to patient selection for watchful waiting management of inguinal hernia. Ann Surg. 2011;253(3):605–10.
4. Hernandez-Irizarry R, Zendejas B, Ramirez T, Moreno M, Ali SM, Lohse CM, et al. Trends in emergent inguinal hernia surgery in Olmsted County, MN: a population-based study. Hernia. 2012;16(4):397–403.

5. Sorensen LT. Wound healing and infection in surgery: the pathophysiological impact of smoking, smoking cessation, and nicotine replacement therapy: a systematic review. Ann Surg. 2012;255(6):1069–79.

6. Monfrecola G, Riccio G, Savarese C, Posteraro G, Procaccini EM. The acute effect of smoking on cutaneous microcirculation blood flow in habitual smokers and nonsmokers. Dermatology. 1998;197(2):115–8.

7. Lindstrom D, Sadr Azodi O, Wladis A, Tonnesen H, Linder S, Nasell H, et al. Effects of a perioperative smoking cessation intervention on postoperative complications: a randomized trial. Ann Surg. 2008;248(5):739–45.

8. Sorensen LT, Friis E, Jorgensen T, Vennits B, Andersen BR, Rasmussen GI, et al. Smoking is a risk factor for recurrence of groin hernia. World J Surg. 2002;26(4):397–400.

9. Burcharth J, Pommergaard HC, Bisgaard T, Rosenberg J. Patient-related risk factors for recurrence after inguinal hernia repair: a systematic review and meta-analysis of observational studies. Surg Innov. 2015;22(3):303–17.

10. Lau B, Kim H, Haigh PI, Tejirian T. Obesity increases the odds of acquiring and incarcerating noninguinal abdominal wall hernias. Am Surg. 2012;78(10):1118–21.

11. Zendejas B, Hernandez-Irizarry R, Ramirez T, Lohse CM, Grossardt BR, Farley DR. Relationship between body mass index and the incidence of inguinal hernia repairs: a population-based study in Olmsted County, MN. Hernia: the journal of hernias and abdominal wall. Surgery. 2014;18(2):283–8.

12. Rosemar A, Angeras U, Rosengren A, Nordin P. Effect of body mass index on groin hernia surgery. Ann Surg. 2010;252(2):397–401.

13. Willoughby AD, Lim RB, Lustik MB. Open versus laparoscopic unilateral inguinal hernia repairs: defining the ideal BMI to reduce complications. Surg Endosc. 2017;31(1):206–14.

14. Ruhling V, Gunnarsson U, Dahlstrand U, Sandblom G. Wound healing following open groin hernia surgery: the impact of comorbidity. World J Surg. 2015;39(10):2392–9.

15. Froylich D, Haskins IN, Aminian A, O'Rourke CP, Khorgami Z, Boules M, et al. Laparoscopic versus open inguinal hernia repair in patients with obesity: an American College of Surgeons NSQIP clinical outcomes analysis. Surg Endosc. 2017;31(3):1305–10.

16. Dunne JR, Malone DL, Tracy JK, Napolitano LM. Abdominal wall hernias: risk factors for infection and resource utilization. J Surg Res. 2003;111(1):78–84.

17. Latham R, Lancaster AD, Covington JF, Pirolo JS, Thomas CS Jr. The association of diabetes and glucose control with surgical-site infections among cardiothoracic surgery patients. Infect Control Hosp Epidemiol. 2001;22(10):607–12.

18. Hellspong G, Gunnarsson U, Dahlstrand U, Sandblom G. Diabetes as a risk factor in patients undergoing groin hernia surgery. Langenbecks Arch Surg. 2017;402(2):219–25.

19. Bode LG, Kluytmans JA, Wertheim HF, Bogaers D, Vandenbroucke-Grauls CM, Roosendaal R, et al. Preventing surgical-site infections in nasal carriers of Staphylococcus aureus. N Engl J Med. 2010;362(1):9–17.

Inguinal and Femoral Anatomy

2

John Mark McLain, Aaron Joseph Arroyave,
Matthew L. Mancini, and Melissa Phillips LaPinska

Inguinal hernia repair is one of the most commonly performed operations by a general surgeon. As is true with most surgical interventions, a majority of the surgical technique is based on the underlying anatomy or disruption of that anatomy. Comprehensive knowledge of the muscles, fascia, nerves, blood vessels, and spermatic cord structures in the inguinal region are needed to provide the best technique with lowest recurrence and complication rates.

Inguinal hernias are classified into either direct or indirect hernias based on the anatomic location. An indirect hernia passes laterally through the internal ring and travels medially through the external ring before exiting down into the scrotum in men. A direct hernia passes medial to the inferior epigastric vessels directly through the abdominal wall. Distinguishing between these two types of hernia may be challenging on physical examination, but repair techniques are commonly applicable to both types. From an embryologic perspective, indirect inguinal hernias are more common than direct inguinal hernias regardless of gender, often with a 2:1 ratio. Men are, however, over 20 times more likely to have an inguinal hernia when compared to female counterparts. Although inguinal hernias are more common than other hernia types in females, women have an increased occurrence of femoral hernias at almost 20:1 when compared to their male counterparts. Both genders have an increased rate of a right-sided inguinal hernia, often attributed to the delay in processus vaginalis closure after slower testicular descent on the right side during fetal development.

Because of the difference in surgical technique between an open and laparoscopic inguinal hernia repair, the anatomy must be differentiated depending on the surgical approach as this "change in view" can often lead to misidentification of normal anatomy. This change in approach to the anatomy of the groin can often be confusing for those less familiar with these two relatively unrelated surgical approaches. It is important to understand from "outside-in" approach, as an open repair, to the "inside-out" approach, as in a laparoscopic repair. For the open approach, delineating the anatomy of the conjoined tendon, the pubic tubercle, and the inguinal (Poupart's) ligament is important for choosing the surgical technique used. Care must be taken in the open approach to identify and avoid injury to the ilioinguinal and iliohypogastric nerves which run anterior to the structures in the inguinal canal and which, if injured, can lead to chronic groin pain following surgery. For the laparoscopic

J. M. McLain (✉) · M. L. Mancini · M. P. LaPinska
Department of Surgery, University of Tennessee
Medical Center, Knoxville, TN, USA
e-mail: JMMcLain@utmck.edu; MMancini@utmck.edu

A. J. Arroyave
General Surgery Resident, Department of Surgery,
University of Tennessee Medical Center,
Knoxville, TN, USA
e-mail: AArroyave1@gmail.com

© Springer International Publishing AG, part of Springer Nature 2018
M. P. LaPinska, J. A. Blatnik (eds.), *Surgical Principles in Inguinal Hernia Repair*,
https://doi.org/10.1007/978-3-319-92892-0_2

or robotic approach, the preperitoneal dissection allows for visualization of the direct, indirect, femoral, and obturator spaces and allows a clear plane of dissection for visualization of the myofascial pectineal orifices, creating space for the eventual mesh overlay. Specifically when looking at the laparoscopic approach, knowledge of the anatomy is critical as recurrence can be higher if the landing zones for the mesh are not created, which may be more common early in the learning curve of this procedure. The difference in view of the anatomy may also lead to unintended injury if understanding the danger areas such as the vascular triangle of doom, and the origins of the cutaneous nerves or triangle of pain are not carefully identified during surgery. Because of the important structures contained so close to the site of inguinal hernia formation, understanding the anatomy of the area – no matter which surgical technique is selected – is essential to prevent injury to the patient.

Understanding the anatomy of the inguinal canal is the basis on which the surgical techniques, detailed in later chapters of this text, are based. The authors believe that knowledge of the details of the anatomy are the key to choosing the right operation for each patient and preventing potential complications of each surgical technique. This chapter will address the basics of the anatomy as well as the specific pearls and pitfalls for each type of surgical technique.

Muscular Anatomy of the Groin

Groin anatomy, from anterior to posterior, includes the skin and subcutaneous tissue, external oblique muscle, internal oblique muscle, and transversus abdominis muscle/fascia which fuse inferiorly to create the inguinal canal. This is best illustrated by Nyhus [1] as shown in Fig. 2.1.

The muscular anatomy of the groin [2] provides a steep learning curve in understanding the complexity of inguinal hernia repair. The importance of understanding this anatomy is underlined when a difficult or complex case presents and necessitates a direct tissue repair without implementation of mesh. The external oblique muscle is the first muscle to be encountered after dissection of the skin and subcutaneous tissue.

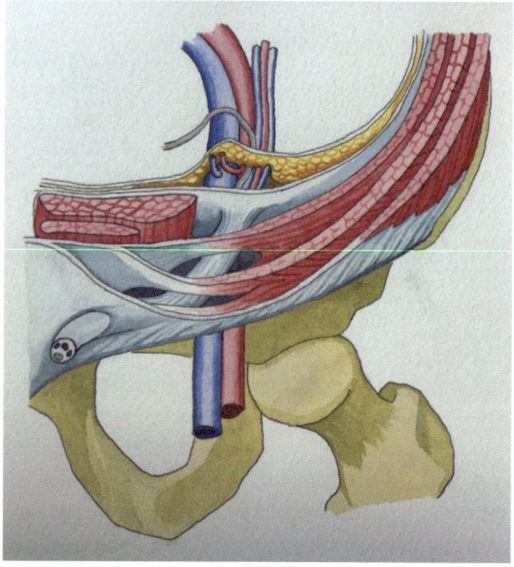

Fig. 2.1 Anterior and posterior fascial fusion of the inguinal canal

The fibers of the external oblique run in an inferior/medial direction, which is commonly referred to as "hands in pockets." The inferior-most portion of the muscle consists of aponeurotic fibers and forms the inguinal (Poupart's) ligament, which is the floor of the inguinal canal. The inferior-medial portion of this ligament consists of a triangular fanning out of the ligament as it joins the pubic tubercle which is referred to as the lacunar (Gimbernat's) ligament.

The internal oblique muscle lies deep to the external oblique muscle, and in contrast to the external oblique, its fibers course in a transverse orientation. The lateral portion of the internal oblique forms the anterior wall of the inguinal canal along with the aponeurosis of the external oblique, while the inferior/medial portion of the muscle forms the superior border/roof of the inguinal canal. The inferior-most portion of the internal oblique forms the cremaster fibers, which dissociate from the main portion of the muscle and course through the spermatic cord.

The transversus abdominis lies deep to the internal oblique and is the innermost of the flat muscles of the abdomen. This muscle forms the posterior wall (floor) of the inguinal canal along with the transversalis fascia, which is a thin aponeurotic membrane between the transverse

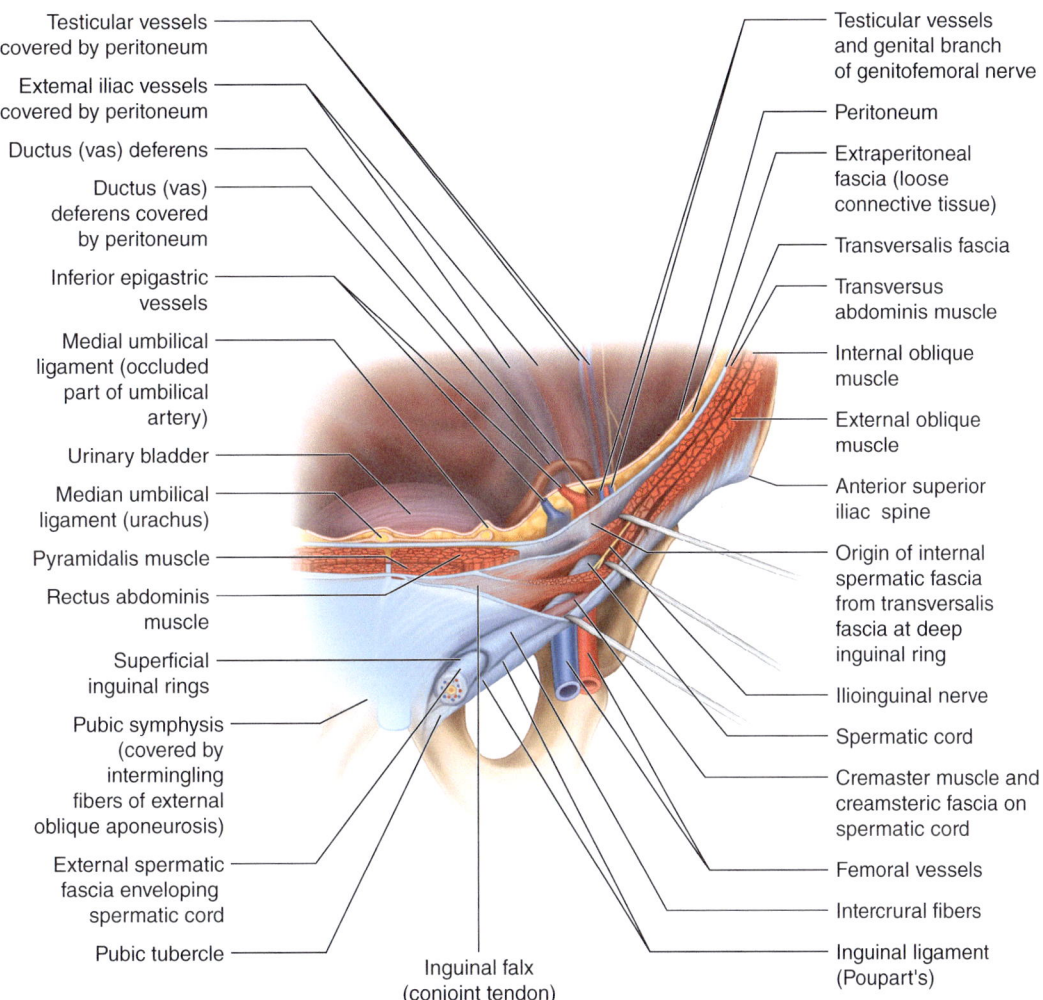

Testicular vessels covered by peritoneum

External iliac vessels covered by peritoneum

Ductus (vas) deferens

Ductus (vas) deferens covered by peritoneum

Inferior epigastric vessels

Medial umbilical ligament (occluded part of umbilical artery)

Urinary bladder

Median umbilical ligament (urachus)

Pyramidalis muscle

Rectus abdominis muscle

Superficial inguinal rings

Pubic symphysis (covered by intermingling fibers of external oblique aponeurosis)

External spermatic fascia enveloping spermatic cord

Pubic tubercle

Inguinal falx (conjoint tendon)

Testicular vessels and genital branch of genitofemoral nerve

Peritoneum

Extraperitoneal fascia (loose connective tissue)

Transversalis fascia

Transversus abdominis muscle

Internal oblique muscle

External oblique muscle

Anterior superior iliac spine

Origin of internal spermatic fascia from transversalis fascia at deep inguinal ring

Ilioinguinal nerve

Spermatic cord

Cremaster muscle and creamsteric fascia on spermatic cord

Femoral vessels

Intercrural fibers

Inguinal ligament (Poupart's)

Fig. 2.2 Fascial layers of the abdominal wall

abdominis and the parietal peritoneum. This relationship is consistent in 75% of patients with the other 25% having only transversalis fascia present in the posterior wall of the canal. This is detailed in Fig. 2.2.

Regardless of the approach (open or laparoscopic) or type of repair (mesh or tissue), the pectineal (Cooper's) ligament is an important landmark [3]. Cooper's ligament is formed primarily of the lateral extension of the lacunar ligament as well as aponeurotic fibers of the internal oblique, transversus abdominis, and pectineus muscles and inguinal falx. The extraordinary strength provided by the combined aponeurotic fibers contributing to Cooper's ligament attributes to its importance as an anchoring structure

in an open tissue repair, such as in the McVay (open non-mesh) repair, or as an anchoring structure in laparoscopic repair.

As mentioned previously, from an open perspective, the floor of the inguinal canal is formed from the inguinal (Poupart's) ligament, which is the thickened lower part of the external oblique aponeurosis running from the anterior superior iliac spine and inserting into the superior pubic ramus. From a posterior view, such as in laparoscopic inguinal hernia repair, the iliopubic tract forms the floor of the canal. This tract is an aponeurotic band, posterior to the inguinal ligament, connecting the superior iliac spine to Cooper's ligament. It forms on the deep side of the inferior border of the transversus abdominis and transver-

Fig. 2.3 Laparoscopic groin anatomy detailing the direct, indirect, and femoral spaces

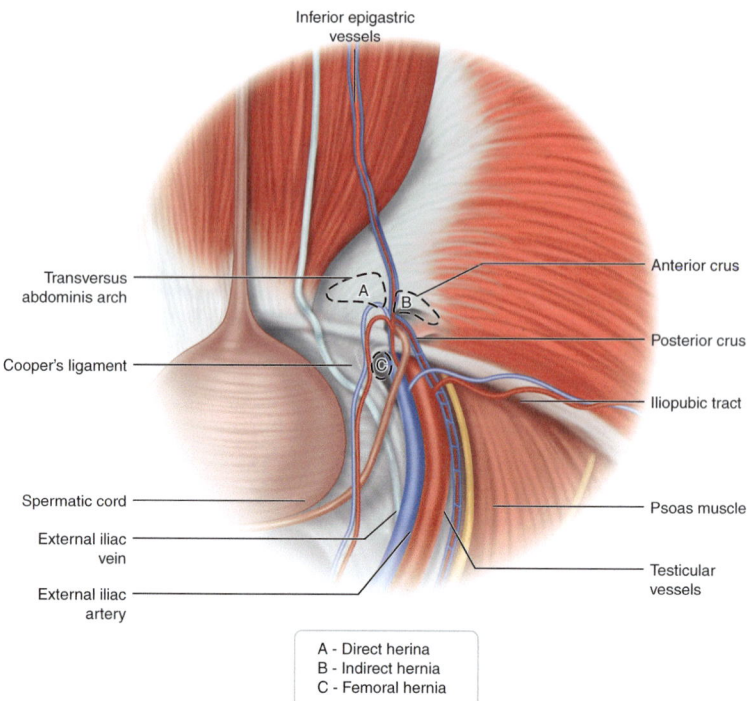

A - Direct herina
B - Indirect hernia
C - Femoral hernia

salis fascia and is an important landmark in a laparoscopic repair. Its identification is key as an avascular plain lies below that where the peritoneum can be pushed cephalad to see the psoas muscle as well as the lateral femoral cutaneous nerve, femoral branch of the genitofemoral nerve, and femoral nerve which are located in the triangle of pain. In a laparoscopic repair, the anatomy is visualized as seen in Fig. 2.3. After Cooper's ligament is exposed, the femoral canal can be identified. The obturator canal is just medial to the vas deferens and can be exposed to make sure the mesh in a laparoscopic repair covers all potential points of weakness.

Vascular Anatomy of the Groin

The classification of a direct or indirect inguinal hernia is dependent on the location of the fascial defect in relationship to the inferior epigastric artery and vein. Direct defects are located medially, while indirect defects are lateral to this vascular bundle. This is illustrated in Fig. 2.4. The inferior epigastric artery arises from the

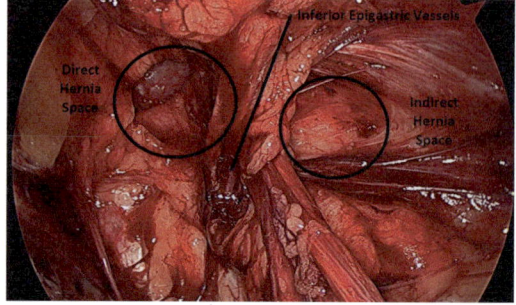

Fig. 2.4 Surgical laparoscopic view of the epigastric vessels and both direct and indirect hernia

external iliac artery and follows the abdominal wall to the linea semilunaris where it runs along the lateral edge of the rectus abdominis, supplying blood flow to the abdominal wall.

In an open repair, the surgeon must also be aware of the superficial epigastric vessels which are often encountered in the subcutaneous dissection above the external oblique. The superficial epigastric artery arises from the femoral artery, approximately 1 cm below the inguinal canal, and provides blood supply for the skin and subcutaneous tissue of the lower abdominal wall.

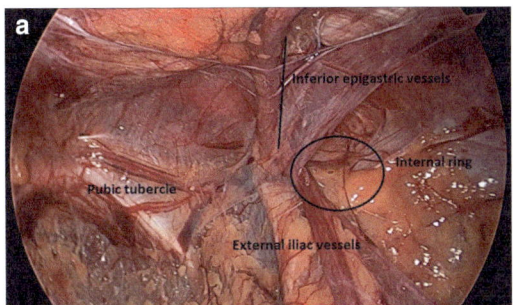

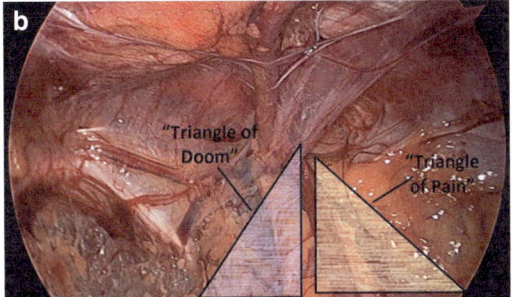

Fig. 2.5 Surgical laparoscopic view of the "triangle of pain" and "triangle of doom"

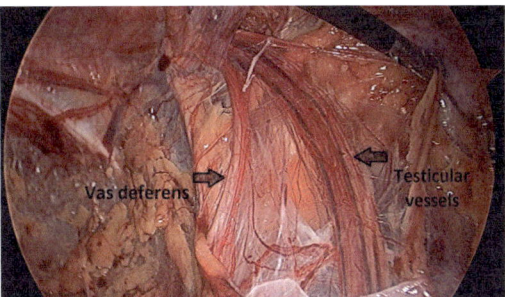

Fig. 2.6 Surgical laparoscopic view of the gonadal vessels and vas deferens

spermatic drainage from the testicle. Care must be taken, particularly in the setting of large indirect inguinal hernias, to preserve these structures without injury. Local trauma to the testicular vessels can result in thrombosis and subsequent testicular ischemia. In women, these structures are replaced by the round ligament which is able to be sacrificed without sequela.

Important Nerves in Groin Anatomy

Knowledge of the anatomy and the course of the nerves of the abdominal wall are important in considering any surgical approach in the groin [4]. Injuries to these nerves can results in chronic postoperative pain which can be disabling to a previously healthy patient. The etiology is often scar tissue which entraps the nerve, leading to the formation of a neuroma which can cause focal point tenderness with radiation along the path of the nerve. Chapters 14 and 15 address treatment options for the management of this. Prevention, however, is the best treatment. The ilioinguinal, iliohypogastric, and genital branch of the genitofemoral nerves are the most commonly encountered nerves in inguinal and femoral hernia repair.

The ilioinguinal and iliohypogastric nerves originate from L1 and pass between the external and internal oblique muscles until an area just medial and superior to the anterior superior iliac spine where they cross through the internal oblique muscle, running under the external oblique muscle and joining the other cord struc-

The external iliac artery and vein are important to recognize and respect during a laparoscopic repair. Because of the ease of evaluation for a femoral hernia as well as the need for posterior dissection back to the psoas to allow adequate room for mesh overlap, these vessels are often skeletonized during the dissection. This must be done with great care to avoid the avulsion of smaller feeding vessels as well as to avoid direct injury. If tacks are placed for mesh fixation, one must also be acutely aware of "triangle of doom" as seen in Fig. 2.5. Tacks placed in this area have a high likelihood of vascular injury and should be avoided.

Similarly, in an open repair, one must remember the close location of the external iliac/femoral vessels just posterior to the inguinal canal. For example, in an open repair with mesh, unintended injury to these vessels can occur if large sutures are taken securing the mesh to the shelving edge of the inguinal ligament.

In men, the testicular artery, which is a direct branch from the aorta, runs through the internal ring and through the inguinal canal as shown in Fig. 2.6 as it supplies blood flow to the testicle. This runs beside the vas deferens which allows

tures in the inguinal canal. These nerves can share distribution of sensory innervation, providing sensation to the skin of the groin, base of the penis/labia, and ipsilateral upper medial thigh. The ilioinguinal nerve is prone to entrapment laterally during the mesh fixation, and, thus, the surgeon must take particular care to isolate and preserve this nerve during dissection of the inguinal canal contents. The iliohypogastric nerve passes cephalad to the spermatic cord, and a normal anatomic variant of the location of this nerve is for it to remain buried within the fibers of the internal oblique muscle. Figure 2.7 shows the ilioinguinal nerve present upon the opening of the external

oblique musculature in an open inguinal hernia repair approach.

Genital branch of the genitofemoral nerve innervates the cremaster muscle and skin on the lateral side of the scrotum/labia. It is the only nerve that travels through the internal ring and accompanies the cremaster vessels in a neurovascular bundle on the backside of the cord. This nerve is often sacrificed in women if surgical dissection requires division of the round ligament. The laparoscopic view of important nerves is shown in Fig. 2.8.

Nerve entrapment is very "patient dissatisfying" complication of inguinal hernia repair despite the relatively low occurrence, reported between 1 and 5% in the surgical literature. If an injury to a nerve were to happen during an open approach for surgical repair of a hernia, the most commonly injured nerve is the ilioinguinal nerve followed by the iliohypogastric nerve. Injury related to an open inguinal hernia repair often results in symptomatology in the distribution over the groin/scrotum as seen in Fig. 2.9. The laparoscopic approach, because of the posterior nature of the dissection, has a much lower risk for injury to the ilioinguinal and iliohypogastric nerve. The most commonly injured nerve during a laparoscopic technique for repair is the genitofemoral nerve. This area of symptomatology is more anterior thigh in nature.

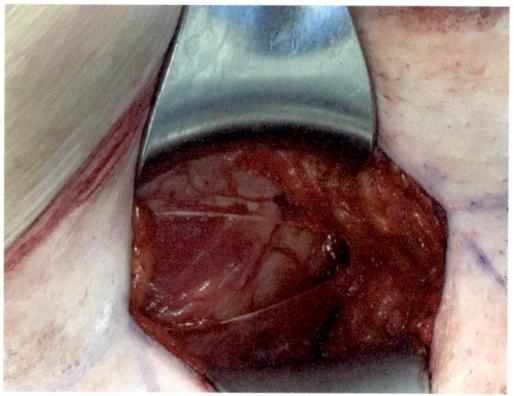

Fig. 2.7 Open surgical view of the ilioinguinal and iliohypogastric nerves

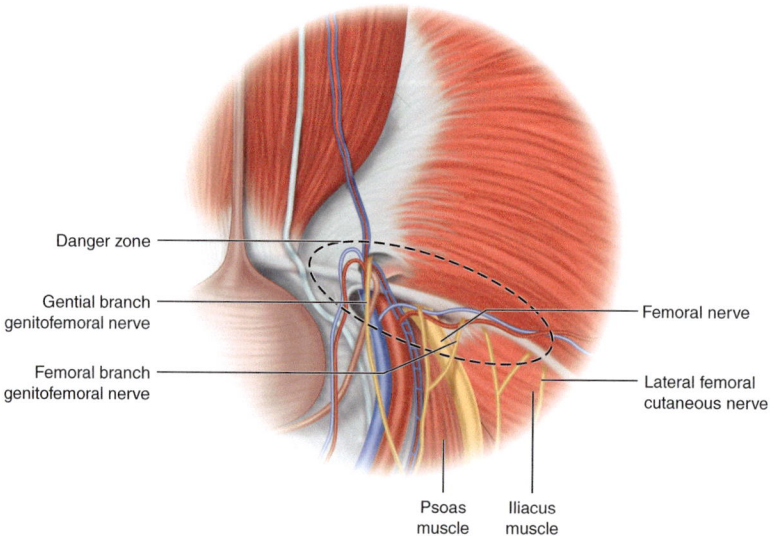

Fig. 2.8 Laparoscopic view of the nerves of the inguinal canal

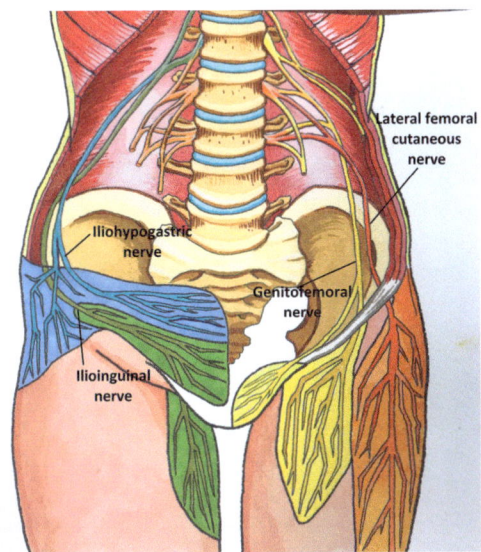

Lateral femoral
cutaneous
nerve

Iliohypogastric
nerve

Genitofemoral
nerve

Ilioinguinal
nerve

Fig. 2.9 Nerves of the inguinal area with associated sensory distribution

Summary

Inguinal hernia repair is one of the most common operations performed by a general surgeon. The anatomy of the groin is viewed quite differently between open and laparoscopic operative approaches. Because of the complexity of the inguinal region with its muscles, fascia, nerves, blood vessels, and spermatic cords, it is essential that the general surgeon be comfortable with the anatomy viewed from the direction of the surgeon's operative choice. Understanding the anatomy for this commonly performed surgery is important in choosing the best, patient-tailored, operative technique with the lowest complications and lowest recurrence rates.

References

1. Nyhus LM. An anatomic reappraisal of the posterior inguinal wall, with special consideration of the iliopubic tract and its relation to groin hernias. Surg Clin North Am. 1960;44:1305.
2. Anson BJ, McVay CB. Inguinal hernia: the anatomy of the region. Surg Gynecol Obstet. 1938;66:186–91.
3. Fitzgibbons RJ Jr, Forse RA. Clinical practice. Groin hernias in adults. N Engl J Med. 2015;372:756–63.
4. Simons MP, Aufenacker T, Bay-Nielsen M, et al. European Hernia Society guidelines on the treatment of inguinal hernia in adult patients. Hernia. 2009;13:343–403.

Inguinal Hernia Repair: Selecting a Repair

Sepehr Lalezari and Gina L. Adrales

Introduction

Inguinal hernia repair is one of the most commonly performed general surgery operations with about 770,000 cases annually in the United States [56]. A hernia can be described simply as a protrusion of preperitoneal fat and peritoneal contents through the myofascial wall that contains it. As this pertains to inguinal hernias, visceral fat or other contents protrude through the myopectineal opening of Fruchaud. Since the first description of hernia repair noted in the ancient Egyptian Ebers Papyrus, there have been countless types of hernia repairs described. Three categories of repair emerge as safe and durable options including primary tissue repair, open mesh repair, and endoscopic mesh repair.

The first feasible primary or tissue inguinal hernia repair was described by Bassini in 1887. Bassini is considered to be the "father of modern inguinal herniorrhaphy" [4]. Since its introduction, many modifications to Bassini's original technique have been described. The most prominent of these are the Halsted repair, the McVay repair, and the Shouldice repair. Bassini's original operation involved high ligation of the hernia sac, opening the cremasteric muscle and transversalis fascia to secure the triple layer of the transversus abdominus, transversalis fascia, and internal oblique muscle to the medial pubic tubercle and the inguinal ligament, thereby reconstructing the posterior inguinal floor. Halsted, who trained with Bassini, modified this technique by adding a fourth layer to the closure with reapproximation of the external oblique aponeurosis deep to the spermatic cord. McVay expanded on the Bassini technique by applying sutures to Cooper's ligament for the medial repair rather than to the inguinal ligament as in the Bassini and Halsted repairs. These concepts ultimately led Shouldice to develop his multilayered closure in 1945. While complication rates between the various tissue repairs are not significantly different, the Shouldice repair is well-accepted among primary hernia repairs due to the lowest reported recurrence rate [2, 10]. Despite this achievement, the Shouldice repair is the least commonly performed hernia repair in the United States with only 55,000 cases performed each year [56]. This repair is a technically demanding operation and requires familiarity with the operation to achieve adequate results. The recurrence rate after Shouldice repair at specialty centers is 0.6–1.4% but rises to 15% at non-specialty centers [2, 7, 42, 64].

S. Lalezari
Johns Hopkins University Bayview Medical Center, Baltimore, MD, USA

G. L. Adrales (✉)
Department of Surgery, Johns Hopkins Hospital, Johns Hopkins University School of Medicine, Baltimore, MD, USA
e-mail: Gadrale1@jhmi.edu

The concept of using a prosthetic to repair hernias in a tensionless manner emerged by the end of the nineteenth century, but a suitable biomaterial was not available until the mid-twentieth century. The "tension-free" mesh repair was first described by Lichtenstein in 1986 [38]. In tensionless hernia repair, mesh can be placed either in the anterior position, posterior position, or a combination of the two. The most popular hernia repair overall is the anterior Lichtenstein repair with a total of 295,000 annual repairs [56]. The frequency of this type of hernia repair is likely related to its reproducibility in regard to recurrence rates and ease of teaching and achieving proficiency with relatively low experience numbers. Other popular anterior mesh repairs include the plug-and-patch repair and the Trabucco sutureless mesh repair. Preperitoneal or retromuscular mesh repair was popularized by Stoppa in 1984 [68]. Combined anterior and posterior repair can also be performed with the Gilbert double-layer mesh system. Since 1990 the preperitoneal technique has been performed via an endoscopic approach, including the transabdominal preperitoneal (TAPP) and the totally extraperitoneal (TEP) mesh repairs.

There is no clear superiority of one laparoscopic technique over the other [10]. Recurrence rates between the two techniques are roughly similar, and studies show no statistical difference between TAPP and TEP [20, 70, 75]. There is also no difference in postoperative pain between the two techniques [20]. Operative times are not statistically different between the two techniques [20, 35, 75]. Visceral injury, seroma, and port site hernias tend to be higher for TAPP than TEP [43, 75], whereas rates of vascular injury and conversion rates to open appear to be higher for TEP repair [75]. While the rate of robotic transabdominal preperitoneal inguinal hernia repair has increased over recent years, there is no prospective longer-term comparative data available to date.

Many factors to consider when selecting the appropriate repair technique are explored herein. These include the recurrence risk, patient characteristics (gender, comorbidities, tolerance for anesthesia), hernia factors (bilaterality, recurrence status, scrotal involvement, and hernia size), economic considerations, level of contamination and acuity, and, importantly, the comfort and skill level of the surgeon in performing the desired technique.

Patient Factors

Female

Indirect inguinal hernias are the most common type of hernias in both males and females. The incidence of femoral hernias is more common in females, and thus, it is imperative to inspect for femoral hernias at the time of inguinal hernia repair. Although the most frequent etiology of the groin hernia in females is an indirect inguinal hernia, femoral hernias are not uncommon. A missed femoral hernia may present as a hernia "recurrence" after initial inguinal repair. In fact, the incidence of a femoral hernia after inguinal hernia repair occurs 15 times more frequently than it does spontaneously [45]. Furthermore, in 41.5% of reoperations in women, a femoral hernia was found as opposed to only 5.4% in males [5]. Additionally, recurrences are more common in females than males after primary inguinal hernia repair [6, 8, 21].

According to the European Hernia Society guidelines, an endoscopic approach should be considered for women because it allows for visualization of the entire myopectineal orifice [46, 63]. The transabdominal approach is a useful technique in cases of longstanding pelvic pain in women to rule out gynecologic occult disease. There is an association between pelvic floor dysfunction such as bladder prolapse and inguinal hernia occurrence in women. The laparoscopic transabdominal approach allows full inspection of the bilateral inguinal, femoral, and obturator spaces. This is also important given the incidence of incarceration at presentation among women and the lack of watchful waiting trial data regarding asymptomatic inguinal hernias in female patients. While there is little known about the impact of inguinal herniorrhaphy on pelvic adhesions and infertility among women, this should be discussed with women of childbearing age desiring pregnancy. The totally extraperitoneal approach may be preferred for this subset of patients unless there is reason to perform pelvic diagnostic laparoscopy.

Male

For men there is no distinct advantage of one technique over another. If there is an elevated prostatic-specific antigen level or a prominent family history of prostate cancer, one should discuss the development of postoperative preperitoneal adhesions after laparoscopic inguinal herniorrhaphy and the potential adverse impact on prostatectomy. Dense adhesions after preperitoneal herniorrhaphy is a reported cause of conversion from laparoscopic or robotic surgery to open prostatectomy [12, 13, 29]. The most concerning aspect of endoscopic hernia repair for future radical prostate surgery is that it may compromise adequate lymph node sampling [16, 22, 67]. Although this should be discussed with patients, safe radical prostatectomy and lymph node dissection are possible after endoscopic hernia repair, and thus the mere possibility of future prostate resection should not limit one from performing an endoscopic mesh repair for the problem at hand.

Alternatively, in the setting of concomitant inguinal hernia and prostate cancer, it is safe to repair the inguinal hernia via a laparoscopic or robotic approach at the time of radical prostatectomy. Inguinal hernias are noted in 15% of patients after radical prostatectomy, and Nielson and Walsh demonstrated that 33% of patients undergoing radical prostatectomy had an existing inguinal hernia [49].

Anesthesia Considerations

It is important to gauge a patients' suitability to undergo general anesthesia. Open approaches can be performed under general, local nerve block, or regional (spinal or epidural) anesthesia. Local anesthesia is associated with lower mortality for both elective and emergency operations [50, 63]. Endoscopic approaches generally are performed under general anesthesia although TEP repair has been described with use of an epidural [33].

According to the European Hernia Society guidelines, primary, reducible, unilateral inguinal hernias approached through an open repair are best performed under local anesthesia [46, 63]. The guidelines note the acceptable alternative of general anesthesia with a combination of local anesthetic. Furthermore, the society recommends against spinal anesthesia and/or long-acting anesthetic agents. Regional anesthetics are associated with prolonged postoperative recovery secondary to increased incidence of urinary retention [26, 53, 63].

Local anesthetics are associated with decreased postoperative pain, faster discharge, decreased operative cost, and decreased urinary complications [16, 26]. Although ideal for elderly patients with significant cardiopulmonary disease that may preclude safe general anesthesia, it has its limitations. Specifically, local anesthesia with sedation may not be ideal for young patients or those with morbid obesity, anxiety, large scrotal hernias, or suspected incarceration or strangulation.

Economic Considerations

The financial impact of inguinal hernia repair includes operational and materials costs as well as the societal economic burden. Open inguinal hernia repair is associated with a lower materials cost compared to minimally invasive repair. The VA Cooperative Study showed that the surgical cost is higher for laparoscopic than open repair, while the postoperative cost to the healthcare system is similar [47]. Additionally, the option of local anesthesia over general anesthesia for open repair, whether primary tissue repair or mesh repair, reduces costs. This has been shown in comparison to either regional or general anesthesia in two randomized control trials [52, 66].

There are other economic considerations that may prove to be important to patients, hospitals, payers, and society over time. The earlier return to work after an endoscopic approach lessens the cost burden from a socioeconomic perspective [20]. Additionally, the laparoscopic repair is more cost effective in terms of incremental cost per quality of adjusted life years gained, and the long-term risk for recurrence is not significantly different [20, 46].

Robotic inguinal hernia repair has become more prominent in recent years. Even without including the acquisition costs of the robot, which are substantial, there is a significantly greater cost of robotic inguinal hernia repair compared to laparoscopic repair. One might argue that the cost of robotic repair may decrease over time with shorter operative times as the longer duration of the robotic repair has been shown to be a contributing factor to the high cost [23]. Even for open inguinal hernia repair, experience and volume matter in terms of cost reduction. In a New York State study of over 155,000 patients, surgeons with <25 annual repairs had greater rates of reoperation, longer operative times, and greater downstream costs [3]. Other centers have noted the favorable finding of decreased recovery time after robotic repair as a mitigating factor for the longer operative time associated with robotic repair [74].

Wound Classification

Inguinal hernia repair is considered a clean operation with a low risk of infection. Preoperative antibiotics generally are not recommended unless the patient is immunocompromised or at a higher than normal risk for infection. However, many surgeons and hospitals continue to administer antibiotic prophylaxis due to hospital guidelines and the planned implantation of permanent mesh. In a clean operation, the surgeon is freer to select an inguinal hernia repair of his or her choosing. Surgical dogma dictates that mesh repair should be avoided in the contaminated field due to the high risk of mesh infection, but various contemporary studies have demonstrated this risk to be lower than once suspected [11]. There are reports of the use of lightweight polypropylene mesh in contaminated fields with low infectious complication rates [11]. Some studies of lightweight

mesh repair for ventral hernias have demonstrated successful mesh salvage with drainage and antibiotic therapy [1, 72]. While this is possible, caution is advisable. The risk-benefit to the patient must be considered thoroughly given the success of non-mesh repair options for inguinal hernia that are more abundant than the repair of the complex, contaminated ventral incisional hernia. In addition, although there are descriptions of the use of biologic mesh in contaminated fields with low infectious complications, a sutured tissue repair is recommended in a contaminated field as a lower-cost and well-studied approach compared to biologic mesh repair [9].

Hernia Factors

Recurrent Hernias

Up to 15% of inguinal hernia repairs are estimated to be for hernia recurrence [8, 51, 55, 58, 62]. Similar to ventral hernia repair, it appears that the risk for hernia recurrence increases with each subsequent repair. Thus, it is imperative to conduct an effective recurrent repair despite the challenges that a preoperative field presents. The recommended approach for a recurrent hernia depends on the initial hernia repair performed. The European Hernia Guidelines recommend that the recurrent repair should be approached in a different manner than the initial hernia repair [63]. There is clear benefit associated with an endoscopic approach to the recurrent inguinal hernia after primary Lichtenstein repair in terms of hernia recurrence, pain, wound complications, and recovery [28, 31, 59, 63]. In particular, laparoscopic repair for the medial recurrence after Lichtenstein repair provides a lower risk of reoperation compared to a repeated anterior repair [48].

In contrast, the recommendation for anterior mesh repair after laparoscopic posterior repair is weak. There are a number of reports of laparoscopic repair after failed laparoscopic inguinal hernia repair and increasing evidence that the benefits of laparoscopic repair extend to recurrent repair such as a lower rate of chronic pain and disability compared to open repair [39, 59, 62, 73].

The laparoscopic transabdominal approach is useful as a diagnostic tool to identify the recurrence as well as the source of groin pain.

Multiply Recurrent Hernias

There is little guidance in the literature regarding the multiply recurrent groin hernia. Avoidance of the same operative site is desirable but not always possible. Reoperations for recurrent inguinal hernias often involve interstitial hernias at the margins of the prior mesh repair and thus require a wider operative field to allow for appropriate mesh overlap. This can be achieved with transabdominal exposure and dissection and placement of a large preperitoneal or sometimes intraperitoneal onlay mesh. Indeed, an 8-year analysis of the Danish Hernia Database supports a laparoscopic reoperation for the recurrent inguinal hernia after Lichtenstein repair with the demonstration of a significantly reduced recurrence rate of 1.3% compared to 11.3% for repeat Lichtenstein repair [8].

Bilateral Hernias

Bilateral inguinal hernias should be repaired laparoscopically. Various studies have shown an advantage of less postoperative pain and earlier return to work with an endoscopic repair with negligible difference in recurrence rates over open repair [40, 61]. Although the cost of a laparoscopic surgery may be greater, this cost is obviated when looking at cost as a quality of adjusted life years (QALY) [44]. This is particularly true for bilateral hernias where operative time and postoperative convalescence may be reduced compared to open anterior repair.

Scrotal and Incarcerated Hernias

Scrotal and incarcerated inguinal hernias are challenging (Fig. 3.1.) These may require a hybrid approach for reduction of the hernia contents, inspection of the incarcerated intestine, and reconstruction of the inguinal floor. The most common complication of laparoscopic scrotal inguinal hernia repair compared to open repair is sero-hematoma [37]. To minimize formation of hematomas, careful hemostasis with electrocautery should be performed [15]. Additionally, ligation and tacking of the distal sac to the posterior inguinal wall decreases the rate of seroma [14]. There have been reports of both TEP and TAPP approaches to safely repair a scrotal hernia [14, 17, 18, 37, 60, 65]. Relaxing incisions may be

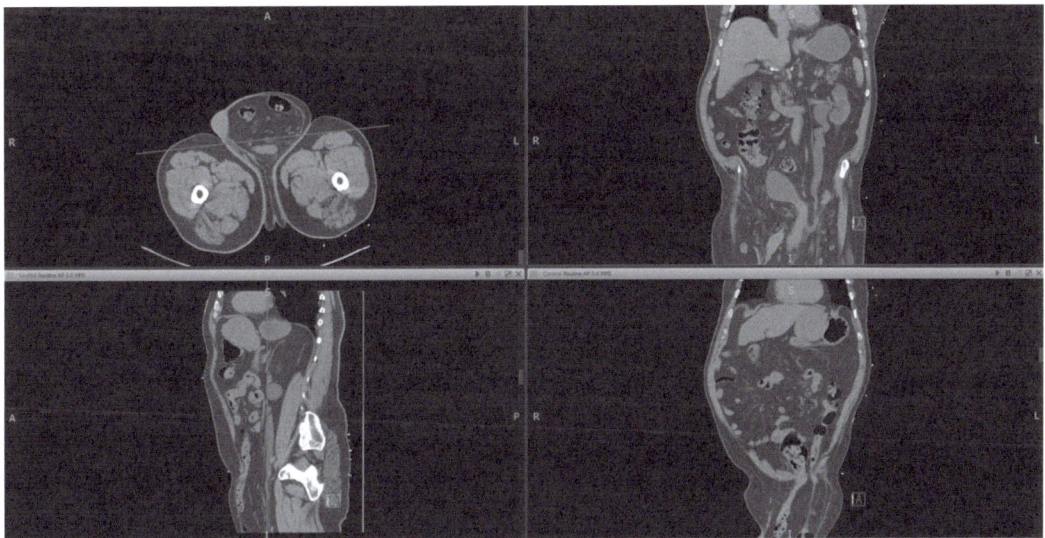

Fig. 3.1 CT scan images of a large scrotal hernia

created laterally in an indirect hernia or medially in a direct hernia [9]. The International Endohernia Society recommends a non-lightweight mesh with large overlap of the defect during endoscopic scrotal hernia repair to reduce the risk of mesh eventration and hernia recurrence [9].

Both anterior Lichtenstein and minimally invasive approaches are used in the care of strangulated hernias. TAPP may be superior to TEP when approaching a strangulated hernia. Several studies demonstrate the feasibility and safety of both TAPP and TEP for the repair of the strangulated hernia repair [17, 25, 34, 36, 41, 60]. The benefit of TAPP is the ability to inspect the bowel under laparoscopic visualization and run the entire length of the small bowel with ease. Bowel or omental resection may be then undertaken completely laparoscopically [54] or via a minilaparotomy.

While open anterior mesh repair is a reasonable and perhaps more straightforward approach, the authors prefer a laparoscopic or robotic transabdominal approach for large scrotal hernias or incarcerated hernias. This technique allows both intraperitoneal and preperitoneal visualization and manipulation of the hernia contents and hernia sac from both anatomic spaces (Fig. 3.2). Alternatively, for patients at high risk for anesthesia complications, open anterior mesh repair with drain placement is a viable option.

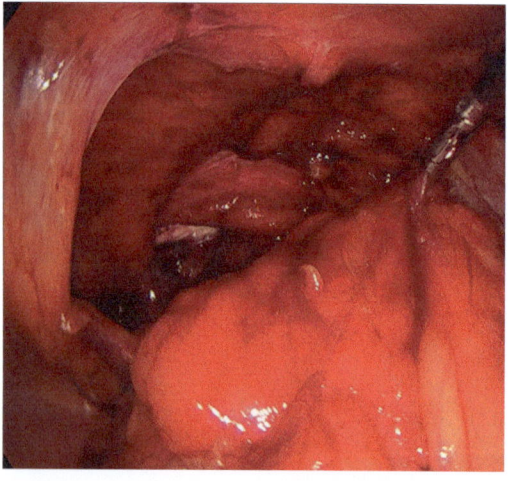

Fig. 3.2 Laparoscopic transabdominal preperitoneal repair of a scrotal hernia. Reduction of intestine and omental hernia contents

Giant Scrotal Hernias

Giant scrotal hernias extend below the midpoint of the inner thigh [24]. These large scrotal hernias may contain a variety of unexpected viscera. As an extreme example, herniation of the stomach into a giant scrotal hernia has been reported [32]. Thus, it is important to approach these hernias with caution. One of the most important considerations to keep in mind when dealing with these hernias is the loss of intraabdominal domain that may make reducing the hernia contents challenging and place the patient at risk for compartment syndrome ([57]). Various approaches to dealing with this have been implemented in the past such as progressive pneumoperitoneum, surgical debulking of viscera, phrenectomy, abdominal wall separation, rotational flaps, and tissue expanders ([27, 69]).

As these giant hernias are often accompanied by significant abdominal wall weakness, open or minimally invasive abdominal wall reconstruction with components separation with mesh reinforcement or flaps may be required. Drain placement is advised as well as management of the excess skin. Immediate or delayed scrotoplasty may be required. Reports of using the scrotal skin as a rotational flap and delayed scrotoplasty are useful adjuncts when respiratory compromise and compartment syndrome are concerns [19, 69].

Surgeon Factors

Surgeon Preferences

A major factor in repair selection is surgeon preference. This preference is often a reflection of surgical residency training, which fosters comfort with a certain inguinal hernia repair or mesh. Other contributing factors may include reimbursement and productivity incentives, patient population, and equipment constraints. It is clear that surgeon preference, in combination with surgeon experience, plays a critical role in the decision-making of choosing the inguinal repair regardless of available evidence. This affects

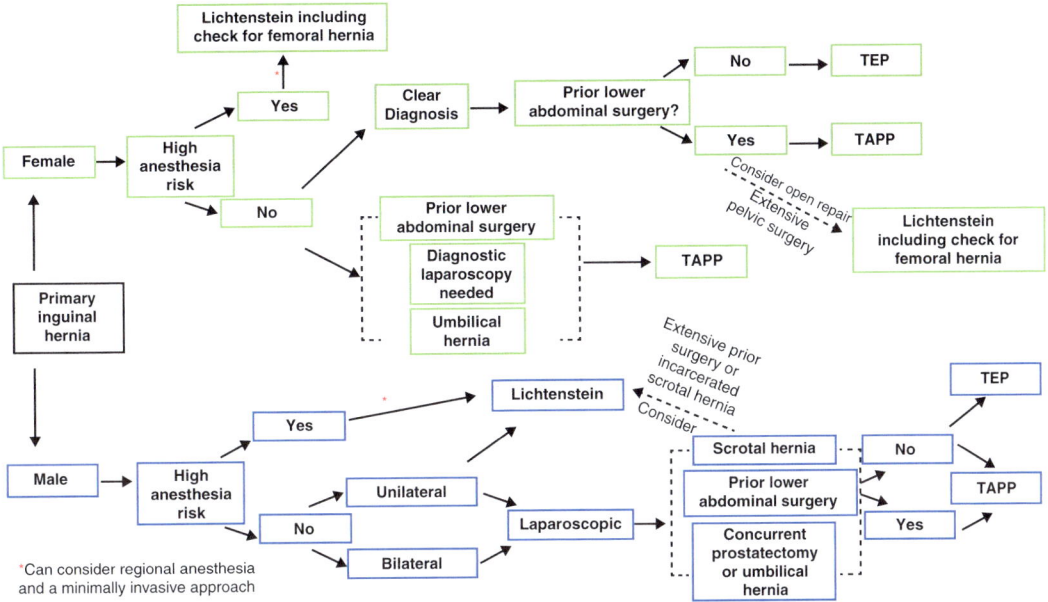

Fig. 3.3 Algorithm for management of the primary inguinal hernia. The authors' algorithm for management of the nonrecurrent inguinal hernia for male and female patients. The experience of the surgeon will impact the approach, particularly for patients with prior lower abdominal surgery and scrotal hernias. Robotic transabdominal repair or robotic or laparoscopic extended-view extraperitoneal repair is an alternative to conventional laparoscopy in patients with prior pelvic surgery, sliding hernias

adoption of recommended best practices. As an example of this, utilization of endoscopic repair in areas where there is substantial evidence to support its use, such as bilateral inguinal hernias or recurrent hernias after anterior repair, is low. This has been demonstrated both in Europe where hernia guidelines are prominent and North America [30, 71].

Experience Level

Various studies have shown unsurprisingly that complication rates decrease with increased experience. One of the most popular studies referenced by surgeons regarding inguinal hernia repair experience is the VA Cooperative Study published in 2004 [47]. In this study recurrence rates between laparoscopic and open were found to be 10.1% and 4.1%, respectively. A criticism of the study was the low entry threshold for surgeon inclusion in the study, performance of 25 open and 25 laparoscopic cases. When the analysis of the same study looked at surgeons who had

performed over 250 laparoscopic cases, the recurrence rates between laparoscopic and open were similar at 5.1% and 4.1%, respectively [70]. The learning curve is definitely a factor in repair technique selection and surgical outcomes [76]. It appears that experience impacts complication rates and operative times more with TEP repair than TAPP. Of note, the operative times for both experienced (30–100 procedures) and novice (<20 procedures) surgeons are lower for TAPP repair than TEP, 70 and 95 min, respectively [75]. The precise number of laparoscopic repairs a novice surgeon needs to ascend the learning curve is unknown, but a Cochrane review by Wake et al. suggests it is between 30 and 100 procedures [75].

Conclusion

There are a number of considerations when selecting the appropriate repair for the primary or recurrent inguinal hernia. Patient and hernia factors play a central role in this decision-making (Fig. 3.3). Ultimately, the experience and comfort level of the surgeon will guide operative management. More contemporary and emerging techniques of robotic repair and laparoscopic enhanced-view extraperitoneal approaches to the complex inguinal hernia are seen with increasing frequency. Comparative analysis via randomized trials as well as registry and quality collaborative data should direct the utilization of any inguinal hernia repair technique. The comprehensive hernia surgeon should have in his or her armamentarium several techniques including primary tissue repair, an open and a minimally invasive mesh repair, and should apply this most effectively with an evidence-based and patient-centered approach.

References

1. Aguilar B, Chapital AB, Madura JA 2nd, Harold KL. Conservative management of mesh-site infection in hernia repair. J Laparoendosc Adv Surg Tech A. 2010;20(3):249–52.
2. Amato B, Moja L, Panico S, Persico G, Rispoli C, Rocco N, et al. Shouldice technique versus other open techniques for inguinal hernia repair. Cochrane Database Syst Rev. 2012;4:CD001543.
3. Aquina CT, Probst CP, Kelly KN, Iannuzzi JC, Noyes K, Fleming FJ, et al. The pitfalls of inguinal herniorrhaphy: surgeon volume matters. Surgery. 2015;158(3):736–46.
4. Awad SS, Fagan SP. Current approaches to inguinal hernia repair. Am J Surg. 2004;188(6, Suppl 1):9–16.
5. Bay-Nielsen M, Kehlet H. Inguinal herniorrhaphy in women. Hernia. 2006;10(1):30–3.
6. BayNielsen M, Kehlet H, Strand L, Malmstrøm J, Andersen FH, Wara P, et al. Quality assessment of 26 304 herniorrhaphies in Denmark: a prospective nationwide study. Lancet. 2001;358(9288):1124–8.
7. Beets GL, Oosterhuis KJ, Go PM, Baeten CG, Kootstra G. Long-term follow-up (12–15 years) of a randomized controlled trial comparing Bassini-Stetten, Shouldice, and high ligation with narrowing of the internal ring for primary inguinal hernia repair. J Am Coll Surg. 1997;185:352–7.
8. Bisgaard T, BayNielsen M, Kehlet H. Rerecurrence after operation for recurrent inguinal hernia. A Nationwide 8year followup study on the role of type of repair. Ann Surg. 2008;247(4):707–11.
9. Bittner R, Arregui ME, Bisgaard T, Dudai M, Ferzli GS, Fitzgibbons RJ, et al. Guidelines for laparoscopic (TAPP) and endoscopic (TEP) treatment of inguinal hernia [International Endohernia Society (IEHS)]. Surg Endosc. 2011;25(9):2773–843.
10. Bittner R, Schwarz J. Inguinal hernia repair: current surgical techniques. Langenbeck's Arch Surg. 2012;397(2):271–82. https://doi.org/10.1007/s00423-011-0875-7. Epub 2011 Nov 25.
11. Carbonell AM, Cobb WS. Safety of prosthetic mesh hernia repair in contaminated fields. Surg Clin North Am. 2013;93(5):1227–39.
12. Cook H, Afzal N, Cornaby AJ. Laparoscopic hernia repairs may make subsequent radical retropubic prostatectomy more hazardous. BJU Int. 2003;91:729.
13. Cooperberg MR, Downs TM, Carroll PR. Radical retropubic prostatectomy frustrated by prior laparoscopic mesh herniorrhaphy. Surgery. 2004;135:452–4.
14. Daes J. Endoscopic repair of large inguinoscrotal hernias: management of the distal sac to avoid seroma formation. Hernia. 2014;18(1):119–22.
15. Deeba S, Purkayastha S, Paraskevas P, Athanasiou T, Darzi A, Zacharakis E. Laparoscopic approach to incarcerated and strangulated inguinal hernias. JSLS. 2009;13(3):327–31.
16. Do HM, Turner K, Dietel A, Wedderburn A, Liatsikos E, Stolzenburg JU. Previous laparoscopic inguinal hernia repair does not adversely affect the functional or oncological outcomes of endoscopic extraperitoneal radical prostatectomy. Urology. 2011;77:963–7.
17. Ferzli G, Shapiro K, Chaudry G, Patel S. Laparoscopic extraperitoneal approach to acutely incarcerated inguinal hernia. Surg Endosc. 2004;18(2):228–31.
18. Ferzli GS, Kiel T. The role of the endoscopic extraperitoneal approach in large inguinal scrotal hernias. Surg Endosc. 1997;11(3):299–302.
19. Gaedcke J, Schaler P, Brinker J, Quintel M, Ghadimi M. Emergency repair of Giant inguinoscrotal hernia in a septic patient. J Gastrointest Surg. 2013;17:837.
20. Gong K, Zhang N, Lu Y, Zhu B, Zhang Z, Du D, et al. Comparison of the open tensionfree meshplug, transabdominal preperitoneal (TAPP), and totally extraperitoneal (TEP) laparoscopic techniques for primary unilateral inguinal hernia repair: a prospective randomized controlled trial. Surg Endosc. 2011;25(1):234–9.
21. Haapaniemi S, Gunnarsson U, Nordin P, Nilsson E. Reoperation after recurrent groin hernia repair. Ann Surg. 2001;234(1):122–6.
22. Haifler M, Benjamin B, Ghinea R, Avital S. The impact of previous laparoscopic inguinal hernia repair on radical prostatectomy. J Endourol. 2012;26(11):1458–62.
23. Higgins RM, Frelich MJ, Bosler ME, Gould JC. Cost analysis of robotic versus laparoscopic general surgery procedures. Surg Endosc. 2017;31(1):185–92.
24. Hodgkinson DJ, McIlrath DC. Scrotal reconstruction for giant inguinal hernias. Surg Clin North Am. 1984;64(2):307–13.
25. Ishihara T, Kubota K, Eda N, Ishibashi S, Haraguchi Y. Laparoscopic approach to incarcerated inguinal hernia. Surg Endosc. 1996;10:1111–3.
26. Jensen P, Mikkelsen T, Kehlet H. Postherniorrhaphy urinary retention--effect of local, regional, and general anesthesia: a review. Reg Anesth Pain Med. 2002;27(6):612–7.

27. Karthikeyan VS, Sistla SC, Ram D, Ali SM, Rajkumar N. Giant inguinoscrotal hernia—report of a rare case with literature review. Int Surg. 2014;99(5):560–4.

28. Karthikesalingam A, Markar SR, Holt PJ, Praseedom RK. Meta-analysis of randomized controlled trials comparing laparoscopic with open mesh repair of recurrent inguinal hernia. Br J Surg. 2010;97(1):4–11.

29. Katz EE, Patel RV, Sokoloff MH, Vargish T, Brendler CB. Bilateral inguinal hernia repair can complicate subsequent radical retropubic prostatectomy. J Urol. 2002;167:637–8.

30. Köckerling F, Bittner R, Kuthe A, Stechemesser B, Lorenz R, Koch A, et al. Laparo-endoscopic versus open recurrent inguinal hernia repair: should we follow the guidelines? Surg Endosc. 2017;31(8):3168–85.

31. Köckerling F, Koch A, Lorenz R, Reinpold W, Hukauf M, Schug-Pass C. Open repair of primary versus recurrent male unilateral inguinal hernias: perioperative complications and 1-year follow-up. World J Surg. 2016;40:813–25.

32. Lajevardi S, Gundara J, Collins S, Samra JS. Acute gastric rupture in a Giant inguinoscrotal hernia. J Gastrointest Surg. 2015;19(12):2283.

33. Lal P, Philips P, Saxena KN, Kajla RK, Chander J, Ramteke VK. Laparoscopic total extraperitoneal (TEP) inguinal hernia repair under epidural anesthesia: a detailed evaluation. Surg Endosc. 2007;21(4):595–601.

34. Legnani GL, Rasini M, Pastori S, Sarli D. Laparoscopic transperitoneal hernioplasty (TAPP) for the acute management of strangulated inguino-crural hernias: a report of nine cases. Hernia. 2008;12(2):185–8.

35. Leibl BJ, Jager C, Kraft B, Kraft K, Schwarz J, Ulrich M, et al. Laparoscopic hernia repair--TAPP or/and TEP? Langenbeck's Arch Surg. 2005;390(2):77–8.

36. Leibl BJ, Schmedt CG, Kraft K, Kraft B, Bittner R. Laparoscopic transperitoneal hernia repair of incarcerated hernias: is it feasible? Results of a prospective study. Surg Endosc. 2001;15(10):1179–83.

37. Leibl BJ, Schmedt CG, Kraft K, Ulrich M, Bittner R. Scrotal hernias: a contraindication for an endoscopic procedure? Results of a singleinstitution experience in transabdominal preperitoneal repair. Surg Endosc. 2000;14(3):289–92.

38. Lichtenstein IL, Shulman SA. Ambulatory outpatient hernia surgery. Including a new concept, introducing tensionfree repair. Int Surg. 1986;71(1):1–4.

39. Lo Menzo E, Spector SA, Iglesias A, Martinez JM, Huaco J, DeGennaro V, et al. Management of recurrent inguinal hernias after total extraperitoneal (TEP) Herniorrhaphies. J Laparoendosc Adv Surg Tech A. 2009;19(4):475–8.

40. Mahon D, Decadt B, Rhodes M. Prospective randomized trial of laparoscopic (transabdominal preperitoneal) vs open (mesh) repair for bilateral and recurrent inguinal hernia. Surg Endosc. 2003;17(9):1386–90.

41. Mainik F, Flade-Kuthe R, Kuthe A. Total extraperitoneal endoscopic hernioplasty (TEP) in the treatment of incarcerated and irreponible inguinal and femoral hernias. Zentralbl Chir. 2005;130:550–3.

42. Malik A, Bell CM, Stukel TA, Urbach DR. Recurrence of inguinal hernias repaired in a large hernia surgical specialty hospital and general hospitals in Ontario, Canada. Can J Surg. 2016;59(1):19.

43. McCormack K, Wake BL, Fraser C, Vale L, Perez J, Grant A. Transabdominal preperitoneal (TAPP) versus totally extraperitoneal (TEP) laparoscopic techniques for inguinal hernia repair: a systematic review. Hernia. 2005a;9(2):109–14.

44. McCormack K, Wake B, Perez J, Fraser C, Cook J, McIntosh E, et al. Laparoscopic surgery for inguinal hernia repair: systematic review of effectiveness and economic evaluation. Health Technol Assess. 2005b;9(14):1. 203, iii–iv

45. Mikkelsen T, BayNielsen M, Kehlet H. Risk of femoral hernia after inguinal herniorrhaphy. Br J Surg. 2002;89(4):486–8.

46. Miserez M, Peeters E, Aufenacker T, Bouillot JL, Campanelli G, Conze J, et al. Update with level 1 studies of the European hernia society guidelines on the treatment of inguinal hernia in adult patients. Hernia. 2014 Apr;18(2):151–63.

47. Neumayer L, GiobbieHurder A, Jonasson O, Fitzgibbons R, Dunlop D, Gibbs J, et al. Open mesh versus laparoscopic mesh repair of inguinal hernia. N Engl J Med. 2004;350(18):1819–27.

48. Öberg S, Andresen K, Rosenberg J. Surgical approach for recurrent inguinal hernias: a Nationwide cohort study. Hernia. 2016;20(6):777–82.

49. Nielsen ME, Walsh PC. Systematic detection and repair of subclinical inguinal hernias at radical retropubic prostatectomy. Urology. 2005;66(5):1034–7.

50. Nilsson H, Stylianidis G, Haapamäki M, Nilsson E, Nordin P. Mortality after groin hernia surgery. Ann Surg. 2007;245:656–60.

51. Nordin P, Haapaniemi S, van der Linden W, et al. Choice of anesthesia and risk of reoperation for recurrence in groin hernia repair. Ann Surg. 2004;240(1):187–92.

52. Nordin P, Zetterström H, Gunnarsson U, Nilsson E. Local, regional, or general anaesthesia in groin hernia repair: multicentre randomised trial. Lancet. 2003;362:853–8.

53. Nordin P, Zetterström H, Carlsson P, Nilsson E. Cost-effectiveness analysis of local, regional and general anaesthesia for inguinal hernia repair using data from a randomized clinical trial. Br J Surg. 2007;94:500–5.

54. Rebuffat C, Galli A, Scalambra MS, Balsamo F. Laparoscopic repair of strangulated hernias. Surg Endosc. 2006;20:13113–4.

55. Rosenberg J, Bisgaard T, Kehlet H, Wara P, Asmussen T, Juul P, et al. Danish hernia database recommendations for the management of inguinal and femoral hernia in adults. Dan Med Bull. 2011;58(2):C4243.

56. Rutkow IM. Demographic and socioeconomic aspects of hernia repair in the United States in 2003. Surg Clin North Am. 2003;83(5):1045–51.

57. Saadi AS, Wadan AH, Hamerna S. Approach to a giant inguinoscrotal hernia. Hernia. 2005;9:277.

58. Saber A, Ellabban GM, Gad M, Elsayem K. Open preperitoneal versus anterior approach for recurrent

inguinal hernia: a randomized study. BMC Surg. 2012;12:22.

59. Saber A, Hokkam EN, Ellabban GM. Laparoscopic transabdominal preperitoneal approach for recurrent inguinal hernia: a randomized trial. J Minim Access Surg. 2015;11(2):123–8.

60. Saggar VR, Sarangi R. Endoscopic totally extraperitoneal repair of incarcerated inguinal hernia. Hernia. 2005;9(2):120–4.

61. Sarli LM, Iusco DRM, Sansebastiano GM, Costi RM. Simultaneous repair of bilateral inguinal hernias: a prospective, randomized study of open, tensionfree versus laparoscopic approach. Surg Laparosc Endosc Percutan Tech. 2001;11(4):262–7.

62. Sevonius D, Montgomery A, Smedberg S, Sandblom G. Chronic groin pain, discomfort and physical disability after recurrent groin hernia repair: impact of anterior and posterior mesh repair. Hernia. 2016;20(1):43–53.

63. Simons MP, Aufenacker T, Bay-Nielsen M, Bouillot JL, Campanelli G, Conze J, et al. European Hernia Society guidelines on the treatment of inguinal hernia in adult patients. Hernia. 2009;13(4):343–403. https://doi.org/10.1007/s00423-011-0875-7. Epub 2009 Jul 28.

64. Simons MP, Kleijnen J, van Geldere D, Hoitsma HFW, Obertop H. Role of the Shouldice technique in inguinal hernia repair: a systematic review of controlled trials and a metaanalysis. Br J Surg. 1996;83(6):734–8.

65. Siow SL, Mahendran HA, Hardin M, Chea CH, Nik Azim NA. Laparoscopic transabdominal approach and its modified technique for incarcerated scrotal hernias. Asian J Surg. 2013;36(2):64–8.

66. Song D, Greilich NB, White PF, Watcha MF, Tongier WK. Recovery profiles and costs of anesthesia for outpatient unilateral inguinal herniorrhaphy. Anesth Analg. 2000;91:876–81.

67. Spernat D, Sofield D, Moon D, Louie-Johnsun M, Woo H. Implications of laparoscopic inguinal hernia repair on open, laparoscopic, and robotic radical prostatectomy. Prostate Int. 2014;2(1):8–11.

68. Stoppa RE, Rives JL, Warlaumont CR, Palot JP, Verhaeghe PJ, Delattre JF. The use of Dacron in the repair of hernias of the groin. Surg Clin North Am. 1984;64(2):269–85.

69. Tahir M, Ahmed FU, Seenu V. Giant inguinoscrotal hernia: case report and management principles. Int J Surg. 2016;6(6):495–7.

70. Takata MC, Duh Q. Laparoscopic inguinal hernia repair. Surg Clin North Am. 2008;88(1):157–78.

71. Trevisonno M, Kaneva P, Watanabe Y, Fried GM, Feldman LS, Andalib A, et al. Current practices of laparoscopic inguinal hernia repair: a population-based analysis. Hernia. 2015;19(5):725–33.

72. Trunzo JA, Ponsky JL, Jin J, Williams CP, Rosen MJ. A novel approach for salvaging infected prosthetic mesh after ventral hernia repair. Hernia. 2009;13(5):545–9.

73. van den Heuvel B, Dwars BJ. Repeated laparoscopic treatment of recurrent inguinal hernias after previous posterior repair. Surg Endosc. 2013;27(3):795–800.

74. Waite KE, Herman MA, Doyle PJ. Comparison of robotic versus laparoscopic transabdominal preperitoneal (TAPP) inguinal hernia repair. J Robot Surg. 2016;10(3):239–44.

75. Wake BL, McCormack K, Fraser C, Vale L, Perez J, Grant A. Transabdominal preperitoneal (TAPP) vs totally extraperitoneal (TEP) laparoscopic techniques for inguinal hernia repair. Cochrane Database Syst Rev. 2005;25(1):CD004703.

76. Wright D, O'Dwyer PJ. The learning curve for laparoscopic hernia repair. Surg Innov. 1998;5(4):227–3.

Prosthetic Options: Advantages and Disadvantages

4

Yuri W. Novitsky and Luis A. Martin-del-Campo

Introduction

Recurrence and postoperative pain are currently the two most important outcomes in groin hernia surgery. Prosthetics are used in surgery to provide a tension-free bridge between fascial defects [1]. When compared to primary repair, the use of mesh for inguinal hernia repair is associated with lower recurrence rates [2]. Therefore, tension-free repair has become the gold standard for inguinal hernia repair [3] and should be used almost routinely [4], while tissue approximation is reserved for cases with questionable viability of hernia contents and operative field contamination [5]. On the other hand, the use of prosthetics is associated with groin pain [6] which has now become the most important complication of hernia repair, affecting at least 10% of patients postoperatively [7].

In recent decades, there has been a substantial increase in the number of available prosthetics. Unfortunately, the "ideal" mesh is yet to be developed, and therefore surgeons must base their choice on intricate knowledge of material properties in order to provide their patient with the best possible hernia repair. Herein we will provide an overview of the common meshes for open and minimally invasive inguinal hernia repairs. The authors' personal algorithm for mesh selection is shown in Fig. 4.1.

Prosthetics Used for Inguinal Hernia

Although there are many properties that can describe every single commercial mesh, they are initially classified as either synthetic or biologic [8].

Synthetic

The most commonly used synthetic material used in hernia surgery is knitted polypropylene (PP) or polyester (POL) and laminar expanded polytetrafluoroethylene (ePTFE). Synthetic meshes are often characterized by their "weight" and porosity [9]. The weight nomenclature was created to compare various constructs of PP-based meshes (Fig. 4.2). While the exact definitions vary in the literature, we utilize the following metrics: Ultralightweight is <30 g/m², lightweight is between 30 and 40 g/m² (Fig. 4.2e, f), mid-weight is 40–70 g/m² (Fig. 4.2c, d), and heavyweight is >90 g/m² (Fig. 4.2a, b) [10]. Another method to decrease the density of prosthetic materials is reducing the number of fibers, thereby increasing the size of the pore [9]: In this regard, there meshes are grouped as microporous, <100 μm; medium pore, 600–1000 μm; large pore, 1000–2000 μm; and very large pore, >2000 μm.

Y. W. Novitsky (✉) · L. A. Martin-del-Campo
Columbia University Medical Center, New York, NY, USA

© Springer International Publishing AG, part of Springer Nature 2018
M. P. LaPinska, J. A. Blatnik (eds.), *Surgical Principles in Inguinal Hernia Repair*,
https://doi.org/10.1007/978-3-319-92892-0_4

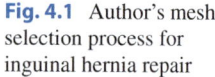

Fig. 4.1 Author's mesh selection process for inguinal hernia repair

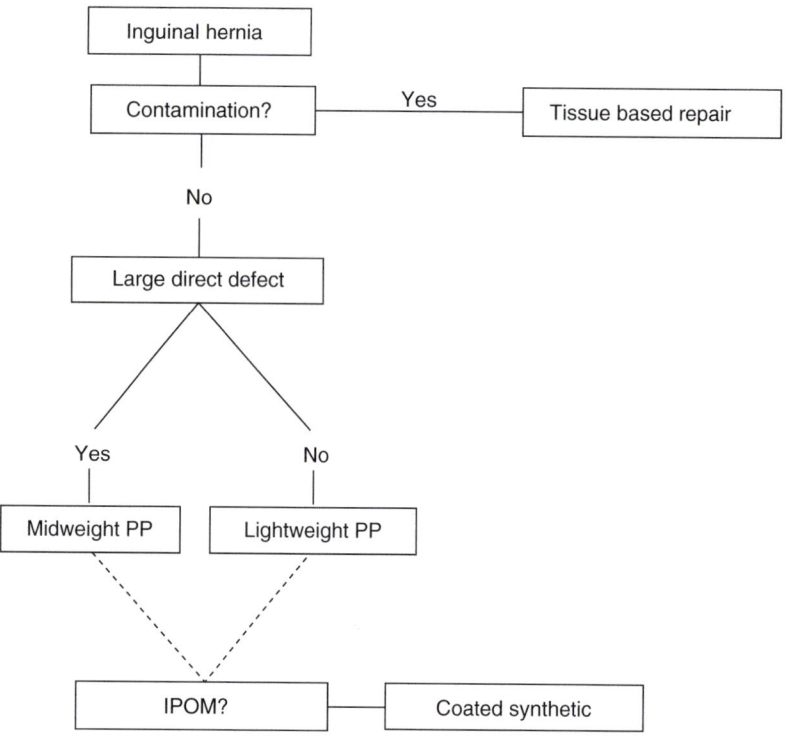

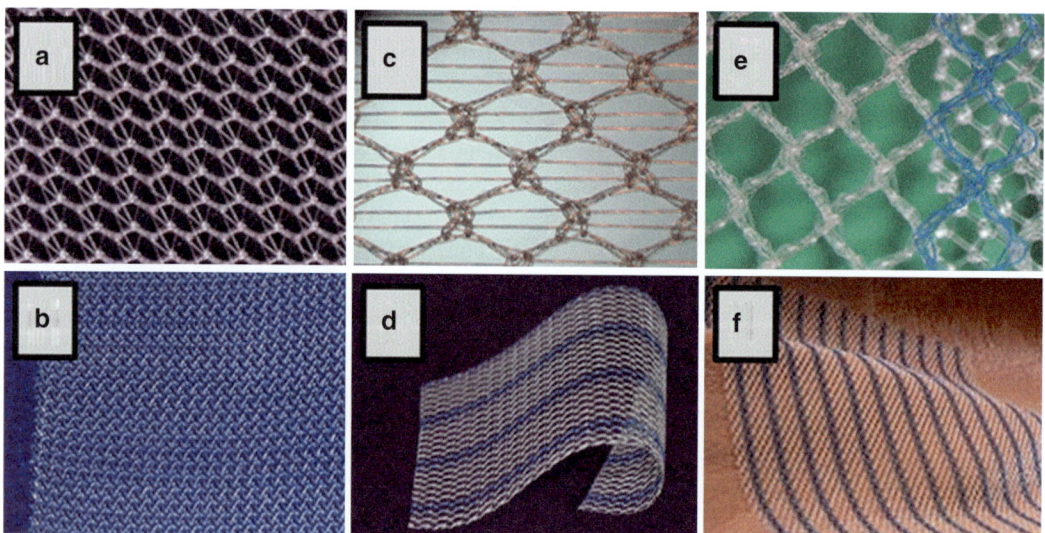

Fig. 4.2 Various constructs of polypropylene mesh: heavyweight (**a**, **b**), mid-weight (**c**, **d**), and light/ultralightweight (**e**, **f**)

Biocompatibility appears to be proportional to the pore size of the mesh.

Every mesh generates an intense host inflammatory reaction that follows a cascading sequence of events (coagulation, inflammation, angiogenesis, epithelialization, fibroplasia, matrix deposition, and contraction) with a resultant formation of dense connective tissue. Although this may have a role in mesh incorporation, the increased amount of connective tissue does not necessarily translate to strength and durability of the repair and can lead to diminished compliance of both the abdominal wall and be associated with patient discomfort. There is no evidence that the inflammatory reaction elicited by mesh implantation significantly increases carcinogenesis.

Prosthetic weight is the subject of constant debate, considering the desire to balance mesh strength with its elicited inflammatory response. Heavyweight PP provides with significantly more strength (up to four times the tensile and burst strength) than the abdominal wall but is associated with an intense foreign body reaction that decreases with lighter PP configurations and larger pores. Lightweight mesh is designed to reduce the amount of synthetic material and its associated tissue reaction, enhancing the formation of a scar "net" instead of a thick "plate" reaction [9]. Accordingly, lightweight PP prosthetics are associated with less shrinkage after implantation in vivo [11].

These modifications have several implications for inguinal hernia repairs. Heavier prosthetics have been generally associated with more groin pain and increased mesh sensation, while ultra-light products have more risk for recurrence because of their reduced material content. Braided POL is very pliable and therefore easier to handle than monofilament PP but is generally considered as less biocompatible and has higher infection rates. In our laboratory experience, we demonstrated that polyester induces the most intense inflammatory reaction among synthetic meshes. When uncoated POL and PP are exposed to the bowel, they both can lead to extensive adhesions and fistula formation [12]. Macroporous meshes have an increased ability to resist infection because of their rapid incorporation. A large-pore PP mesh could sometimes be salvaged after infection, while ePTFE will almost always need to be explanted.

In an effort to minimize fibrotic response and to prevent adhesions, PP and POL meshes have been coated with anti-adhesive barriers using absorbable or nonabsorbable materials such as omega-3 fatty acids, polyglactin, polydioxanone, poliglecaprone, hyaluronic acid, collagen, or titanium. These layers are intended to persist until neoperitoneum has covered the implant, typically within 10–14 days after surgery.

Biologic Mesh

Biologic mesh typically consists of decellularized matrix derived from porcine, bovine, or human cadavers. Their theoretical use would be in the infected field [13]; nevertheless there is no data supporting this statement for inguinal hernia. Randomized controlled trials have not shown any clear advantages of biologics over synthetics for elective groin hernia repair [14, 15], and therefore their routine use has not been adopted.

Scenarios for Synthetic Mesh Selection

PP is the most frequently used prosthetic in groin hernia repairs. The use of flat POL has been associated with significantly higher "catching or pulling" sensation at short-term follow-up (34.3% vs 5.7%) when compared to PP in traditional Lichtenstein repairs [16], without improving any other mesh-related outcome.

Lightweight or Heavyweight Mesh in Open Surgery?

Meta-analysis [17, 18] has found that the use of lightweight PP mesh is associated with less chronic pain and foreign body sensation while having recurrence rates as heavyweight PP mesh. A systematic review with similar findings noted that although overall pain is lower in the lightweight group, there are no differences when accounting for severe pain between groups [19]. Animal studies have shown that the use of lighter prosthetics may reduce the rates of vas deferens obstructions [20], and therefore its use could be preferred in young male patients.

Considering these benefits, published guidelines support the use of lightweight meshes for most open inguinal hernias but add a word of caution for large direct hernias where there may be a role for heavier prosthetics [21]. This is because of bulging and mesh failure in cases where lightweight implants were used to bridge very large defects.

Lightweight or Heavyweight in Minimally Invasive Repairs?

Two meta-analyses have shown that the weight of synthetics used in minimally invasive inguinal hernia repair does not affect the recurrence rate, but when analyzing chronic pain, they reported either no difference between groups [22] or a reduced rate favoring lightweight group [23]. Although many individual studies reported modest benefits for lightweight mesh, a more recent double-blinded randomized trial on TEP repairs showed that lightweight mesh group had higher rates of significant postoperative pain (2.9% vs 0.7%) and higher recurrence rates (2.7% vs 0.8%) [24]. Although the HerniaSurge guidelines do not report relevant differences for this type of repair, we believe that the choice of mesh should also be individualized in laparoendoscopic repairs. Patients who will most benefit from lightweight mesh are thin, athletic men and women, those with indirect or small direct defects, as well as patients with femoral hernias. To prevent bulging and recurrences, we advocate for using midweight in patients with large direct and recurrent hernias.

Composite Mesh

The use of coating in synthetic prosthetics has been associated to less postoperative pain both in short- and long-term follow-up. Nevertheless, this difference could be potentially attributed to the use of heavyweight PP in the control group and not necessarily to the coating in the lightweight composite. A systematic review addressing this found no significant benefit in pain reduction between nonabsorbable and composite prosthetics but highlights the advantages of light-

weight in pain and foreign body sensation when compared to heavyweight synthetics [25].

Self-Gripping and Preformed Mesh

The use of suture-based mesh fixation has been associated with adverse patient outcomes in hernia surgery, especially postoperative pain. This has led to developing of several novel fixation mechanisms for PP and POL prosthetics, such as self-gripping synthetic mesh with microhooks. Atraumatic mesh fixation has been associated with reduced early postoperative pain scores. As it would be expected, the use of non-suture fixation techniques in open groin repairs generally reduces the operative time but does not improve chronic postoperative pain [26, 27]. The use of self-gripping mesh in open surgery has not changed hernia recurrence rates, postoperative complications, or hospital stay. Small comparative studies and cohorts have shown that self-gripping mesh is feasible and safe in TAPP and TEP repairs [28, 29] and have highlighted the potential benefits over other fixation methods; but this remains to be elucidated with higher quality evidence.

In an effort to accommodate abdominopelvic contours during repair, preformed meshes are available. Products with a three-dimensional structure mimic the anatomy of the inguinal floor in an attempt to cover the entire myopectineal orifice and reduce or eliminate the need for fixation [30], which may be the principle for their theoretical advantage. Nevertheless, the clinical benefits of pre-shaped meshes have not been established to date.

Intraperitoneal Onlay Mesh (IPOM)

Traditional laparoscopic ventral hernia repairs require placement of a mesh intraperitoneally, and this requires prosthetics that promote tissue ingrowth on one side (peritoneal side) and impede adhesion formation on the other (visceral) side. Historically, two-sided ePTFE with a macroporous corrugated surface and a microporous surface was used for intraperitoneal onlay mesh (IPOM) repair for inguinal hernias; nevertheless this technique is used very infrequently now; intraperitoneal placement of ePTFE and other composite prosthetics has been reported where it was judged that IPOM was needed [31, 32].

Conclusions

The vast majority of patients with inguinal hernias will require prosthetic reinforcement. Mesh selection influences clinical outcomes in hernia surgery. The use and choice of mesh for inguinal hernia repairs must be guided by hernia characteristics (contamination, size, and anatomy), patient factors (age, body habitus, level of function, and expected activity), and the surgeon's operative approach and experience. Knowledge of the characteristics of commercially available prosthetics is paramount for their appropriate use in the groin hernia population.

References

1. Ramshaw B, Grant S. Biology of prosthetics. In: Kingsnorth ALK, editor. Abdominal hernias. London: Springer; 2013.
2. Scott NW, McCormack K, Graham P, Go PM, Ross SJ, Grant AM. Open mesh versus non-mesh for repair of femoral and inguinal hernia. Cochrane Database Syst Rev. 2002;2002:CD002197.
3. Pickett L. Prosthetic choice in open inguinal hernia repair. In: Jacob B, Ramshaw B, editors. The SAGES manual of hernia repair. New York: Springer; 2013. p. 19–26.
4. Rosenberg J, Bisgaard T, Kehlet H, et al. Danish hernia database recommendations for the management of inguinal and femoral hernia in adults. Dan Med Bull. 2011;58:C4243.
5. O'Neill SM, Chen DC, Amid PK In: Novitsky YW, editor. Hernia Surgery: Current Principles. Switzerland: Springer; 2016. p437–49
6. Hernia Repair JM. Now and in the future. In: Campanelli G, editor. Inguinal hernia. Philadelphia: Springer; 2017. p. 37–42.
7. Nguyen DK, Amid PK, Chen DC. Groin pain after inguinal hernia repair. Adv Surg. 2016;50:203–20.
8. Cobb WS, Peindl RM, Zerey M, Carbonell AM, Heniford BT. Mesh terminology 101. Hernia. 2009;13:1–6.
9. Earle DB, Mark LA. Prosthetic material in inguinal hernia repair: how do I choose? Surg Clin North Am. 2008;88:179–201. x
10. Coda A, Lamberti R, Martorana S. Classification of prosthetics used in hernia repair based on weight and biomaterial. Hernia. 2012;16:9–20.
11. Silvestre AC, de Mathia GB, Fagundes DJ, Medeiros LR, Rosa MI. Shrinkage evaluation of heavyweight and lightweight polypropylene meshes in inguinal hernia repair: a randomized controlled trial. Hernia. 2011;15:629–34.
12. Orenstein S, Novitsky YW. Synthetic mesh choices for surgical repair. In: Rosen MJ, editor. Atlas of abdomial wall reconstruction: Philadelphia: Elsevier; 2012. p. 322–9.
13. Novitsky YW. Biology of biological meshes used in hernia repair. Surg Clin North Am. 2013;93:1211–5.
14. Bochicchio GV, Jain A, McGonigal K, et al. Biologic vs synthetic inguinal hernia repair: 1-year results of a randomized double-blinded trial. J Am Coll Surg. 2014;218:751–7.
15. Bellows CF, Shadduck P, Helton WS, Martindale R, Stouch BC, Fitzgibbons R. Early report of a randomized comparative clinical trial of Strattice reconstructive tissue matrix to lightweight synthetic mesh in the repair of inguinal hernias. Hernia. 2014;18:221–30.
16. Sadowski B, Rodriguez J, Symmonds R, et al. Comparison of polypropylene versus polyester mesh in the Lichtenstein hernia repair with respect to chronic pain and discomfort. Hernia. 2011;15:643–54.
17. Uzzaman MM, Ratnasingham K, Ashraf N. Meta-analysis of randomized controlled trials comparing lightweight and heavyweight mesh for Lichtenstein inguinal hernia repair. Hernia. 2012;16:505–18.
18. Sajid MS, Leaver C, Baig MK, Sains P. Systematic review and meta-analysis of the use of lightweight versus heavyweight mesh in open inguinal hernia repair. Br J Surg. 2012;99:29–37.
19. Smietanski M, Smietanska IA, Modrzejewski A, Simons MP, Aufenacker TJ. Systematic review and meta-analysis on heavy and lightweight polypropylene mesh in Lichtenstein inguinal hernioplasty. Hernia. 2012;16:519–28.
20. Junge K, Binnebosel M, Rosch R, et al. Influence of mesh materials on the integrity of the vas deferens following Lichtenstein hernioplasty: an experimental model. Hernia. 2008;12:621–6.
21. Miserez M, Peeters E, Aufenacker T, et al. Update with level 1 studies of the European hernia society guidelines on the treatment of inguinal hernia in adult patients. Hernia. 2014;18:151–63.
22. Currie A, Andrew H, Tonsi A, Hurley PR, Taribagil S. Lightweight versus heavyweight mesh in laparoscopic inguinal hernia repair: a meta-analysis. Surg Endosc. 2012;26:2126–33.
23. Sajid MS, Kalra L, Parampalli U, Sains PS, Baig MK. A systematic review and meta-analysis evaluating the effectiveness of lightweight mesh against heavyweight mesh in influencing the incidence of

chronic groin pain following laparoscopic inguinal hernia repair. Am J Surg. 2013;205:726–36.

24. Burgmans JP, Voorbrood CE, Simmermacher RK, et al. Long-term results of a randomized double-blinded prospective trial of a lightweight (Ultrapro) versus a heavyweight mesh (Prolene) in laparoscopic total extraperitoneal inguinal hernia repair (TULP-trial). Ann Surg. 2016;263:862–6.

25. Markar SR, Karthikesalingam A, Alam F, Tang TY, Walsh SR, Sadat U. Partially or completely absorbable versus nonabsorbable mesh repair for inguinal hernia: a systematic review and meta-analysis. Surg Laparosc Endosc Percutan Tech. 2010;20:213–9.

26. Sanders DL, Nienhuijs S, Ziprin P, Miserez M, Gingell-Littlejohn M, Smeds S. Randomized clinical trial comparing self-gripping mesh with suture fixation of lightweight polypropylene mesh in open inguinal hernia repair. Br J Surg. 2014;101:1373–82. discussion 82

27. Chatzimavroudis G, Papaziogas B, Koutelidakis I, et al. Lichtenstein technique for inguinal hernia repair using polypropylene mesh fixed with sutures vs. self-fixating polypropylene mesh: a prospective randomized comparative study. Hernia. 2014;18:193–8.

28. Fumagalli Romario U, Puccetti F, Elmore U, Massaron S, Rosati R. Self-gripping mesh versus staple fixation in laparoscopic inguinal hernia repair: a prospective comparison. Surg Endosc. 2013;27:1798–802.

29. Bresnahan E, Bates A, Wu A, Reiner M, Jacob B. The use of self-gripping (Progrip) mesh during laparoscopic total extraperitoneal (TEP) inguinal hernia repair: a prospective feasibility and long-term outcomes study. Surg Endosc. 2015;29:2690–6.

30. LeBlanc K. Meshes for inguinal hernia repair. In: Campanelli G, editor. Inguinal hernia surgery: Philadelphia: Springer; 2017. p. 143–9.

31. Tran H, Tran K, Zajkowska M, Lam V, Hawthorne WJ. Single-port onlay mesh repair of recurrent inguinal hernias after failed anterior and laparoscopic repairs. JSLS. 2015;19:e2014 00212.

32. Hyllegaard GM, Friis-Andersen H. Modified laparoscopic intraperitoneal onlay mesh in complicated inguinal hernia surgery. Hernia. 2015;19:433–6.

Part II

Open Surgical Techniques

Open Non-mesh Inguinal Hernia Repair

5

Bruce Ramshaw and Sherard Chiu

Introduction

Inguinal hernias remain one of the most common indications for surgery worldwide. About 27% of males and 3% of females will develop an inguinal hernia during their lifetime. Because of the prevalence and the complexity of the inguinal anatomy, many different repair techniques have been described. However, the goal of all these techniques remains the same: to improve quality of life by providing long-lasting closure of the groin defect. With modern techniques, recurrence rates remain very low, below 5% in most reported series. Although lately, chronic pain has become more of a concern. The etiology of chronic pain is multifactorial and difficult to understand using a reductionist mind-set. In this chapter, we will discuss the open tissue-based repair and issues associated with these repairs. We will also discuss the complex issue of chronic groin pain and mesh-related complications which have raised the awareness about non-mesh repairs in recent years.

B. Ramshaw (✉)
Department of Surgery, University of Tennessee Medical Center and Graduate School of Medicine, Knoxville, TN, USA
e-mail: BRamshaw@utmck.edu

S. Chiu
Department of Surgery, University of Tennessee Graduate School of Medicine, Knoxville, TN, USA

Complexity of the Inguinal Anatomy

There are many textbooks, anatomic illustrations, and published manuscripts describing the inguinal anatomy and specific tissue repair techniques for inguinal hernia repair. As more and more descriptions of techniques and the anatomy are published, it has become clear that this area of the body is one of the most complex. In the descriptions of chronic musculoskeletal groin injury, Bill Meyers, a world expert in the field, has described at least 17 different injury types or variants resulting in the same athletic pubalgia syndrome. This does not include chronic groin pain with etiologies from the hip and/or spine. There is almost no other region of our body where more things come together – the perineum, lower extremity, lower abdomen, etc. Due to this anatomic complexity, it can be difficult to follow anatomic descriptions of the specific tissue repairs described in this chapter. We will attempt to explain each description based on available references and try to minimize anatomic terms that may be controversial or that are rarely used. After these descriptions, we will present a section describing the general principles of open tissue repair techniques using common anatomic language, not the specific named structures that can sometimes make it difficult for learners attempting to understand these techniques. Also, if a tissue repair is performed as a re-operative procedure, as is sometimes done as a part of the procedure for chronic pain, many specific named anatomic structures are either not recognizable of significantly altered due to the prior operation(s).

Techniques

There are many methods to repairing inguinal hernias, from traditional open tissue-based repairs to laparoscopic mesh repairs. In the United States, as in most other developed countries, mesh repair has become the standard. While in less developed countries, tissue-based repairs are still the primary technique used. There are many types of tissue-based repairs, and although these repairs are considered by some to be superior to mesh repair in terms of the risk of developing chronic pain, they have been shown to have a higher recurrence rate compared to techniques in which a mesh is used. There are two main categories of tissue-based repairs: tension and tension-free. We will discuss the more popular techniques of both.

Bassini

The Bassini repair is performed by opening the pelvic floor and reducing all the preperitoneal and hernia contents back into the abdominal cavity and then sewing the conjoint tendon to the inguinal ligament. In his repair, Bassini opened the transversalis fascia, but this step may be replaced by placing sutures between the conjoint tendon and the deeper transversalis fascia to the inguinal ligament. Care must be taken to ensure the incorporation of all three anatomic layers medially: internal oblique muscle, transversus abdominis muscle, and transversalis fascia. Single interrupted permanent sutures are traditionally used to perform the repair. The repair should start medially, securing the lateral edge of the rectus sheath/conjoint tendon to the fascia overlying the pubic tubercle. Subsequent sutures laterally should be placed from the conjoint tendon to the inguinal ligament. Laterally, each suture should incorporate few fibers of the

inguinal ligament to avoid injuring the femoral vessels. The internal ring should be reconstructed allowing the tip of your finger or an instrument to pass through the ring to avoid constriction of the cord structures. In order to decrease tension on the repair, a vertical incision can be made on the anterior rectus sheath. This type of "relaxing incision" would modify the Bassini repair into a more tension-free tissue repair.

Shouldice

The Shouldice repair is another popular tissue-based repair. The transversalis fascia is opened from the medial aspect of the internal ring to the fascial thickening of Cooper's ligament being careful not to injure the inferior epigastric vessels. This incision allows identification of the transversalis abdominis muscle, internal oblique muscle, and transversalis fascia. Flaps of the transversalis fascia are developed medially and laterally. The lateral flaps should be carried out to Cooper's ligament to expose the iliopubic tract. A four-layer repair is performed as follows with nonabsorbable suture, traditionally stainless steel wire: the first layer anchors the transversalis fascia to the fascia overlying the periosteum of the pubic tubercle. This is run laterally, approximating the posterior rectus sheath to the iliopubic tract. After this is run as laterally as possible, it is then continued on the posterior transversalis fascia and is run superiorly and laterally until the internal ring is recreated. This suture is then reversed and brought back medially, approximating the three layers (transversalis fascia, internal oblique, and transversus abdominis) to the inguinal ligament. This will continue to the tail of the first suture, and these will be tied to each other. The first layer should be imbricated at this point. The third layer is completed in a similar fashion starting at the internal ring and run medially, approximating the internal oblique and transversus abdominis to the posterior external oblique aponeurosis just above the inguinal ligament. The fourth layer is then run back toward the internal ring, reinforcing the third layer by approximating the internal oblique and transversus abdominis to the external oblique aponeurosis, thus reconstructing the external ring.

McVay

The McVay/Cooper's is a repair that can be used to repair femoral, indirect, and direct hernias. The posterior wall of the inguinal canal is opened, exposing the internal oblique muscle, transversus abdominis muscle aponeurosis, and transversalis fascia. Simple interrupted sutures are used to approximate the internal oblique aponeurosis, transversus abdominis aponeurosis, and transversalis fascia to Cooper's ligament starting medially. Laterally, this will transition to suturing the internal oblique aponeurosis, transversus abdominis aponeurosis, and transversalis fascia to the inguinal ligament in order to recreate the internal ring. Care must be taken not to injure the femoral vein. This repair may result in tension for which a relaxing incision may be performed. The rectus sheath is exposed and incised vertically along its edge from the tubercle and cephalad longitudinally 5–6 cm. It is a good idea to create the relaxing incision first, if performed, before tying the repair sutures. Today, this repair is mainly used for repair of femoral hernias. The previously discussed repairs are all tension repairs, unless a relaxing incision is utilized.

Desarda

The Desarda repair may be considered a tension-free tissue repair. In the case of an indirect hernia, the sac is excised. However, with a direct hernia, the sac is inverted into the abdominal cavity using a purse-string suture. The upper leaf of the external oblique aponeurosis is sutured to the inguinal ligament from the pubic tubercle to the abdominal ring using absorbable suture in a continuous fashion. The first two medial stitches are taken through the anterior rectus sheath, and the last two are taken to slightly narrow the abdominal ring. A splitting incision is then made in the upper leaf of the external oblique aponeurosis. This incision is started from the pubic symphysis and taken 1–2 cm beyond the abdominal ring laterally. The upper border of this incision is sutured to the internal oblique with absorbable suture. This results in the formation of a new posterior wall of the inguinal canal. The spermatic cord is placed in the canal, and the lateral leaf of the external oblique aponeurosis is sutured to the newly formed medial leaf of the external oblique in front of the cord using absorbable suture.

Guarnieri

The Guarnieri technique may also be considered a tension-free tissue-based repair that begins similarly to other open techniques. The external oblique is opened, and flaps are created. The cord is then isolated. The internal oblique muscle is separated from the cremasteric fibers. A plane is developed between the internal oblique muscle and the aponeurosis of the transversus abdominus. Retracting the internal oblique muscle fully exposes the transversalis fascia medial to the deep ring. An incision at the proximal portion of the tunica vaginalis including the internal ring is carried medially and cephalad to the transversalis fascia and aponeurosis of the transversus. The sac is isolated and can be ligated or pushed back into the preperitoneal space. The cord structures are then dissected out of the tunica vaginalis and cremasteric muscles. The incision of the transversalis fascia is extended a few centimeters up to the rectus sheath. The cord structures are then transposed to the medial opening of the incised transversalis fascia. Suture is then used to create this new deep inguinal ring, and the transversalis fascia is closed transversely in a running fashion. This will close off the original deep inguinal ring opening. A second layer is created using the same suture bringing the layer of the cremasteric muscles together with the tunica vaginalis. The external ring will be transposed to where the internal oblique muscle meets the rectus muscle sheath. The lateral border of the external oblique aponeurosis is then sutured to the rectus sheath behind the cord. Then another continuous suture is used to approximate the lateral border of the external oblique aponeurosis to the rectus sheath above the cord, forming the new external ring. A releasing incision is made on the lateral border of the rectus sheath. The last suture line starts at the pubis to the new external ring and then from there toward the anterior iliac spine overlapping the medial border of the external oblique aponeurosis to the lateral surface of the lateral oblique aponeurosis.

General Principles

The general principles for an open tissue repair for an inguinal hernia include opening the external oblique musculofascia to expose the cord structures, isolating the cord structures to attempt to protect them and retracting them, usually with a Penrose drain, to better expose the deeper structures. The external oblique can be opened by identifying the external ring and opening it from medial to lateral. The next step is to identify the hernia contents and hernia defect. An indirect hernia travels with the cord structures through the internal ring. The herniated contents, with a lipoma of the cord if identified, can be dissected free from the cord structures and replaced back into the abdominal cavity. If a direct defect is present, there is disruption of the inguinal floor comprised of the internal oblique, transversus abdominus, and/or transversalis fascia layers. A direct defect is likely to be acquired – more related to poor collagen and/or repetitive increase in abdominal pressure, such as a chronic cough – where an indirect defect is often more likely to be congenital. However, there are usually many factors involved in the development of any inguinal hernia. An indirect hernia is more likely to be successfully repaired with a tissue-only repair than is a direct hernia. Some patients will have both an indirect and direct hernia, often referred to as a pantaloon defect. Once the hernia contents are reduced, the repair can begin. The reconstruction of the transversalis, transversus abdominus, and internal oblique will recreate the internal ring and reconstruct the inguinal floor. This can be done with or without approximation to Cooper's ligament. Approximation to Cooper's ligament

will reinforce the femoral space. This would be necessary if a femoral hernia was present. After the deeper tissues are reconstructed to recreate the internal ring, the external oblique musculofascia is reapproximated to reconstruct the external ring. The subcutaneous tissue and skin are then reapproximated. The general difference between tissue repairs that may be considered tension reduced include those that propose relaxing incisions and those that divide one musculofascial layer and approximate it to a different musculofascial layer. Based on evidence in the literature, it appears that open tissue-based inguinal hernia repairs are more alike than different. Outcomes are much more likely to be due to the skill and experience with any one tissue repair than the specific tissue repair itself.

Outcomes

The outcomes for open non-mesh inguinal hernia repair demonstrate a higher recurrence rate, increased short-term pain, and a longer recovery time compared with open and laparoscopic mesh hernia repairs. However, the differences are generally quite small, with differences in recurrence rates in single digit percentages, and recovery time difference is typically only a matter of days. In fact, there are also studies of high-volume hernia centers, specifically the Shouldice Clinic, where recurrence rates have been documented to be as low as or even lower than mesh-based inguinal hernia repairs. The challenge for the Shouldice technique is that these excellent results have generally not been reproducible for other surgeons. Chronic pain after inguinal hernia repair has been a growing concern with hernia mesh considered by some a contributing factor in the development and severity of chronic pain after inguinal hernia repair. A more detailed discussion of this topic will be discussed in the next section.

A recent systematic review published in the Cochrane Database looked at mesh and non-mesh hernia repairs. The review suggested that although the Shouldice repair had a higher recurrence rate than repair that utilized mesh, it demonstrated a lower recurrence rate than other non-mesh repairs. There are numerous studies that demonstrate the equivalence and/or superiority between mesh and non-mesh repairs. This confusion of outcomes in the literature reflects the complexity of this issue. There are many factors at each local environment that will impact the outcomes for any specific inguinal hernia repair technique. For example, the outcome for a hernia surgeon or practice where the experience is many hundreds or thousands of procedures will be different than for a surgeon or practice at another local environment where the experience is less than 100 procedures with a specific repair technique. There are also patient factors that will impact outcomes. If a surgeon or practice in one local environment applies strict criteria, such as smoking cessation, a BMI range requirement, and exclusion of types of hernias (e.g., scrotal hernias) and another surgeon or practice at another local environment does not apply these criteria similarly, the outcomes will be different using the same specific technique.

Because of this complexity, and the fact that many variables are not controllable, we will need to apply systems and data science principles in the future to better match specific inguinal repair options to specific patient subpopulations in each local environment where the procedures are performed. We have demonstrated over the past many decades that reductionist science tools, such as prospective, randomized controlled trials, have been inadequate to give insight into the best possible inguinal hernia repair option for various patient subpopulations. It is time to apply the tools of systems and data science, such as continuous quality improvement and nonlinear analytics, to complex healthcare problems such as an inguinal hernia. This would not only apply to the appropriate application of mesh and non-mesh inguinal hernia repair techniques for various identified patient subpopulations but also for the application of watchful waiting strategies for appropriate other patient subpopulations for whom that approach would result in the best outcome.

Why We Should Rethink Open Non-mesh Repair for Inguinal Hernia

For the past quarter of a century, most surgeons in the Western world have utilized a mesh repair for inguinal hernias in adults, either through an open of laparoscopic approach. This likely developed for several reasons. One is that a patient generally has less acute pain and a quicker recovery after an inguinal hernia repair with mesh. It is also easier to learn and perform a mesh repair compared with a tissue repair because detailed familiarity with the anatomy may be less important for a mesh repair. However, as mesh became more prevalent, increasing concern about chronic pain after inguinal hernia repair has surfaced. Although the rate of severe postoperative inguinodynia is low (less than 5–10%), the number of patients impacted is significant because of the number of inguinal hernia repairs performed each year. Based on this percentage and the number of inguinal hernia repairs, there are at least hundreds of thousands of people suffering from this problem in the United States alone.

It has become public knowledge, primarily through advertisements by plaintiffs' lawyers, that hernia mesh is the cause of this problem (as well as other complications) after hernia repair. But this is a simplistic, incomplete understanding of a complex problem. Mesh does not cause chronic pain. Chronic pain does occur in patients who undergo non-mesh repair and in patients who have other surgical procedures that do not implant mesh or other medical implants. The rate of chronic pain can even be higher after other operations such as thoracotomy and mastectomy. However, mesh may be a contributing factor, among many others, in the development of chronic pain after inguinal hernia repair. As mentioned above, we will need to apply the tools from systems and data science to begin to identify these factors and develop predictive algorithms that can give insight to patient subpopulations that will be at risk for developing chronic pain after inguinal hernia repair if a mesh is used.

In the future, we should also be able to bring more advanced materials science solutions to the development of potentially more biocompatible hernia mesh devices. Until January 2017, the FDA regulatory process inhibited any attempt to bring a newer, potentially better, material for hernia mesh to the US market. This was because any new material would have required a premarket approval (PMA) process. The time and expense required and the uncertainty in gaining approval resulted in no company attempting to obtain regulatory approval for a hernia mesh manufactured using a newer, potentially more biocompatible, material. The materials available today, all plastic polymers, were "grandfathered" in and were not required to go through a regulatory approval process because they had been used as surgical implants before the Medical Device Regulation Act became law in 1976. Modern plastic polymer technology, developed by Carothers in 1935, is almost a century old. Materials science has generated a wealth of possible materials that could be more biocompatible and result in less complications. Plant-based bioplastics and newly discovered materials, such as graphene, are just two examples of items that may show this potential.

Summary

Open, non-mesh inguinal hernia repair techniques are gaining interest for several reasons. These tissue repairs eliminate one potential contributing factor, hernia mesh, to the development of chronic groin pain after inguinal hernia repair.

However, this complication, as devastating as it can be, is a complex problem. Eliminating hernia mesh from the operation will not completely eliminate the problem of chronic groin pain after inguinal hernia repair and might lead to an increase in the rate of hernia recurrence. To better understand complex problems and identify appropriate treatment options based on factors related to patient subpopulations, the principles and tools from systems and data science will be necessary.

Selected References

Amato B, Moja L, Panico S, et al. Shouldice technique versus other open techniques for inguinal hernia repair. Cochrane Database Syst Rev. 2012;18(4):CD001543.

Bendavid R, Lou W, Grischkan D, et al. A mechanism of mesh-related post-herniorrhaphy neuralgia. Hernia. 2016;20(3):357–65.

Bulbuller N, Kirkil C, Godekmerdan A, et al. The comparison of inflammatory response and clinical results after groin hernia repair using polypropylene or polyester meshes. Ind J Surg. 2015;77(Suppl 2):S283–7.

Fischer JE. Hernia repair: why do we continue to perform mesh repair in the face of the human toll of inguinodynia? Am J Surg. 2013) Oct;206(4):619–23.

Iakovlev VV, Guelcher SA, Bendavid R. Degradation of polypropylene in vivo: a microscopic analysis of meshes explanted from patients. J Biomed Mater Res B Appl Biomater. 2017;105(2):237–48.

Malik A, Bell CM, Stukel TA, Urbach DR. Recurrence of inguinal hernias repaired in a large hernia surgical specialty hospital and general hospitals in Ontario, Canada. Can J Surg. 2016;59(1):19–25.

Szopinski J, Dabrowiecki S, Pierscinski S, et al. Desarda versus Lichtenstein technique for primary inguinal hernia treatment: 3-year results of a randomized clinical trial. World J Surg. 2012;36:984–92.

Open Inguinal Hernia Repair

Wen Hui Tan and Jeffrey A. Blatnik

Introduction

The open inguinal hernia repair remains one of the most common procedures performed by general surgeons today. An estimated 20 million inguinal hernia repairs are performed yearly worldwide; 800,000 of them are in the United States [1, 2]. Despite advancements in minimally invasive techniques, the majority of these repairs are still performed with an open approach. In our practice, we prefer to utilize a minimally invasive approach for most patients. However, those with a recurrence after laparoscopic approach, prior pelvic surgery, inability to tolerate general anesthesia, or known hostile abdomen are better served by an open repair.

A number of open, tissue-based repairs exist and will be covered in a separate chapter, but they rely on relieving tension on the native tissue to repair the hernia defect. A higher recurrence rate is often reported in tissue-based repairs, and as such a majority of surgeons have transitioned to a tension-free, mesh-based repair. Specifically, for open repairs the Lichtenstein tension-free mesh repair has become the standard of care and will be described in the subsequent paragraphs [3]. Other mesh based repairs will also be covered

W. H. Tan · J. A. Blatnik (✉)
Section of Minimally Invasive Surgery, Department of Surgery, Washington University School of Medicine in St. Louis, St. Louis, MO, USA
e-mail: JBlatnik@wustl.edu

including plug and patch as well as preperitoneal hernia systems.

Preprocedure

Though an uncomplicated inguinal hernia repair is considered a clean procedure, several meta-analyses suggest that prophylactic antibiotics reduce the incidence of surgical site infections [4–6]. Preoperative antibiotics, such as cefazolin, should be given within 1 h before a skin incision is made and should cover normal skin flora. The choice of anesthesia depends on multiple patient factors including comorbidities and hernia size, but repairs can be safely performed under general, regional, or local anesthesia [7].

Operative Steps: Lichtenstein Repair

A mix of long- and short-acting local anesthetic (such as 1% lidocaine and 0.5% bupivacaine with epinephrine) should be infiltrated along the line of the incision and into the subcutaneous adipose tissue as preemptive analgesia. Some data has shown a reduction in the rate of postoperative pain, nausea, vomiting, and opioid use in patients who receive preemptive analgesia [8].

An incision should be made approximately 1 cm above the pubic tubercle, parallel to the inguinal ligament, and extending 5–6 cm laterally.

© Springer International Publishing AG, part of Springer Nature 2018
M. P. LaPinska, J. A. Blatnik (eds.), *Surgical Principles in Inguinal Hernia Repair*,
https://doi.org/10.1007/978-3-319-92892-0_6

Dissection is carried down through the subcutaneous tissue and Camper's and Scarpa's fascia, exposing the aponeurosis of the external oblique (Fig. 6.1a). Care should be taken to properly divide the superficial epigastric veins, as failure to do so may result in superficial postoperative hematomas. Local anesthetic should also be injected immediately beneath the external oblique aponeurosis to anesthetize all three major nerves in the inguinal canal (Fig. 6.1b). The external oblique aponeurosis is then opened along the line of its fibers through the external inguinal ring, and both the upper and lower leaves are freed from the spermatic cord (Fig. 6.1c). The ilioinguinal nerve is visible below the external oblique aponeuroses and should be safeguarded (Fig. 6.1d). Controversy remains as to the role of routine division of the ilioinguinal nerve and/or iliohypogastric nerve during surgery to minimize the risk of postoperative pain. A double-blinded randomized controlled trial evaluating over 800

patients demonstrated that pain is not affected by elective division of the ilioinguinal nerve during hernia repair [9]. It is our practice to preserve the nerve when possible at the time of repair. However, should it be under increased tension or if we have concern for possible traction injury, we will prophylactically divide the nerve with bipolar cautery where it exits the abdominal wall musculature.

The spermatic cord, including the genitofemoral nerve, spermatic vessels, and ilioinguinal nerve, is encircled with a Penrose drain (Fig. 6.2a) and separated from the floor of the inguinal canal for roughly 2 cm beyond the pubic tubercle. In larger inguinal hernias that extend into the scrotum, this can be a challenging part of the procedure. Once the cord is encircled, the cremaster fibers surrounding the spermatic cord are separated circumferentially from the spermatic cord and if necessary can be divided longitudinally. This will expose an indirect hernia sac (Fig. 6.2b),

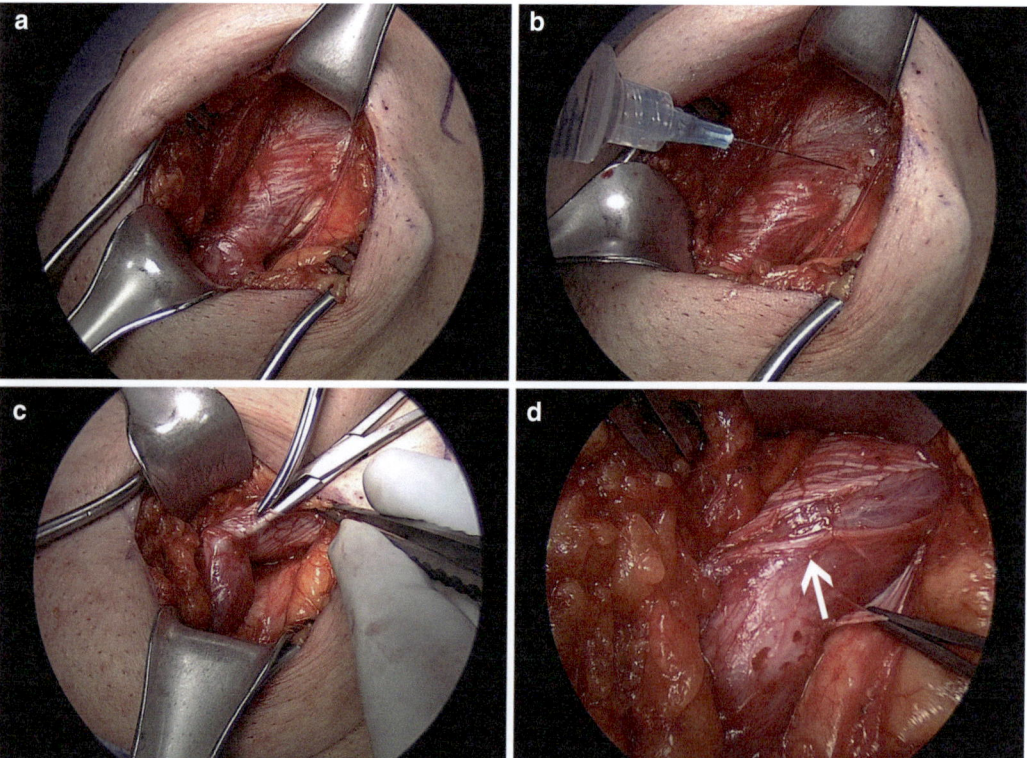

Fig. 6.1 (**a**) Aponeurosis of the external oblique. (**b**) Injection of local anesthetic. (**c**) Opening of the external oblique aponeurosis. (**d**) Ilioinguinal nerve (indicated by the white arrow)

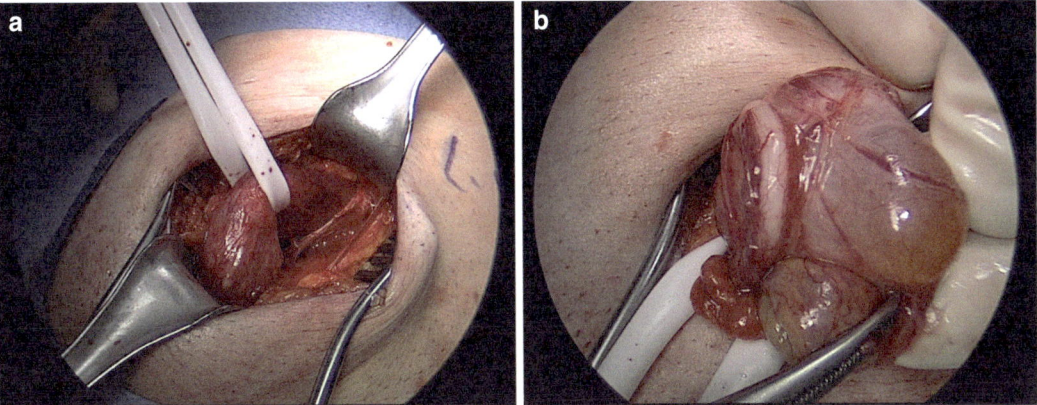

Fig. 6.2 (**a**) Penrose encircling cord contents. (**b**) Indirect hernia sac and vas deferens

if present, usually positioned anteromedially to the cord. An indirect hernia sac should be separated from the cord down to the internal inguinal ring. The sac can then be inverted or ligated (Fig. 6.2b) depending on surgeon preference. We prefer to open the sac to ensure there are no abdominal contents and then suture ligate it at the internal ring. If present, a direct inguinal hernia lies posteromedial to the cord structures. Completely skeletonizing the cord of cremasteric fibers is unnecessary and can lead to injury to the nerves, vas deferens (Fig. 6.2b), or a low-hanging testicle. In the setting of a large direct defect, we will on occasion loosely reconstruct the floor of the canal with interrupted absorbable sutures to facilitate easier mesh placement.

An 8 × 16 cm piece of polypropylene mesh is cut in the shape depicted in Fig. 6.3, with a slit in the lateral aspect of the mesh, creating two tails: a wider superior tail (about two-thirds the width of the mesh) and a thinner inferior tail. The spermatic cord should be retracted cephalad and the mesh placed such that there is roughly 2 cm of overlap medially over the pubic tubercle and 2–3 cm of overlap over the internal oblique muscle edge. To secure the mesh, an initial stitch is placed at the pubic tubercle, taking care to incorporate the rectus sheath above but not periosteum, as this may be a source of post-herniorrhaphy pain. As most hernia recurrences after open inguinal hernia repair occur medially, this stitch is vital to a successful repair. The spermatic cord

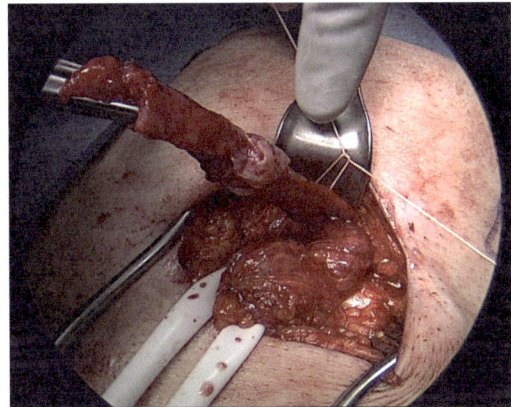

Fig. 6.3 Ligation of hernia sac

is then placed between the two tails of the mesh. Subsequently, the lower edge of the mesh is secured in either a continuous or interrupted fashion using a nonabsorbable suture to the iliopubic tract or shelving edge of the inguinal ligament (Fig. 6.4a), ending just lateral to the internal inguinal ring. Proceeding further laterally risks injury to the femoral nerve. Another stitch is placed at the pubic tubercle, superior to the initial stitch. Care should be taken not to injure or incorporate the iliohypogastric nerve. It is our practice to do this with absorbable sutures, placed in parallel orientation to the nerve and to not over tighten the suture. A new internal inguinal ring is formed by suturing the lower edges of the tails of the mesh to the inguinal ligament just lateral to

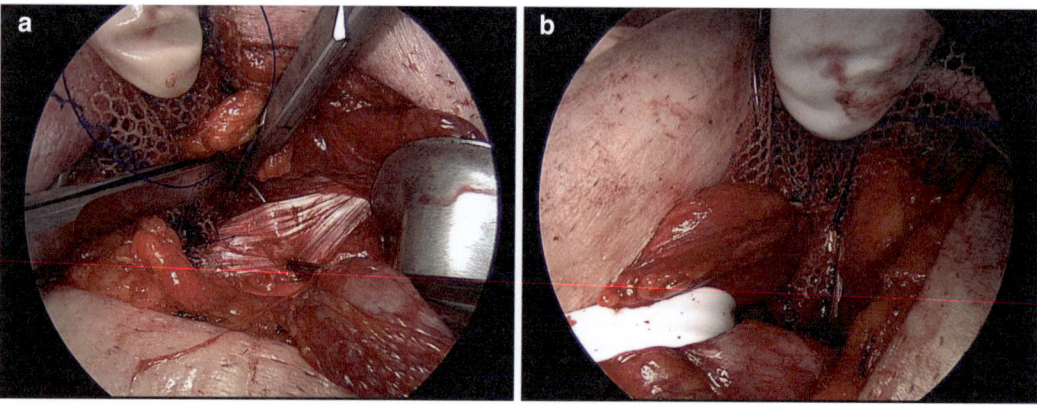

Fig. 6.4 (**a**) Mesh is secured to the shelving edge of the inguinal ligament. (**b**) Formation of the new internal inguinal ring

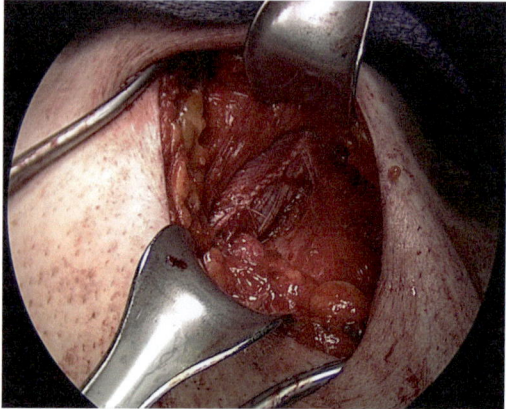

Fig. 6.5 Closure of the external oblique aponeurosis

where the suture securing the lower edge of the mesh to the inguinal ligament ends (Fig. 6.4b). The excess mesh is trimmed, leaving roughly 5 cm of mesh lateral to the internal inguinal ring that will be tucked under the external oblique aponeurosis. The mesh should not be taut or completely flat, in order to accommodate increased abdominal pressure when the patient is no longer supine. However, we do not want to have excess wrinkles or bunching in the mesh either. Following mesh placement, the external oblique aponeurosis is closed using a running absorbable suture (Fig. 6.5). Scarpa's fascia and the subcutaneous tissues are reapproximated using interrupted absorbable sutures, and the skin is closed with a running subcuticular absorbable suture [10–13].

Other Mesh-Based Repairs

Beyond the Lichtenstein style of repair, there are other mesh-based techniques utilized for open inguinal hernia repair. The plug-and-patch style of repair utilizes a prosthetic plug that is placed within the internal ring to reduce the risk for recurrence. Although this is still commonly used for repair, many surgeons have moved away from this technique as the potential for chronic pain may potentially be higher with this style of repair [14]. There are numerous case reports describing migration of the plug from the internal ring into the peritoneal cavity requiring surgical removal.

Beyond the plug-and-patch system is the prolene hernia system. This approach utilizes a bilayered mesh device in which one layer is placed in the preperitoneal plane, and the second layer is placed above the transversalis fascia and secured similarly to a Lichtenstein style repair. The idea behind this style of repair is to reduce the recurrence rate as well as reducing hernia repair time.

Postoperative Care

Elective open inguinal hernia repairs are typically outpatient procedures, and patients can be discharged with appropriate analgesic medications. Patients should be instructed to refrain from heavy lifting and strenuous exercises for a few weeks. The exact period of time is left up to the surgeon's discretion.

Outcomes

Potential complications include seroma, hematoma, infection, urinary retention, groin pain, ischemic orchitis, and recurrence. Approximately 13% of all groin hernia repairs are for recurrent hernias [1]. The recurrence rates for tissue-based repairs were often as high as 25%; however, since the introduction of tension-free, mesh-based repairs, that rate is now 0–1.7% [15]. Overall, the incidence of cardiovascular, intraoperative, or serious adverse surgical events after inguinal hernia surgery is low [16]. In contrast, chronic postherniorrhaphy groin pain is very common, in some series, affecting 10–12% of patients undergoing open mesh-based repairs, and in others, as high as 37%. Factors that may be predictive of chronic inguinodynia include recurrence, complication, mesh weight, preoperative pain score, and age [17]. Some of these patients will eventually require subsequent selective neurectomy and/or mesh removal if they do not respond to conservative pain management [18].

Comparative studies looking at the three primary mesh-based inguinal hernia repair techniques (Lichtenstein, plug-and-patch, and Prolene Hernia System) in general show similar rates in outcomes including pain, quality of life, and recurrence rates [19, 20].

References

1. Aquina CT, Probst CP, Kelly KN, et al. The pitfalls of inguinal herniorrhaphy: surgeon volume matters. Surgery. 2015;158:736–46.
2. Sajid MS, Leaver C, Baig MK, Sains P. Systematic review and meta-analysis of the use of lightweight versus heavyweight mesh in open inguinal hernia repair. Br J Surg. 2012;99:29–37.
3. Fitzgibbons RJ Jr, Richards AT, Quinn TH. Open hernia repair. In: Harken AH, Soper NJ, Cheung LY, Meakins JL, Holcroft JW, Wilmore DW, editors. ACS surgery: principles and practice. New York: WebMD Professional Publishing; 2003.
4. Mazaki T, Mado K, Masuda H, Shiono M. Antibiotic prophylaxis for the prevention of surgical site infection after tension-free hernia repair: a Bayesian and frequentist meta-analysis. J Am Coll Surg. 2013;217:788–801. e1–4
5. Zamkowski MT, Makarewicz W, Ropel J, Bobowicz M, Kakol M, Smietanski M. Antibiotic prophylaxis in open inguinal hernia repair: a literature review and summary of current knowledge. Wideochir Inne Tech Maloinwazyjne. 2016;11:127–36.
6. Li JF, Lai DD, Zhang XD, et al. Meta-analysis of the effectiveness of prophylactic antibiotics in the prevention of postoperative complications after tension-free hernioplasty. Can J Surg. 2012;55:27–32.
7. Nordin P, Zetterstrom H, Gunnarsson U, Nilsson E. Local, regional, or general anaesthesia in groin hernia repair: multicentre randomised trial. Lancet. 2003;362:853–8.
8. Nesioonpour S, Akhondzadeh R, Pipelzadeh MR, Rezaee S, Nazaree E, Soleymani M. The effect of preemptive analgesia with bupivacaine on postoperative pain of inguinal hernia repair under spinal anesthesia: a randomized clinical trial. Hernia. 2013;17:465–70.
9. Picchio M, Palimento D, Attanasio U, Matarazzo PF, Bambini C, Caliendo A. Randomized controlled trial of preservation or elective division of ilioinguinal nerve on open inguinal hernia repair with polypropylene mesh. Arch Surg. 2004;139:755–8. discussion 9
10. Amid PK. Lichtenstein tension-free hernioplasty: its inception, evolution, and principles. Hernia. 2004;8:1–7.
11. Amid PK, Chen DC. Lichtenstein tension-free hernioplasty. In: Fischer JE, Jones DB, Pomposelli FB, Upchurch GR, et al., editors. Fischer's mastery of surgery. 6th ed. Philadelphia, PA: LWW; 2011.
12. Malangoni MA, Rosen MJ. Hernias. In: Townsend CM, Beauchamp RD, Evers BM, Mattox KL, editors. Sabiston textbook of surgery: the biological basis of modern surgical practice. 19th ed. Philadelphia, PA: Saunders; 2012.
13. Cox DD, Bhanot P. Open inguinal hernia repair with plug and patch technique. In: Evans SR, editor. Surgical pitfalls: prevention and management. 1st ed. Philadelphia, PA: Saunders; 2009. p. 501–9.
14. Hallen M, Sevonius D, Westerdahl J, Gunnarsson U, Sandblom G. Risk factors for reoperation due to chronic groin postherniorrhaphy pain. Hernia. 2015;19:863–9.
15. Gopal SV, Warrier A. Recurrence after groin hernia repair-revisited. Int J Surg. 2013;11:374–7.
16. Nilsson H, Angeras U, Sandblom G, Nordin P. Serious adverse events within 30 days of groin hernia surgery. Hernia. 2016;20:377–85.
17. Pierides GA, Paajanen HE, Vironen JH. Factors predicting chronic pain after open mesh based inguinal hernia repair: a prospective cohort study. Int J Surg. 2016;29:165–70.
18. Zwaans WA, Perquin CW, Loos MJ, Roumen RM, Scheltinga MR. Mesh removal and selective neurectomy for persistent groin pain following Lichtenstein repair. World J Surg. 2017;41:701–12.

19. Magnusson J, Nygren J, Gustafsson UO, Thorell A. UltraPro hernia system, Prolene hernia system and Lichtenstein for primary inguinal hernia repair: 3-year outcomes of a prospective randomized controlled trial. Hernia. 2016;20:641–8.

20. Nienhuijs SW, Rosman C. Long-term outcome after randomizing prolene hernia system, mesh plug repair and Lichtenstein for inguinal hernia repair. Hernia. 2015;19:77–81.

Preperitoneal (Stoppa) Open Inguinal Hernia Repair

7

Arielle J. Perez and David M. Krpata

No disease from the human body, belonging to the domain from the surgeon, demands in its treatment, a better mixture of precise, anatomical knowledge along with surgical skill compared to hernia in most its variations.
— Sir Astley Paston Cooper (1804)

History

Posterior preperitoneal repair of the inguinal hernia was first introduced by Cheatle in 1920 [1, 2]. This same exploitation of the preperitoneal space along with closure of the hernia defect for repair was popularized by Nyhus [2]. In 1969, Rene Stoppa abandoned the need for closing the hernia defect when he introduced a novel technique for inguinal hernia repair with the "giant prosthetic reinforcement of the visceral sac" [2–4]. This approach repaired the hernia by occluding the myopectineal orifice with a large piece of mesh placed on top of the peritoneum but deep to the abdominal wall muscles. By doing so, the force generated on the mesh by the intra-abdominal pressure was exploited to provide physical stabilization and ultimately maintaining the mesh in position [5] (Fig. 7.1).

The myopectineal orifice was first described by Henry Fruchaud in 1956 as the area of weakness in the abdominal wall from which the origin of all groin hernias stem [6]. This space is separated in two by the inguinal ligament – the superior space, the origin for direct and indirect hernias, and the inferior space, the origin for

A. J. Perez · D. M. Krpata (✉)
Cleveland Clinic Comprehensive Hernia Center, Digestive Disease and Surgery Institute, Cleveland Clinic Foundation, Cleveland, OH, USA
e-mail: krpatad@ccf.org

femoral hernias. The boundaries of the orifice are created superiorly by the internal oblique and transversus muscles, inferiorly by the superior pubic ramus, medially by the rectus muscle sheath, and laterally by the iliopsoas muscle (Fig. 7.2).

The method of the preperitoneal placement of mesh used by Stoppa is the foundation for the same planes exploited in modern laparoscopic transabdominal preperitoneal (TAPP) and totally extraperitoneal (TEP) techniques. The difference in access to the space and fixation of the mesh are the only comparable differences.

Preoperative Considerations

With multiple methods of inguinal hernia repair in the arsenal of today's surgeon, the Stoppa repair should be reserved for certain patients. The morbidity of the repair by placing a large prosthetic over bilateral groins and requiring an extensive dissection in delicate tissue planes should be undertaken by a surgeon well acquainted with the anatomy of the area. Gainant published a prospective, nonrandomized study of laparoscopic TEP vs Stoppa repair of bilateral inguinal hernias. Recurrence rates were similar, 2% in the Stoppa and 1.1% in the laparoscopic group, and complications occurred in 3% of the Stoppa and 4% of the laparoscopic group [7].

© Springer International Publishing AG, part of Springer Nature 2018
M. P. LaPinska, J. A. Blatnik (eds.), *Surgical Principles in Inguinal Hernia Repair*,
https://doi.org/10.1007/978-3-319-92892-0_7

45

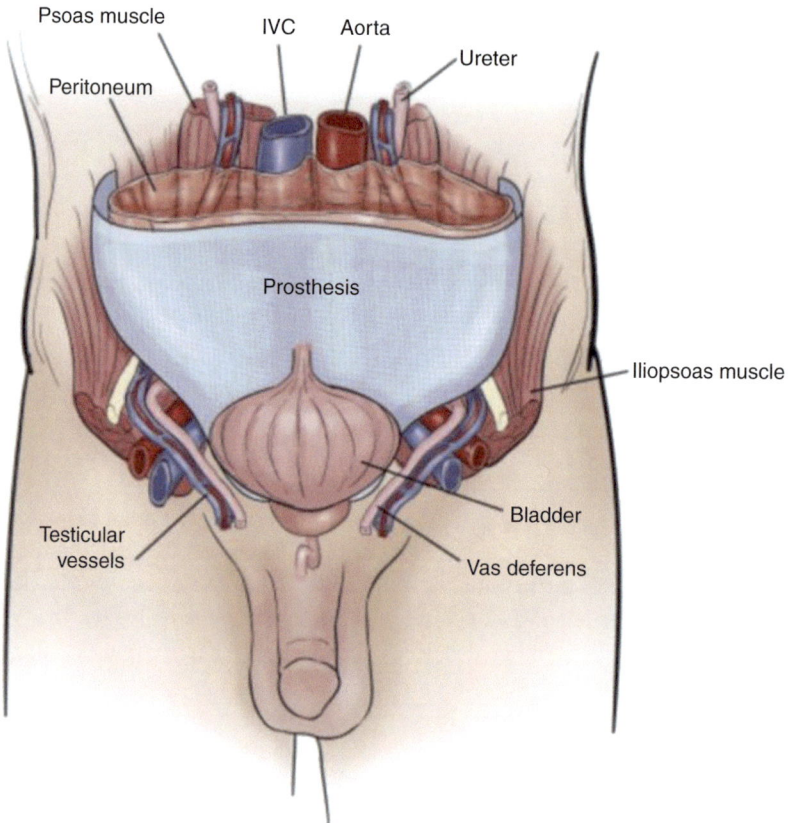

Fig. 7.1 Stoppa's giant prosthetic reinforcement of the visceral sac exploits a preperitoneal space which excludes all viscera and allows for coverage of bilateral inguinal and femoral regions. (Chapter 82 Atlas of Abdominal Wall Reconstruction: e2)

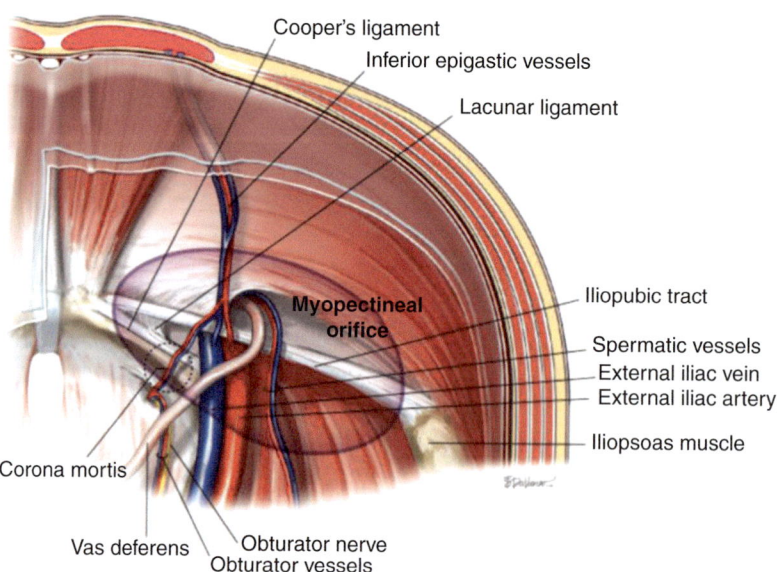

Fig. 7.2 Myopectineal orifice which includes the direct and indirect inguinal space along with the femoral space. (TEP chapter from Rosen's Atlas)

The advantages of the Stoppa repair, covering the large myopectineal orifice, addressing bilateral sides, and exploiting the preperitoneal space, is what dictates the ideal patient selection. Patients who can withstand general anesthesia with recurrent hernias, prior anterior repairs, or large and/or bilateral inguinoscrotal hernias should be considered for the Stoppa hernia repair. However, if it is felt that an initial anterior approach or laparoscopic repair would be sufficient, those methods should be pursued first.

Absolute contraindications for the Stoppa repair are the same for other pelvic surgeries in which a prosthetic will be placed: intra-abdominal infection and active coagulopathy. Relative contraindications are based on the comfort of the surgeon and patient history: prior pelvic radiation, prior operations in which the space of Retzius has been explored, and prior lower abdominal surgeries with extensive dissection.

All skin infections in the operative area should be treated prior to elective surgery. Patients who are actively smoking should be encouraged to quit smoking at least 6 weeks prior to operation to reduce wound morbidity and improve healing. Neither mechanical nor antibiotic bowel preparation is necessary prior to a Stoppa repair.

Preoperatively, clippers are used to remove all hair from the surgical field. A single dose of perioperative antibiotics should be given based on hospital protocol for clean skin and soft tissue cases within 1 h prior to skin incision. Due to the extent of the pelvic dissection, our preference is to place a Foley catheter. While a Foley catheter may not be necessary for all Stoppa repairs, the patient should at minimum void prior to surgery.

Choice of prosthesis should be left to the operating surgeon. In our practice, a heavy weight monofilament polypropylene mesh is most commonly used; however, this is also our practice for open, anterior (Lichtenstein) hernia repairs and laparoscopic hernia repairs. These meshes come in various sizes and can easily be trimmed to the size of the preperitoneal pocket that is created.

Technique

Positioning: Patients should be prepped and draped in the supine position. The surgical table is often placed in the Trendelenburg position which uses gravity to displace the bowels and improves exposure.

Incision: A lower midline incision is made from navel to pubis. Entrance into the peritoneal cavity should be made through the linea alba and carried down inferiorly, taking care to avoid injury to the bladder (Fig. 7.3).

Intraperitoneal: All adhesions to the abdominal wall should be taken down with care to preserve the peritoneum. Once all omentum and intestines are free, a countable surgical towel should be placed inside the abdomen to exclude the viscera from the abdominal wall

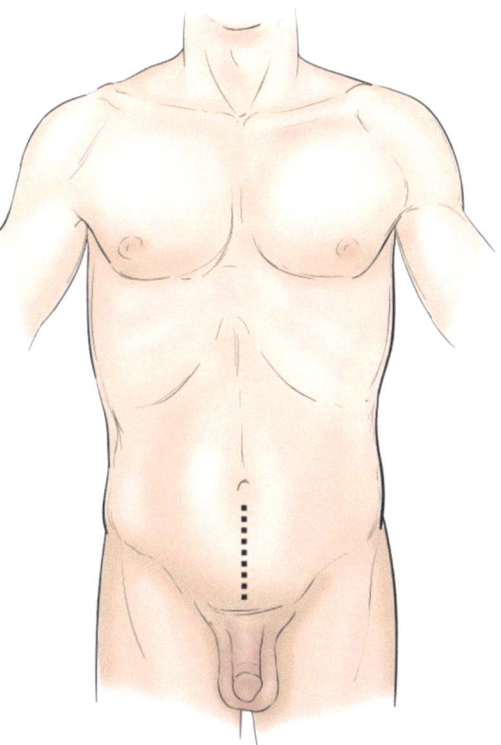

Fig. 7.3 Initial incision should be made in the midline from pubis to navel. If needing to repair an umbilical hernia, the incision can be extended more superiorly. (Chapter 82 Atlas of Advanced Operative Surgery)

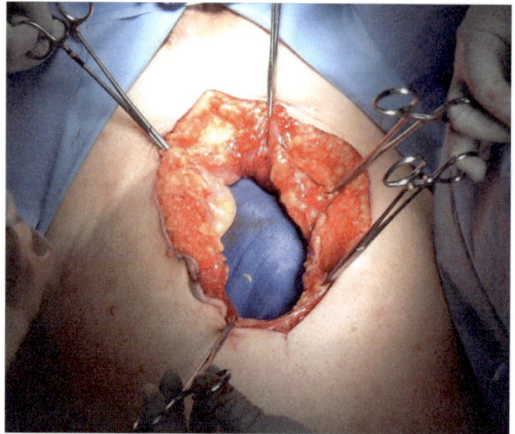

Fig. 7.4 Once all adhesions are taken down from the abdominal wall, a blue countable towel should be placed to aid in dissection

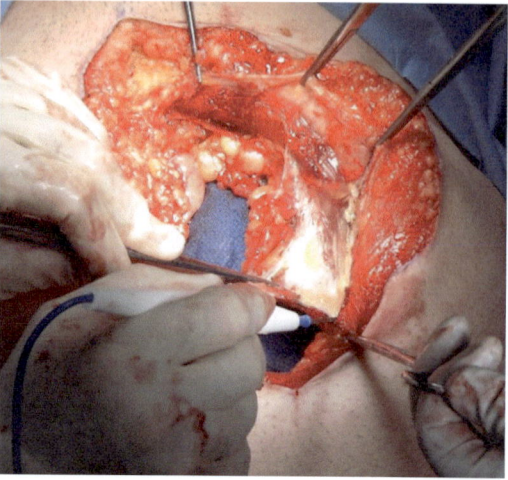

Fig. 7.5 A retromuscular flap is made by taking down the posterior rectus sheath superior to the arcuate line and the transversalis fascia inferior

to allow for a safer dissection in the next steps (Fig. 7.4). For some cases, the operation can be performed by staying completely extraperitoneal if the peritoneum is not violated during transection of the linea alba. In our experience, a Stoppa repair is reserved for more complex inguinal hernias, and as a result we find it beneficial and possibly safer to go intraperitoneal and exclude the viscera with a surgical towel.

Dissection of the preperitoneal space begins by first creating a retromuscular flap on one side. This is done by taking down the posterior rectus sheath superior to the arcuate line and the transversalis fascia inferior to the arcuate line (Fig. 7.5). Care should be taken to preserve the inferior epigastric vessels and maintain them in close adherence to the rectus muscle (Fig. 7.6).

Superior to the arcuate line, the posterior rectus sheath is incised 1 cm medial to the linea semilunaris similar to the inferior dissection of a posterior component separation (Fig. 7.7). This dissection will allow for wide mesh overlap with lateral access to the psoas muscle and mesh coverage up to the umbilicus if necessary. The preperitoneal/retroperitoneal space is then dissected out further laterally to expose the iliopsoas muscles and iliac vessels (Fig. 7.8).

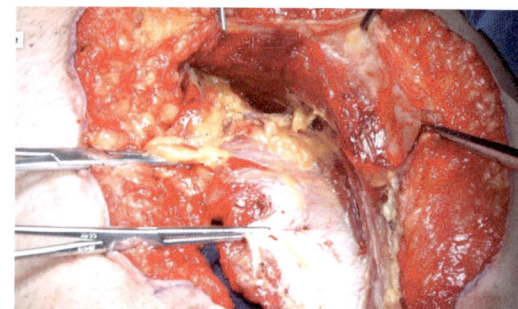

Fig. 7.6 Creating the retromuscular flap and taking care to leave the inferior epigastric vessels up to the muscle

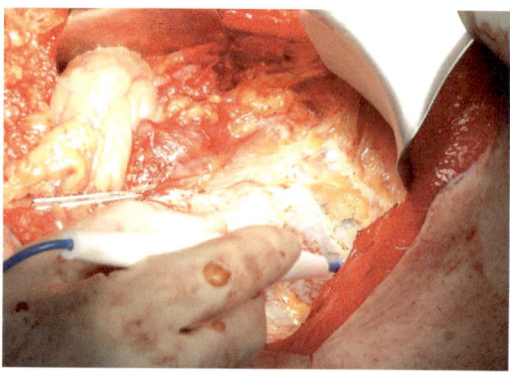

Fig. 7.7 Incision of the posterior rectus sheath medial to the linea semilunaris while maintaining the peritoneum intact

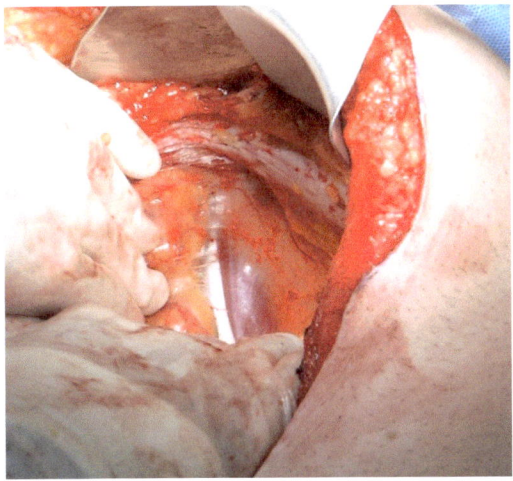

Fig. 7.8 Dissection should be carried out laterally to the point where the iliopsoas muscle is exposed

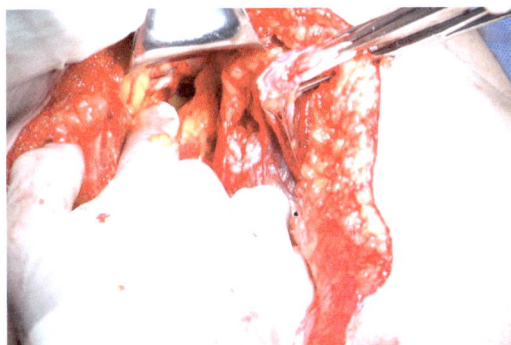

Fig. 7.9 Cooper's ligament exposed medially to the spermatic cord and epigastric vessels

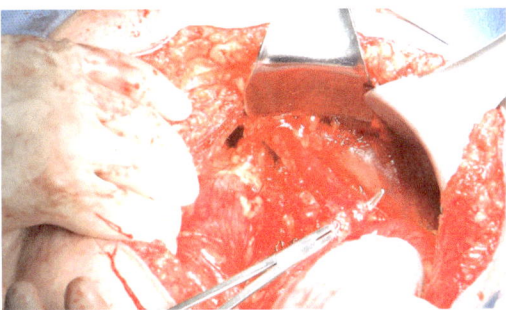

Fig. 7.10 Cord structures isolated off the hernia sac

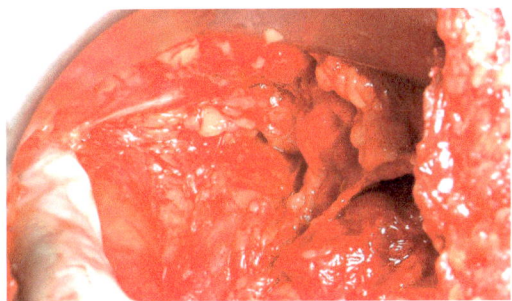

Fig. 7.11 Bilateral Cooper's ligaments and pubis exposed to develop the space of Retzius

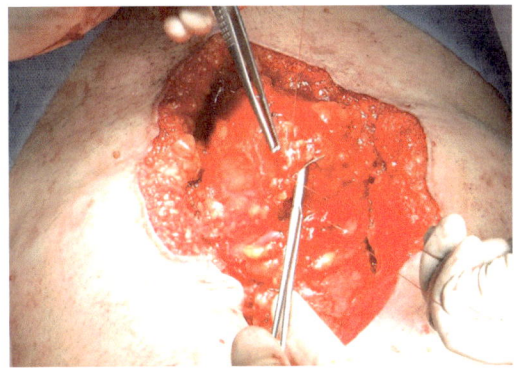

Fig. 7.12 Posterior rectus sheath closed to exclude the internal viscera from the mesh

Medial to the epigastric vessels and spermatic cord/round ligament, Cooper's ligament should be exposed to find the inferomedial landmark of the dissection (Fig. 7.9).

Once both lateral and medial dissections have taken place, the spermatic cord and hernia can be isolated and the hernia sac carefully dissected away from the cord structures (Fig. 7.10).

The contralateral side can then be addressed in a similar fashion. Both sides should be dissected down to the inferomedial aspect of both Cooper's ligaments with the pubis exposed and the space of Retzius displayed to prove sufficient space in which the mesh can lay and overlap both the obturator and femoral canal (Fig. 7.11).

Once both sides have sufficiently been dissected, the hernias reduced, and a large preperitoneal/retroperitoneal pocket created, the surgical towel is removed and the posterior fascia/peritoneum closed with absorbable suture. All peritoneal defects should be closed to ensure no visceral herniation and possible creation of an internal hernia below the mesh (Fig. 7.12).

Prosthesis Insertion

A sufficiently large mesh should be used. The mesh size is typically a minimum of 24 cm × 16 cm which provides coverage between both iliac spines and from umbilicus to pubis [8] (Fig. 7.13). The mesh is cut to size to fit in the preperitoneal/retroperitoneal pocket which should extend laterally past the anterosuperior iliac spines, superiorly up to (if not above) the umbilicus, and inferiorly past the pubis and into the space of Retzius (Fig. 7.14).

Theoretically and according to Stoppa's description of the procedure, no fixation of the mesh is needed. If fixation is desired, the mesh can be fixated using absorbable suture at the level of the pubis (we prefer fixation to Cooper's ligaments) and also transfacially in the lateral and medial aspects taking care to avoid injury to nerves and vessels (Fig. 7.15).

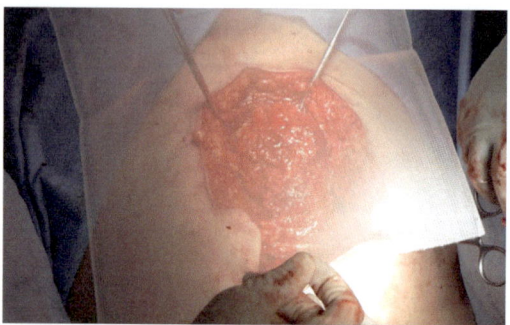

Fig. 7.13 Large mesh size is used to ensure sufficient coverage. The mesh can be trimmed as needed

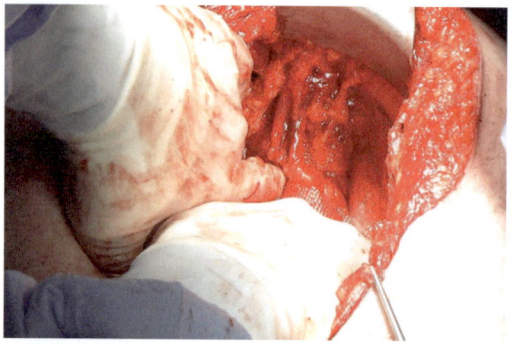

Fig. 7.14 Mesh coverage needs to be sufficient to extend to the cord structures and iliopsoas laterally

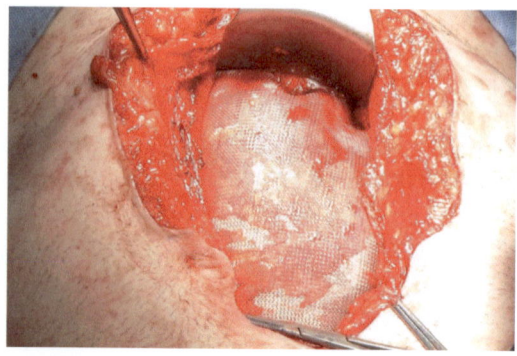

Fig. 7.15 Mesh in the preperitoneal space

The overlying fascia is then closed over the mesh. If suction drainage tubes are desired, they should be placed anterior to the mesh prior to fascial closure.

Postoperative Management

Suction drains may not be necessary, but this is left to the discretion of the operating surgeon. Diet are typically advanced quickly based on the degree of bowel manipulation during surgery. Early ambulation should be encouraged and activity resumed early based on the patient's comfort.

Pitfalls

Recurrence is usually due to insufficient prosthetic coverage which can be the result of an incomplete dissection or inappropriate mesh size.

Prior to closing the peritoneum, all bowel should be carefully inspected for any injury and repaired prior to carrying on with the operation.

References

1. Cheatle GL. An operation for inguinal hernia. Br Med J. 1921 Dec 17;2(3181):1025–6.
2. Read RC. British contributions to modern herniology of the groin. Hernia. 2005 Mar;9(1):6–11.
3. Stoppa R, Quintyn M. [Deficiencies of the abdominal wall in aged persons]. Sem Hop. 1969 Jul 10;45(31):2182–2184. French.

4. Stoppa R, Petit J, Abourachid H, Henry X, Duclaye C, Monchaux G, Hillebrant JP. [Original procedure of groin hernia repair: interposition without fixation of Dacron tulle prosthesis by subperitoneal median approach]. Chirurgie. 1973 Feb;99(2):119–123. French.
5. Carter PL. Lloyd Nyhus and Rene Stoppa: preperitoneal inguinal pioneers. Am J Surg. 2016 May;211(5):836–8.
6. Fruchaud H. Anatomie chirurgicale des hernies de l'aine. Paris: Doin; 1956. p 299–303 and 336–342.
7. Gainant A, Geballa R, Bouvier S, Cubertafond P, Mathonnet M. [Prosthetic treatment of bilateral inguinal hernias via laparoscopic approach or Stoppa procedure]. Ann Chir. 2000 Jul;125(6):560–565. French.
8. Stoppa R. Groin Hernia repair by bilateral extraperitoneal mesh prosthesis. In: Zurker M, et al., editors. Surgical management of abdominal wall hernias, vol. 16. London: Martin Dunitz Ltd; 1999. p. 203–14.

Part III

Laparoscopic Repair Techniques

Transabdominal Preperitoneal (TAPP) Repair

8

Vamsi V. Alli and Eric M. Pauli

Abbreviations

MPO	Myopectineal orifice
rTAPP	Robotic transabdominal preperitoneal
TAPP	Transabdominal preperitoneal
TAR	Transversus abdominis release
TEP	Total extraperitoneal

Introduction

Minimally invasive approaches to hernias of the myopectineal orifice (MPO) of Fruchaud build upon historic posterior approaches to the preperitoneal space such as those of Nyhus and Read [1] as well as Rives, Stoppa, Wantz, and Rignault's addition of widely overlapping mesh, resulting in the so-called giant prosthetic reinforcement of the visceral sac [2]. Both the retromuscular (pre-transversalis) plane and the preperitoneal plane can be entered to accomplish a minimally inva-

sive repair of an MPO hernia. In the case of a total extraperitoneal (TEP) repair (see Chap. 9), the desired plane is accessed directly, generally in the periumbilical region, thus avoiding any violation of the peritoneal cavity. Conversely, in a TAPP repair, the peritoneal cavity is accessed to visualize the MPO bilaterally. Laparoscopic instrumentation is then used to develop the desired plane (generally the preperitoneal plane) to afford repair.

Understanding the difference between the pre-transversalis/retromuscular and the preperitoneal planes, learning to correctly dissect one or the other, and developing the skill to comfortability (and knowingly) transition between the two are critical for any surgeon attempting to master minimally invasive inguinal hernia surgery. Similarly, posterior approaches to abdominal wall hernias, particularly the transversus abdominis release (TAR) method of component separation, rely on understanding the difference between the retro-muscular and preperitoneal planes [3]. As such, familiarity with the anatomy of a TAPP repair will facilitate performance of both open and minimally invasive TAR herniorrhaphy (and vice versa).

Laparoscopic TAPP repairs are also the foundation upon which robotic surgical repairs of MPO hernias (so-called rTAPP repairs) are founded. Because of the recent and quite rapid rise in the adoption of robotic techniques, an understanding of laparoscopic TAPP methods is critical for any surgeon seeking to perform the

Electronic Supplementary Material The online version of this chapter (doi:10.1007/978-3-319-92892-0_8) contains supplementary material, which is available to authorized users.

V. V. Alli · E. M. Pauli (✉)
Division of Minimally Invasive and Bariatric Surgery, Department of Surgery, Penn State Hershey Medical Center, Hershey, PA, USA
e-mail: valli@pennstatehealth.psu.edu;
epauli@pennstatehealth.psu.edu

© Springer International Publishing AG, part of Springer Nature 2018
M. P. LaPinska, J. A. Blatnik (eds.), *Surgical Principles in Inguinal Hernia Repair*,
https://doi.org/10.1007/978-3-319-92892-0_8

operation with robotic assistance. Please see Chap. 10 for further details on rTAPP.

There are innumerable manuscripts comparing TAPP and TEP methodology and expounding upon the virtues of each. Such comparisons are more thoroughly reviewed elsewhere in this book. In this "technique" chapter, we would like to highlight two technical advantages offered by the TAPP approach. First is the ability to view the entire lower abdomen prior to performing any dissection over the MPO. This affords the surgeon the ability to accurately inspect both MPOs for evidence of hernias in the direct, indirect, and/or femoral spaces. This is particularly useful in the cases with a clear unilateral hernia diagnosis but an unclear contralateral one. Secondly, in cases of incarcerated hernias, the abdominal access afforded by the TAPP approach is useful not only to facilitate manual reduction of incarcerated contents but also for inspection and resection (if necessary) of the recently freed viscera.

The primary technical disadvantage of the TAPP approach is that the need to enter the abdominal cavity requires the ability to navigate and safely manage intra-abdominal adhesions (Fig. 8.1). Patients with prior extensive intraperitoneal surgery or significant risk of adhesions below the level of the umbilicus are not ideal candidates for a TAPP repair. In these instances a TEP or an open anterior approach should be considered.

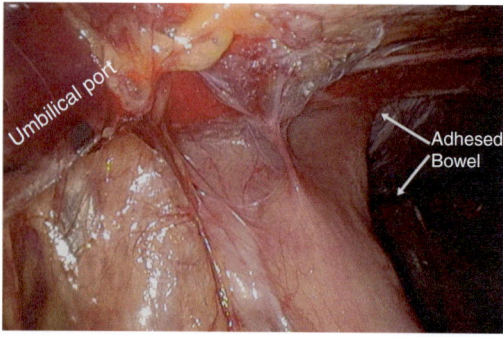

Fig. 8.1 Intra-abdominal adhesions encountered during TAPP repair. Bowel (indicated by arrows) adherent to the anterior abdominal wall as a result of prior midline laparotomy

Operative Technique

Anesthesia

Laparoscopic TAPP hernia repairs typically require general anesthesia and neuromuscular blockade. We routinely infiltrate local anesthetic at port site locations to minimize postoperative pain and reduce early narcotic requirements. We utilize a low-volume intravenous fluid protocol to avoid significant distention of the urinary bladder during the course of the operation. Following best practice guidelines [4], all patients receive prophylactic antibiotics immediately prior to surgical incision (although recent literature suggests that the administration of antibiotics for inguinal hernia repair is not only unnecessary but potentially detrimental [5]).

Patient Preparation and Positioning

The patient is instructed to void immediately before transportation to the operative theater. Upon arrival to the room, they receive prophylactic subcutaneous anticoagulation (5000 units of unfractionated heparin) and serial compression devices to reduce the risk of venous thromboembolism. Following induction of anesthesia, the patient is positioned in a supine position on the operative table with both arms tucked. This positioning permits both surgeon and assistant to comfortably stand toward the head of the bed (generally at the level of the patients shoulder) without leaning backward over outstretched arm boards. Because steep head-down positioning is utilized during the case, the patient must be secured to the bed in a reliable and robust fashion. We preferentially eschew the use of a Foley catheter unless there is a reasonable expectation that bladder distention will interrupt the progress of the case (e.g., anticipated difficult bilateral dissection leading to a lengthy operation, prior mesh in situ, active symptoms of bladder outlet obstruction most typically from benign prostatic issues, or patients who perform self-catheterization at home).

The hair on the abdomen and groin are clipped, and a chlorhexidine-based preparation is used to cleanse the skin. Preparation should take into consideration the need for management of both intra-abdominal complications as well as the need to convert to an open approach. We typically prep from the xyphoid to the upper thigh but generally do not include the genitals in the prep unless there are some additional mitigating circumstances (such as an incarcerated hernia that may require external counterpressure to free).

A single laparoscopic tower (including light source, video processor, insufflator, electrosurgical generator, and video monitor) is placed at the foot of the bed (Fig. 8.2a). Alternatively, the tower can be positioned off the patient's head (generally to the patient's left, opposite the anesthesia machine) with a secondary monitor placed at the foot of the bed (Fig. 8.2b). The assistant stands ipsilateral to the side of interest and is responsible for camera navigation. The surgeon stands contralateral to the hernia with a monopolar cautery foot pedal positioned for easy access during the procedure.

Port Placement

For TAPP hernia repairs, we prefer to make initial entry using a 12 mm Hasson cannula utilizing a curvilinear incision above the umbilicus, although other entry methods may be used based on surgeon's comfort and experience. The larger umbilical port provides a great deal of versatility for this operation including the easy introduction of large pieces of mesh to complete the repair. An open access method also permits repair of any umbilical hernia defects which are often found in conjunction with inguinal hernias [6]. A 5 mm, 30° laparoscope is utilized to allow maximal flexibility in operative visualization. Pneumoperitoneum is established using a carbon dioxide (CO_2) insufflator set to 15 mm of mercury (mmHg) pressure; the patient is placed in a steep head down (Trendelenburg) position to allow gravity-based retraction of the viscera away from the MPO. Visual inspection of the MPO is then undertaken to confirm the diagnosis.

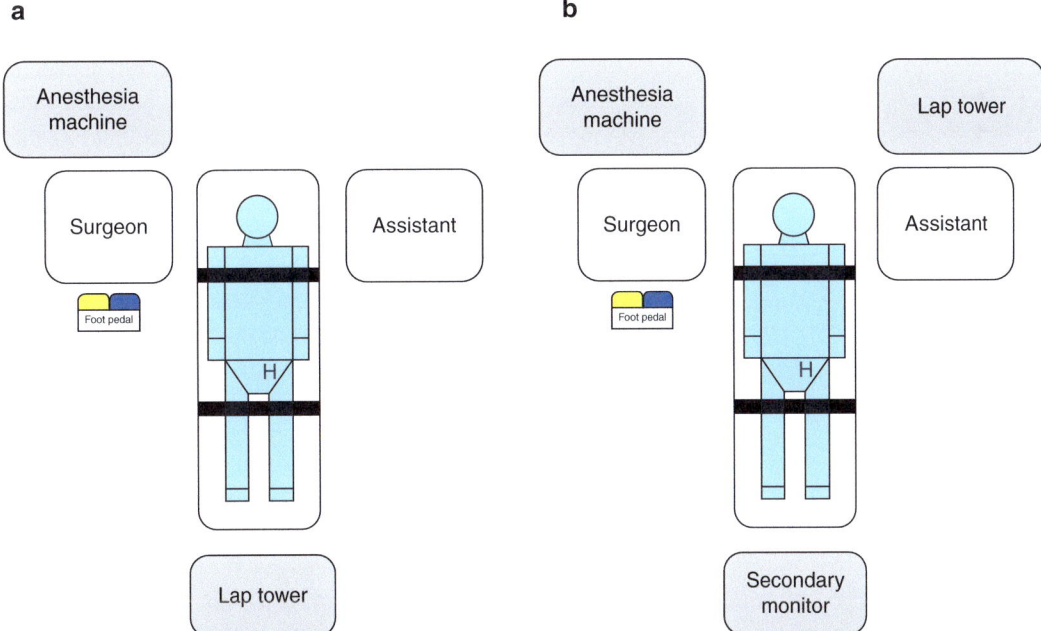

Fig. 8.2 Room setup for laparoscopic TAPP repair of a left inguinal hernia. (**a**) Standard setup utilizes a laparoscopic tower positioned at the foot of the table. (**b**) Alternative setup places a secondary monitor at the foot of the table, with the laparoscopic tower positioned at the head of the bed

Two additional 5 mm ports are placed laterally, their location varying slightly based on the visual inspection of the MPO. For patients undergoing bilateral repairs, ports are placed symmetrically: each several centimeters lateral to the *linea semilunaris* (lateral border of the rectus muscle) and each just superior to the level of the umbilical port (Fig. 8.3). For patients undergoing a unilateral repair, the ports are shifted slightly to improve the ergonomics of a unilateral operation. The 5 mm port contralateral to the side of the defect is shifted toward the side of the hernia, occupying a position now just lateral to the *linea semilunaris*. The 5 mm port ipsilateral to the hernia is shifted slightly more cephalad, occupying a position more superior to the umbilical port but still lateral to the linea semilunaris. Figure 8.4a and b illustrate port placement for unilateral right and left repairs, respectively.

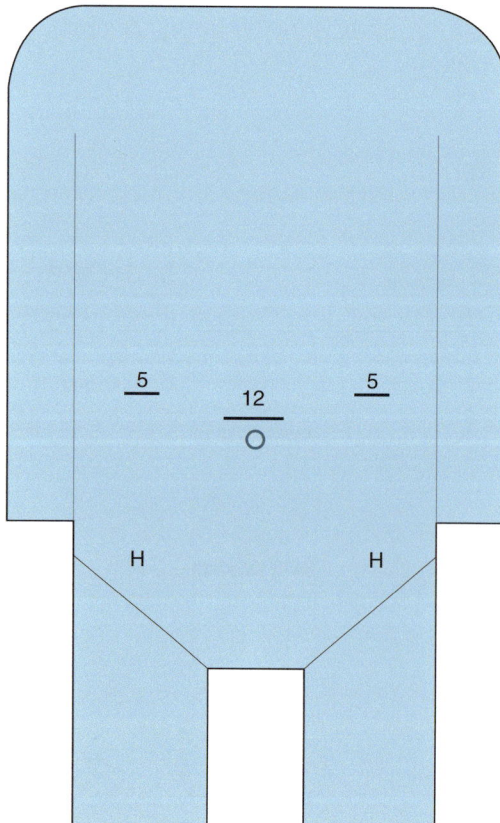

Fig. 8.3 Port placement diagram for bilateral TAPP inguinal repair

Utilizing smaller (5 mm), non-cutting (radially dilating) trocars and avoiding port placement through the *linea semilunaris* are all maneuvers intended to reduce the risk of postoperative port site hernia formation.

Ergonomic and Operative Flow Considerations

One of the common criticisms of TAPP repair is that port placement is non-ergonomic and requires the surgeon to lean across the table to perform the operation. This position results from the use of the two lateral ports as the working ports and the umbilical port for the camera (generally a 10 mm lens assembly). The operating surgeon fatigues quickly and can develop back pain from leaning across the table, while collisions with the assistant's camera arm slow the repair and result in an unsteady view of the operative field (Fig. 8.5a and Video 8.1 illustrate these issues associated with this port utilization scheme).

The use of a high-definition 5 mm, 30° laparoscope and shifting its position to the 5 mm port ipsilateral to the hernia entirely eliminate these ergonomic concerns. The high-definition camera and 30° lens allow the assistant to provide a view of the operative field virtually identical to that obtained by the use of a 10 mm laparoscope placed centrally. However, shifting the camera laterally permits the surgeon to operate through the umbilical and contralateral 5 mm port (the two ports closest to the surgeon) while maintaining an upright and ergonomically correct position (Fig. 8.5b and Video 8.1 illustrate more ergonomic port utilization).

We preferentially utilize instruments passed through the midline umbilical port as the primary dissection tools. Only instruments passed through the midline are attached to the monopolar cautery cable. Instruments passed through the 5 mm port contralateral to the hernia generally serve retraction and counter traction purposes. This system of port utilization means that when two similar instruments are present in the operative field (e.g., two Maryland dissectors), there is no

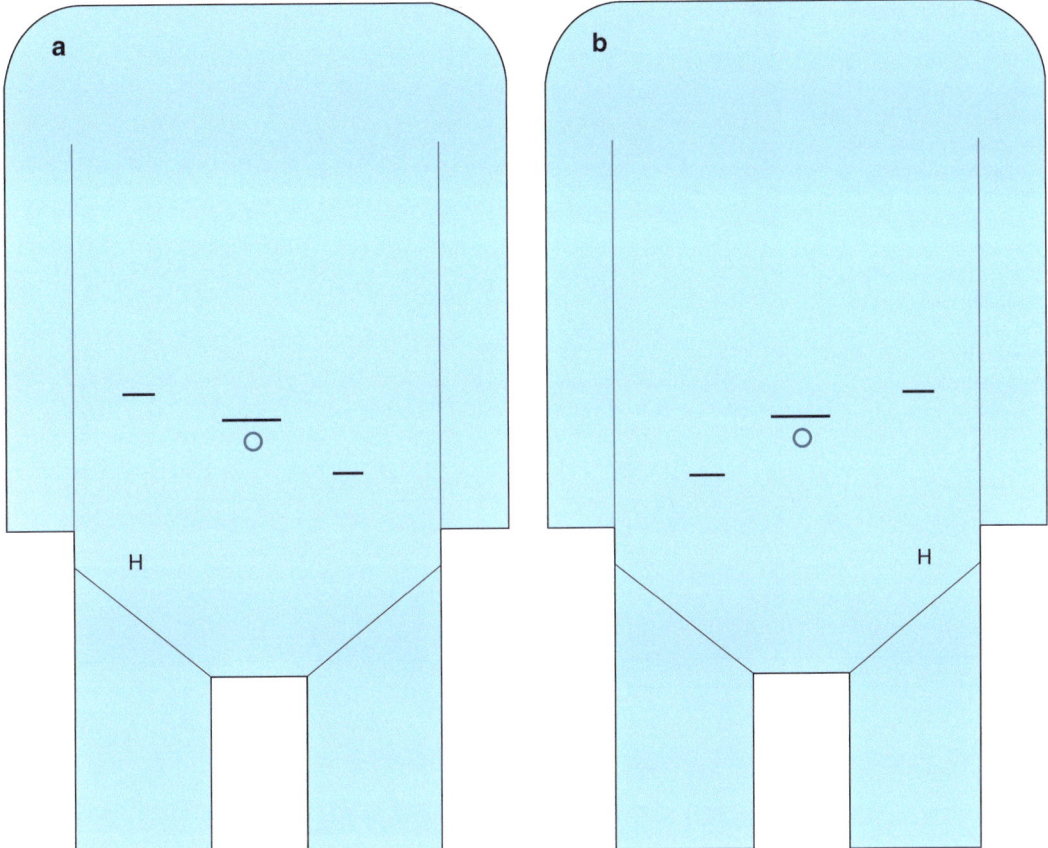

Fig. 8.4 Diagram of port placement for unilateral right (**a**) and left (**b**) TAPP inguinal hernia repair

confusion about where energy is going to be delivered. Since the retraction hand is often out of the field of view of the camera and often retracts downward toward the bowel, this convention also reduces the risk of inadvertent thermal injury to the bowel.

To improve the flow of the case, we have available both a laparoscopic scissors and a Maryland dissector with cautery attachments. Switching between these two primary dissection devices therefore requires no more than instrument withdrawal and a simple switch of the monopolar cord from one to the other. Tool change does not require the removal and replacement of instrument handles. Many standard laparoscopic instrument trays include only one handle capable of attachment to a monopolar cautery cable, so an extra handle may need to be added to the TAPP instrument set.

Procedure Steps

Video 8.2 demonstrates all of the operative steps of a bilateral TAPP repair as detailed below. By convention, the umbilical port is the primary working port used for dissection, and the only port through which electrosurgical devices are placed. The contralateral 5 mm port is utilized for retraction of the peritoneal flap and hernia sac during the dissection. There are, however, occasions where the opposite configuration is utilized for retraction, most notably during reduction of a large indirect sac and/or large lipoma of the cord.

After port placement, peritoneoscopy is performed to assess for trocar site or access injuries and to confirm the diagnosis of hernia/herniae. Atraumatic graspers can be used to reduce any incarcerated contents and to manually reposition any adjacent bowel that did not clear the MPO

Fig. 8.5 Ergonomic considerations of port utilization. (**a**) Surgeon must lean over the patient and collides with the assistants arm when the umbilical port is utilized for the laparoscopic camera/lens assembly. (**b**) Placing the camera/lens assembly ipsilateral to the hernia allows upright posture for both surgeon and assistant

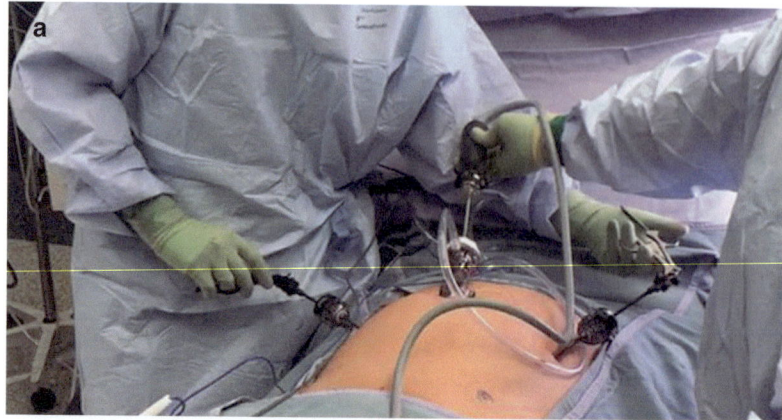

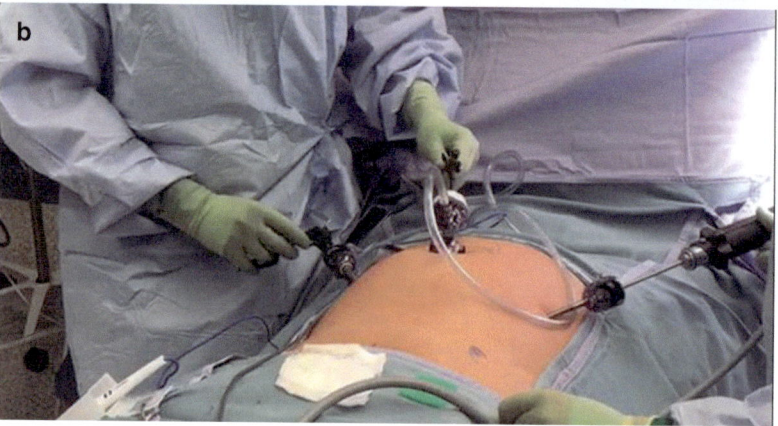

with Trendelenburg positioning. Adhesions in the region of the MPO should be taken down sharply with minimal use of surgical energy. The goals of adhesiolysis are to free any points of tension that may tear or preclude easy flap closure and to move bowel away from the anticipated location of preperitoneal dissection. Care must be taken to avoid injury not only to the viscera but also to the peritoneum which should ideally be intact or readily closed at the conclusion of the preperitoneal dissection.

Peritoneal Flap Creation

We typically create a very large peritoneal flap, beginning the dissection well above the hernia defect. Preperitoneal access begins just below the umbilicus and just lateral to the medial umbilical ligament. When bilateral repairs are performed, the peritoneum is left uncut and undissected from medial umbilical ligament to medial umbilical ligament to permit easier flap alignment and closure at the end of the procedure.

From this medial starting position, endoscopic sheers and monopolar coagulation current are utilized to create a peritoneal incision directed straight lateral (not inferior-lateral) from the starting point. This requires upward torque on the scissors from the midline port that results in the instrument tips being aimed for a point just below the 5 mm port on the side ipsilateral to the defect. Care is taken to remain in the true preperitoneal plane (posterior or deep to the transversalis fascia) as this is an avascular plane and minimal (if any) energy is required for dissection. The transversalis fascia should remain in apposition to the rectus muscle. Exposed muscle fibers are an indication that dissection has extended into the wrong plane (Fig. 8.6). Care must also be taken to avoid inadvertent injury to the inferior epigastric vessels which run between the transversalis

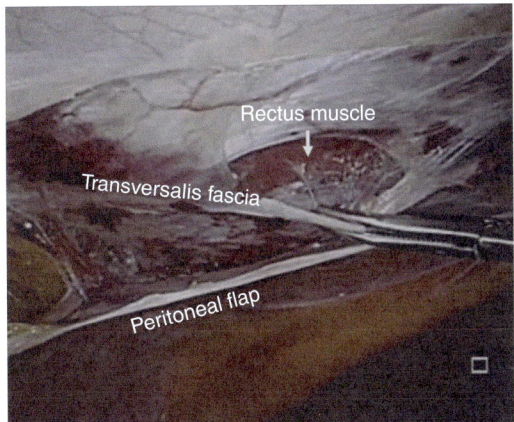

Fig. 8.6 TAPP dissection should occur between the peritoneum and the transversalis fascia. Identification of bare muscle fibers indicates incorrect entry in the pre-transversalis plane

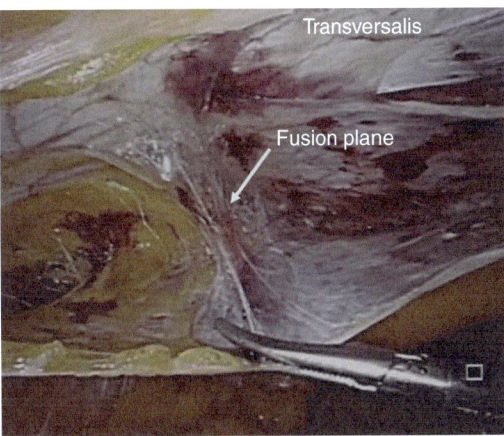

Fig. 8.8 Fusion plan between peritoneum and transversalis that occurs near the linea semilunaris

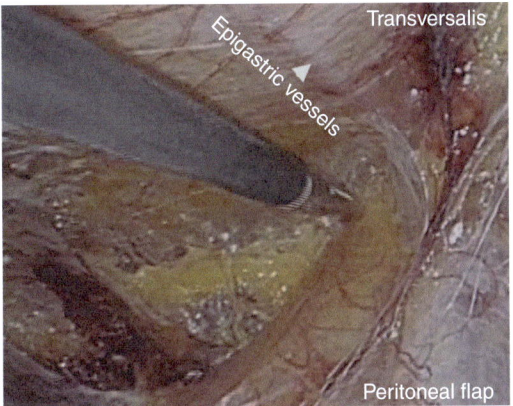

Fig. 8.7 The inferior epigastric vessels are visible through the intact transversalis fascia

fascia and the rectus muscle itself. While not directly visualized during this part of the dissection, the epigastric vessels are clearly identifiable through the intact transversalis fascia (Fig. 8.7). Throughout the dissection, firm posterior and cephalad traction of the flap is critical for separation of the peritoneum and transversalis fascia. This pull should also be directed medial (during lateral dissection) or lateral (during medial dissection) to facilitation flap creation. One of the hardest elements of a TAPP repair to learn/teach is the required force and tension vector for retraction. The surgeon must learn from on-screen visual cues and from subtle haptic feedback

whether their off-screen counter-tension is appropriate (facilitating dissection) or inappropriate (resulting in tears in the thin peritoneal flap or ineffectual/inefficient dissection).

In virtually all patients, there is a fusion plane between the peritoneum and transversalis fascia that occurs at the lateral 1/3 of the rectus muscle near the linea semilunaris (Fig. 8.8). This plane runs in a cranio-caudal direction along the length of the rectus muscle. Identification of this fusion is important for several reasons:

1. Due to the fusion, there is a tendency to inadvertently enter the pre-transversalis plane or to tear holes in the peritoneum. Correct dissection may require sharp dissection using scissors or cautery, in addition to altering the traction/countertraction maneuvers to safely release the peritoneum.
2. The fusion generally happens within 1 cm (medial/lateral) of the location of the epigastric vessels. Finding the fused segment should therefore alert the surgeon to their proximity to the vessels.
3. The remainder of the operative dissection can be divided into three distinct zones of dissection relative to the fused section of the peritoneal flap (representing the location of the epigastric vessels). We describe these as the medial, lateral, and middle zones of the peritoneal flap.

Medial Dissection

Medial dissection will open the space of Retzius and permit identification of the pubic symphysis in the midline, followed by identification of Cooper's ligament. For bilateral repairs, dissection can be continued across the midline at this point due to the ease with which the space of Retzius opens. The most efficacious maneuver here is a posterior/medial push directed downward toward the bladder. When direct defects are present, they can often be reduced with a simple downward push from the Maryland dissector entering from the midline port. For larger direct defects, a two-handed maneuver is often required. Here, the midline Maryland grasper is used to grab the "pseudosac" (the bulging transversalis fascia), and the Maryland retractor is moved into the dissection plane to push downward on the peritoneum. By working hand over hand in this fashion, the peritoneum over the direct defect can be easily reduced (generally much easier than indirect sac reduction). The plane should be opened inferior enough to permit identification of the inferior pubic ramus (and the obturator space) as well as the retropubic space in the midline.

Because the fused middle part of the dissection has not been completed, medial dissection is facilitated by navigating the laparoscope into a position between the fused peritoneum/transversalis fascia (laterally) and the medial umbilical ligament (medially) and utilizing the 30° lens to look directly inferiorly, toward the bony pelvis. This maneuver requires a camera operator capable of navigating into the preperitoneal plane, past undissected parts of the flap and around working instruments without dirtying the lens or colliding with working instruments.

During medial dissection, several critical structures should be identified. As mentioned above, the urinary bladder is left in continuity with the peritoneal flap as the dissection approaches (and ultimately crosses) the midline. Early medial dissection (including contralateral medial dissection in patients undergoing bilateral repairs) may help avoid injury to the bladder if no Foley catheter is used as the bladder will increasingly distend with urine as the case progresses

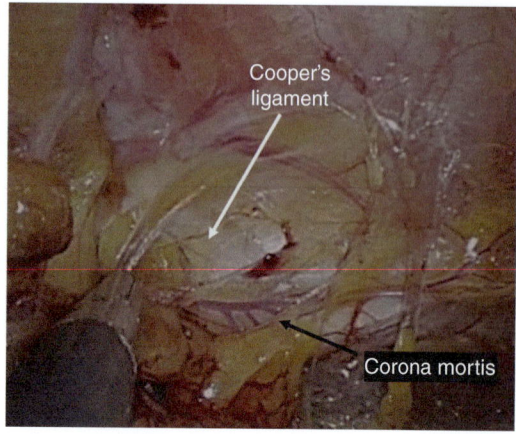

Fig. 8.9 Corona mortis vessels along the pubis. Also visible is Cooper's ligament superior to the bone

even when a low volume resuscitation strategy in employed. The lateralmost aspect of the medial dissection is the femoral and obturator spaces, and care must clearly be taken to avoid the neurovascular structures found here.

Running to/from the iliac vessels are small vascular branches that supply the bony pelvis (the so-called *corona mortis* vessels). These branches are often encountered running along the pubic rami toward the symphysis (Fig. 8.9). They need to be avoided during dissection and their position noted so that they are not injured during mesh placement and/or fixation. Small amounts of bleeding from these vessels can result in the development of a large postoperative hematoma because of the ease with which the space of Retzius opens. This is particularly critical in patients requiring anticoagulation or antiplatelet agents for medical comorbidities or in whom nonsteroidal anti-inflammatory agents that alter platelet function (such as ketorolac) will be given.

Lateral Dissection

During the lateral dissection, the primary goals are to identify and preserve the neurovascular structures of the lateral abdominal sidewall while identifying the lateral aspect of any indirect hernia sac. Both of these goals are most easily accomplished by ensuring that dissection leaves

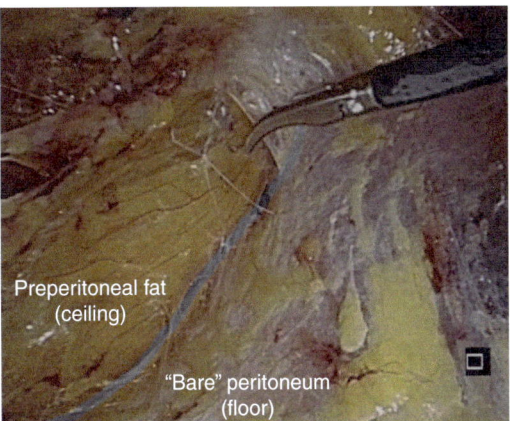

Preperitoneal fat
(ceiling)

"Bare" peritoneum
(floor)

Fig. 8.10 The "floor" of dissection should be bare perito-neum; all preperitoneal fat has been lifted up to the "ceiling," leaving all critical structures against the pelvic sidewall

all preperitoneal fat against the abdominal and pelvic sidewall (i.e., on the "ceiling" of dissec-tion) and that only the peritoneum is being retracted medially (i.e., the "floor" of the dissec-tion is bare peritoneum) (Fig. 8.10). The lateral dissection should be undertaken with care to avoid damage to the lateral femoral cutaneous, anterior femoral cutaneous, femoral branch of genitofemoral, and femoral nerves within the so-called triangle of pain. This zone is bounded by gonadal vessels medially, ileopubic tract superi-orly, and the peritoneal reflection laterally.

If at any point the surgeon questions the direc-tion or extent of the lateral dissection, the camera can be backed away from the dissection and out of the preperitoneal space. The retraction hand is used to raise the peritoneal flap back to its native position. This gives a clear overview of the entire dissection flap and is one of the advantages offered by TAPP repair. At some point in the lateral dissec-tion, further inferior and lateral dissection is hin-dered by the fusion plane in the middle zone, prohibiting adequate counter traction. At this point it is time to perform the middle dissection.

Middle Dissection and Sac Reduction

Working carefully under the epigastric vessels, the middle of the flap can be created. Blunt and sharp

dissection are utilized along with judicious elec-trocautery to separate the peritoneum from the transversalis fascia by following the fusion plane between the two inferiorly. Once the medial edge of the hernia sac has been identified, the counter traction hand can be shifted into the preperitoneal plane and used to grasp the proximal hernia sac. The sac is separated from the cord structures by working on the lateral edge and pulling the sac out of the indirect defect. Complete sac reduction can be achieved in almost all cases. Occasionally a longer sac poses a difficult dissection and may be more safely divided with cautery. As the sac is being reduced, the final portion of the dissection separates the inferior sac wall from the retroperito-neal structures. It is at this point that the vas defer-ens is encountered. The sac is separated from the vas and the dissection continued taking the perito-neum off of the retroperitoneal structures beyond the area where the vas deferens crosses medially over the iliac vessels. Dissection in the so-called triangle of doom completes the circumferential mobilization of the indirect sac from the cord structures and creates room for inferior overlap of the mesh. Despite the proximity to the iliac ves-sels, it is critical to be thorough in completing the inferior dissection as the inferior location is the most common site of hernia recurrence following laparoscopic inguinal herniorrhaphy.

Cord Lipoma Management

The cord should be inspected for any retroperito-neal fat that accompanied the hernia sac (the so-called lipoma of the cord) (Fig. 8.11a). Any lipomas encountered should be reduced to elimi-nate symptoms related to the bulging fat and to avoid symptoms (pain and a bulge) that may mimic a hernia recurrence. The blood supply of these lipomas runs adjacent to the cord along the pelvic sidewall in the retroperitoneum. They can generally be reduced back beyond the area where the inferior edge of the mesh will be positioned (Fig. 8.11b). If the lipoma cannot be satisfactorily reduced back to this level, removal of the lipoma should be considered to permit appropriate mesh positioning.

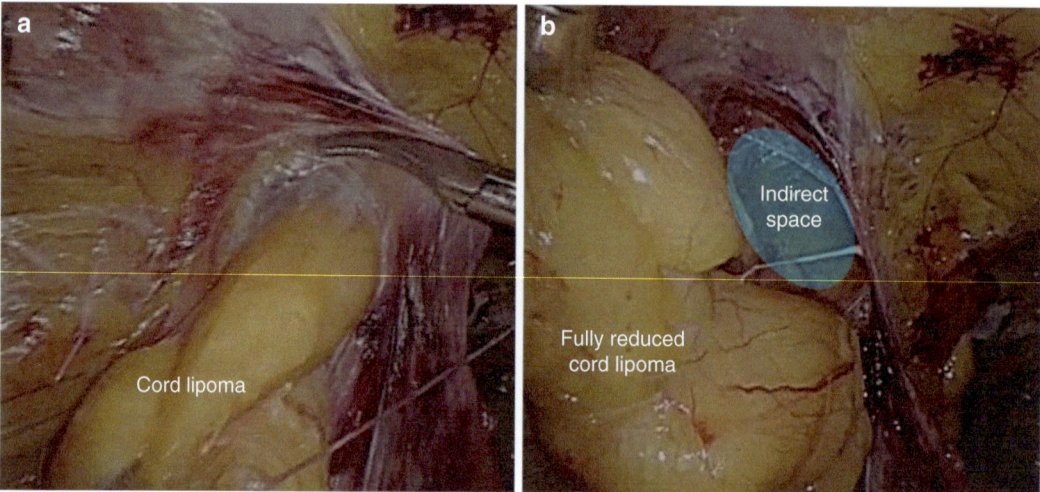

Fig. 8.11 (**a**) A large lipoma is identified running along the cord structures in an indirect defect and (**b**) the lipoma is reduced and separated from the cord structures via manual traction

Confirmation of the "Critical View" of the MPO

Prior to mesh introduction, we review the entire dissection to ensure the adequacy of the preperitoneal space that has been created, to ensure that all fat has been reduced from defects, to inspect for bleeding, and to gauge the size and anticipated anatomical lay of the mesh. Some authors have described this as assessing the "critical view" of the myopectineal orifice, and we have adopted this method as a surgical pause in the case that serves to confirm the dissection is complete [7].

Mesh Placement

A wide array of mesh types are available for inguinal repair including flat and anatomically shaped sheets. Our personal preference is for anatomically shaped, reduced-weight polypropylene. The mesh is introduced through the midline umbilical port with using a blunt tipped grasper holding the medial edge of the mesh. It is quickly passed through the valve mechanism of the trocar to prevent loss of pneumoperitoneum and dragged into the preperitoneal space and medially. A second blunt-tipped grasper is used

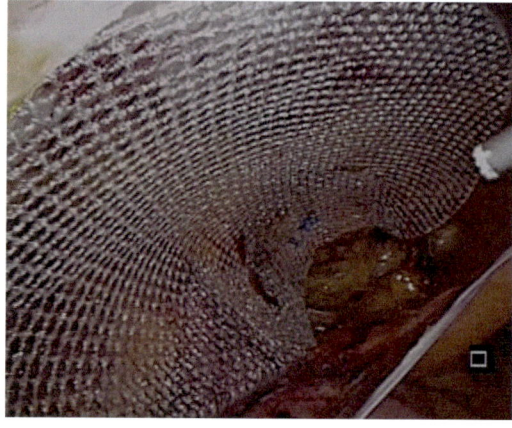

Fig. 8.12 Final positioning of mesh, immediately prior to placement of mechanical fixation

to assist in mesh positioning. We typically avoid grasping the mesh, as the mesh can be more easily shifted using the closed blunt tips of the instruments than by grasping it.

The mesh should reach the midline (pubic symphysis) in order to cover all three of the potential spaces of the MPO (direct, indirect, and femoral). The inferior edge must be positioned such that it lays flat and is immediately along the junction of the peritoneum and retroperitoneum in the inferiormost aspect of the dissection. The mesh should not have any folds, bends, or ripples (Fig. 8.12).

Mesh can be secured in place to prevent migration, or the surgeon can rely only on intra-abdominal pressure to hold the mesh against the abdominal wall. In the case of mechanical fixation either via tacks, staples, or suture, appropriate placement above the ileopubic tract is necessary to reduce the risk of nerve injury and postoperative pain syndromes. This means that lateral fixation should occur in a palpable area of the abdominal wall medial and superior to the anterior superior iliac spine. Inferior medial fixation is generally placed into Cooper's ligament whereas superior fixation utilizes the transversalis fascia and rectus muscle. The epigastric vessels should again be identified before placing mechanical fixation to avoid vascular puncture.

Tissue sealants can be used to secure the mesh as well (either in conjunction with mechanical fixation or as a stand-alone method). Not only is there no tissue penetration with glues (and a potential reduced risk of chronic pain), but adhesives permit fixation of the inferior edge of the mesh directly to the retroperitoneum in the triangle of doom and the triangle of pain. This is the area of mesh that is most critical to the success of the repair as rolling of the edge during flap closure (or simple migration early in the postop period) is suspected as the cause of inferior recurrence.

Our preference is to secure the mesh with three absorbable tacks in the following positions: (1) inferior medial (to Cooper's ligament), (2) superior medial (medial to the epigastric vessels), and (3) laterally above the level of the anterior superior iliac spine. We habitually secure the inferior edge of the mesh using fibrin sealant.

Closure of the Peritoneal Flap

The goal of flap closure is to ensure the entire mesh surface is covered by soft tissue, preventing bowel and mesh interaction. This can be accomplished using several methods, including tacks, staples, or suture. Care must be taken to avoid injury to the epigastric vessels while ensuring that there are no gaps in the closure that will permit bowel to slip into the preperitoneal flap and

obstruct. For bilateral repairs, the alignment and re-approximation are facilitated by leaving the midline intact during the dissection (i.e., two smaller flaps, not one large flap) (Fig. 8.13).

While some surgeons have shown the safety of flap closures that rely only on abdominal pressure to hold the flap in place (the abdomen is desufflated while the flaps are held in position with instruments and then instruments are removed), we choose to always close the flap (Fig. 8.14).

Any incidental defects in the peritoneal flap should be identified for the same reasons outlined above. They can be closed with clips, staples,

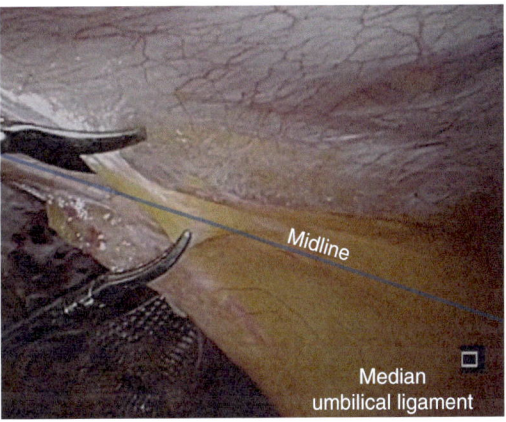

Fig. 8.13 Maintaining the continuity of the peritoneum in the midline at the time of flap creation for bilateral repairs

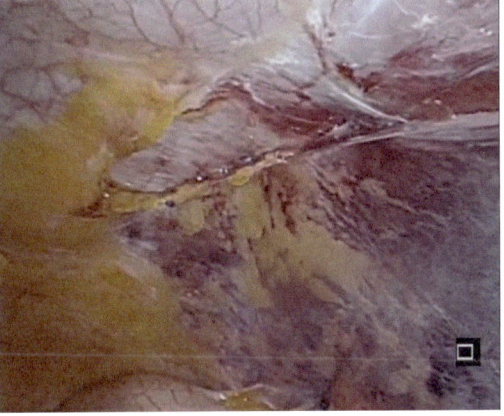

Fig. 8.14 Final view of the completed tack closure of the peritoneal flap

endoloops, or free needle suturing. Such closures should only include the peritoneum and not the mesh and critical structures that lay beneath. Tacks cannot be used below the ileopubic tract to close these defects, but a large hernia sac can be pulled up to cover such holes and the distal end of the sac tacked to the abdominal wall at the level of the flap closure.

Case Completion

The pneumoperitoneum is slowly evacuated, while peritoneal flap and mesh are observed to ensure no resultant mesh migration, kinking, or exposure. Ports are then removed, and the midline port is closed using the previously placed stay sutures to approximate fascia.

For cases involving an umbilical hernia warranting mesh repair, the mesh can be introduced though the midline defect and secured with tacks under visualization using the two 5 mm lateral ports. The fascia can be closed over the mesh completing a hybrid intraperitoneal onlay patch (IPOM) repair.

Post-Procedure Care

Patients proceed through standard postoperative recovery pathways and are generally discharged the same day. Pain is managed with oral nonsteroidal anti-inflammatory agents and oral narcotics if necessary. No formal restrictions on weight lifting or activity are made; however, patients are counseled to limit physical activities when they feel minimal discomfort. They are seen back in the clinic after 4–6 weeks for routing postoperative examination.

References

1. Novitsky YW, Czerniach DR, Kercher KW, Kaban GK, Gallagher KA, Kelly JJ, et al. Advantages of laparoscopic transabdominal preperitoneal herniorrhaphy in the evaluation and management of inguinal hernias. Am J Surg. 2007;193(4):466–70.
2. Wantz GE. Giant prosthetic reinforcement of the visceral sac. Surg Gynecol Obstet. 1989;169(5):408–17.
3. Jones CM, Winder JS, Potochny JD, Pauli EM. Posterior component separation with transversus abdominis release: technique, utility, and outcomes in complex abdominal wall reconstruction. Plast Reconstr Surg. 2016;137(2):636–46.
4. Bratzler DW, Dellinger EP, Olsen KM, Perl TM, Auwaerter PG, Bolon MK, et al. Clinical practice guidelines for antimicrobial prophylaxis in surgery. Am J Health Syst Pharm. 2013;70(3):195–283.
5. Köckerling F, Bittner R, Jacob D, Schug-Pass C, Laurenz C, Adolf D, et al. Do we need antibiotic prophylaxis in endoscopic inguinal hernia repair? Results of the Herniamed registry. Surg Endosc. 2015;29:3741–9.
6. Ruhl CE, Everhart JE. Risk factors for inguinal hernia among adults in the US population. Am J Epidemiol. 2007;165(10):1154–61.
7. Daes J, Felix E. Critical view of the myopectineal orifice. Ann Surg. 2017 Jul;266:e1–2. https://doi.org/10.1097/SLA.0000000000002104.

Totally Extraperitoneal (TEP) Repair (with Video)

David J. Berler and Brian P. Jacob

Introduction

Together, inguinal and femoral hernias are categorized as groin hernias. It is estimated that the prevalence of inguinal hernias is between 5% and 10% and that the lifetime risk of developing an inguinal hernia is up to 27% in men and 3% in women [1]. As a result, groin hernias are among the most common diagnoses leading to referral to a general surgeon, with approximately 800,000 inguinal hernioplasties performed annually in the United States [2].

The tension-free repair utilizing prosthetic mesh popularized by Lichtenstein in the 1980s has become the standard open repair. However, the rising popularity of laparoscopic surgery in the early 1990s presented the general surgeon with a new approach in hernia repair. Specifically, laparoscopic inguinal hernia repair was refined into the two predominant techniques that are currently employed, transabdominal preperitoneal

Electronic Supplementary Material The online version of this chapter (doi:10.1007/978-3-319-92892-0_9) contains supplementary material, which is available to authorized users.

D. J. Berler
Resident in General Surgery, Icahn School
of Medicine at Mount Sinai, New York, NY, USA

B. P. Jacob (✉)
Icahn School of Medicine at Mount Sinai,
New York, NY, USA

repair (TAPP) and total extraperitoneal repair (TEP). The benefits of laparoscopic repair include similar recurrence rates, decreased rates of seroma and hematoma formation, and easier examination for other coexisting abdominal wall defects when compared to open repair. Reduced incidence of acute, postoperative pain and quicker return to work and daily activities have also been demonstrated; the benefits of laparoscopic repair include similar recurrence rates, decreased rates of seroma and hematoma formation, and easier examination for other defects when compared to open repair. The drawbacks of the laparoscopic approach include lengthier operating time, the requirement of general as opposed to regional or local anesthesia, and its steeper learning curve [3].

This chapter will discuss the indications, technique, current trends, potential complications, pitfalls, and outcomes from TEP.

Historical Perspective

Tait was the first to employ a transabdominal approach in the repair of abdominal wall hernias. He recognized and repaired inguinal hernias during laparotomy for other primary indications. Inguinal hernia repair became a potential frontier in the world of minimally invasive surgery once laparoscopic surgery gained widespread acceptance and refinement in the 1980s and 1990s. Ger and colleagues published a paper describing successful laparoscopic, stapled closure of the patent processus vaginalis in 15 animals with indirect inguinal hernias in 1990 [4]. Later that year Velez and Klein published similar data and Schultz performed the first known TAPP. McKernon and Laws expanded the concept of preperitoneal mesh placement and performed the first TEP in 1993.

The TAPP approach is based on a technique that was analogous to the Rives-Stoppa repair, in which peritoneal flaps are created and mesh is laid in the retromuscular space to cover the entire myopectineal orifice [5]. The TEP approach similarly places a preperitoneal mesh, but the entire dissection is extraperitoneal. Both TAPP and TEP are acceptable laparoscopic techniques in the repair of inguinal hernias, and approach selection is determined by surgeon experience and patient history and preference.

Indications and Contraindications

Laparoscopic inguinal hernia repair is conventionally indicated for hernias that are bilateral or recurrent following open repair [6]. The laparoscopic approach avoids the morbidity associated with bilateral groin incisions and allows for bilateral repair with one operation. It also obviates the need to dissect in the anterior space where the planes may be obliterated from prior repairs and mesh. Increasingly, surgeons have been offering laparoscopic repair upfront, even in the setting of unilateral, previously unrepaired hernias due to the reduction in postoperative acute pain and time away from work and daily activities, as well overall improved quality of life [7]. This is particularly true for surgeons who are comfortable with the laparoscopic technique.

There are several contraindications to laparoscopic repair. The most notable are a patient's inability to tolerate general anesthesia or pneumoperitoneum due to cardiopulmonary disease. Relative contraindications include a history of or future plans for preperitoneal surgery. Large, chronically incarcerated scrotal hernias and strangulated inguinal hernias that will require bowel resection are additional relative contraindications.

TEP vs. TAPP vs. Open Repair

The decision of whether to proceed with an open or laparoscopic approach to inguinal hernia repair is highly patient specific. Once committed to a laparoscopic repair, the choice between the TEP and TAPP techniques should also be tailored to each patient as well as surgeon experience. Both procedures have their merits and disadvantages as well as relative indications and contraindications.

Adequately powered randomized clinical trials comparing the open and laparoscopic approaches are quite sparse. Schrenk et al. compared 86 patients who underwent inguinal hernia with the Shouldice technique ($n = 34$), laparoscopic TAPP ($n = 28$), and laparoscopic TEP ($n = 24$) [8]. Postoperative pain was significantly less in the TAPP patients on postoperative days 0 (4.8 vs. 6.5, 6.2 $p = 0.02$) and 1 (4 vs. 6, 6 $p = 0.01$). There was no significant difference in visual analogue scale scores for pain between the patients in up to 30 days. There was no significant difference between the three groups with respect to patient satisfaction, time to return to work and daily activities, analgesic use, or length of stay. Cosmesis was significantly better in the TEP and TAPP groups compared to the open repair group.

A 2005 Cochrane review identified ten total studies comparing TAPP to TEP (though the Schrenk paper was the only RCT that was included). All studies were prospective with a mean follow-up time of 3 months. The authors found that both visceral injuries and port site hernias were more likely in patients undergoing TAPP repair. Conversions were more likely in the TEP group. There were no differences in cost between TAPP and TEP in any of the included papers [9].

Furthermore, the literature demonstrates no significant difference in operative time between TEP and TAPP. Although it might seem logical that TEP is a quicker operation since the balloon dissector creates the preperitoneal space and there are no peritoneal flaps to be closed at the case's conclusion, the literature does not support this. The mean operating time was 46 vs. 52.3 min for TAPP and TEP, respectively, in the Schrenk study. More recent prospective trials have shown no difference in mean operating times between TEP and TAPP [10, 11].

One might expect that postoperative bowel obstructions are more common in patients undergoing a TAPP repair since the abdominal cavity is entered during this approach while the peritoneal cavity is not breached in the TEP approach. A 2005 Swedish retrospective study of over 33,000 patients found that the risk for postoperative intestinal obstruction is increased following TAPP inguinal hernia repair when compared to open (Lichtenstein) and TEP repair (RR (2.79, 95% CI 1.01–7.42) [12]. Some of these patients (a minority), however, had had a history of prior abdominal surgery thereby rendering it difficult to attribute postoperative adhesive bowel obstructions to the TAPP technique alone.

TAPP is much more intuitive then TEP since the approach uses more commonly accessed planes. It is generally accepted that TAPP is conceptually and anatomically easier to both learn and teach. The literature confirms that the steep learning curve for TEP approaches up to 50 cases, when considering operative times and the incidence of complications [13].

TEP Technique

The following is the technique for TEP inguinal hernia repair currently used by the authors.

Preoperative prophylactic antibiotics are given in accordance with SCIP protocol. A 10-mm curvilinear, infraumbilical incision is made, deepened through the subcutaneous tissue and separated to expose the anterior rectus sheath. We prefer to place to stay stitches in the anterior fascia. The anterior rectus sheath is incised longitudinally, slightly off midline. This is an important point as incising in the midline where the anterior and posterior rectus sheaths merge might lead to inadvertent entry into the peritoneal cavity. The rectus abdominis fibers are retracted laterally with an S retractor to reveal the white posterior rectus sheath below. The dissecting balloon is placed through the incision, just superficial to the

posterior sheath, and advanced in a parallel motion along the anterior abdominal wall toward the pubis. The laparoscope is inserted, and the balloon dissector is inflated under direct vision to create the preperitoneal space. When no further movement is observed with sequential pumping, the balloon is deflated and removed.

A Hasson trocar may then be placed in the umbilical incision, and the preperitoneal space is insufflated to a pressure of 15-mmHg. A laparoscope is reinserted, and if the space has been created correctly, the underside of the rectus muscle will be in the superior portion of the field; the inferior epigastric vessels will be visible. The patient is placed in Trendelenburg position, and two additional 5-mm ports are placed: one two fingerbreadths above the pubis and another midway between this port and the umbilical port.

Identification and clearing of the anatomic landmarks is key prior to beginning dissection and the repair of the hernia. First, Cooper's ligament and the pubic tubercle are identified and cleared of any overlaying fat. This is easiest to perform with two blunt-ended graspers, by placing their ends firmly against the bones and then gently spreading them apart. The space of Retzius is thus developed, with the bladder moving downward out of the field in doing so. The direct space is often exposed as well with this maneuver.

The inferior epigastric vessels are then identified running superiorly along the anterior abdominal wall. They are compressed in an anterior direction with one grasper while another grasper may be used to develop the dissection plane between the transversalis fascia and the peritoneum. These two layers typically separate with fairly little force; however, care must be taken especially when there is any amount of fusion, as inadvertent rents may be created in the peritoneum, leading to pneumoperitoneum and loss of the preperitoneal space.

There is typically areolar tissue in this area, making the dissection relatively hemostatic. The plane is developed laterally to the pelvic sidewall, just medial to the anterior superior iliac spine – the position of which may be laparoscopically confirmed by external palpation. The correct plane of dissection is the junction of the transversalis muscle fibers and the peritoneum. In this manner, the space of Bogros is developed.

Once sufficient medial and lateral dissection have clarified, the relevant anatomic landmarks, identification, reduction, and repair of inguinal hernias are feasible. The direct space is examined first, where a defect may already be visible; the dissecting balloon often reduces these hernias on its own. In males, the spermatic cord structures are identified lateral to the epigastric vessels; in females, the round ligament is seen and may be ligated. The approximate position of the external iliac artery and vein should be identified and all dissection in this area avoided.

An indirect inguinal hernia sac is typically located on the superolateral aspect of the cord, as it enters the deep inguinal ring. The cord bundle is grasped, and the sac is gently separated from the cord structures, with the vas deferens typically being in the posterior position. While one grasper is elevating the cord structures, another, in open position, is used to gently sweep the cremasteric muscle fibers downward in an effort to skeletonize the cord, and in doing so form a posterior window between peritoneum and cord. This assists in identifying the edge of the hernia sac. The cord should be handled gently, and with open instruments as much as possible, to avoid crushing injuries to its contents. The sac is then pulled cephalad and laterally, away from the cord. The apex of the sac may then be grasped and pulled cephalad, effectively reducing the hernia. In a similar fashion, lipomas of the cord may (and should) be reduced as well. The femoral space may be visualized and any hernias within it addressed at this point.

Indirect inguinal hernias may be more challenging to fully reduce than direct ones. Should complete reduction ultimately be technically impossible, the hernia sac may be ligated. This is typically done with a laparoscopic stapler though may also be completed with an Endoloop or laparoscopically placed clips. The proximal portion of the sac is thus ligated. Care must be taken when doing this, such that no intraabdominal contents or viscera are within the hernia sac. The distal sac (the part of the sac remaining within

deep ring and allowed to persistently herniate) should be left open to drain, thus avoiding hydrocele formation.

Once the dissection, exposure of necessary anatomic points of fixation, and hernia reduction are complete (with nothing entering the deep inguinal ring other than the cord), a piece of prosthetic mesh is shaped, folded, and introduced through the umbilical trocar. The size of the mesh will be dictated by the size of the defect; however, it should generally measure at least 10×15 cm. The prosthesis is laid flush against the myopectineal orifice and flattened to overlay the cord structures. Importantly, all defects and the entire myopectineal orifice must be covered or there is risk for recurrence. It is often easiest to place the rolled up mesh superiorly, and then roll it downward. A single "anchoring" tack is deployed at the pubic tubercle to allow for relative mesh fixation in the tight preperitoneal space. Subsequently, manipulation and fixation of the prosthesis are more feasible and achieved with tacks at Cooper's ligament and anteriorly. Importantly, tacks should be avoided lateral to the inferior epigastric vessels; should they be absolutely necessary, it is important that they be above a line connecting the pubic tubercle to the anterior superior iliac spine. This avoids the development of chronic pain syndromes, which have been associated with tacks placed in this area (the so-called triangle of pain).

Attention may then be paid to the contralateral side and the above processes repeated for hernias that are identified. The mesh/meshes should cross midline and in the case of bilateral repairs, should overlap each other.

As the preperitoneal space is allowed to desufflate, a grasper is placed on the lateral edge of the mesh (where no fixation has been performed), thus compressing it against the pelvic sidewall. This prevents the mesh from folding or migrating as the preperitoneal space collapses. We recommend reinsufflation of the space prior to closure to verify mesh positioning and ensure adequate hemostasis.

The trocars are then removed and the umbilical port site closed with a figure-of-eight suture. In males, the testes should be examined to assure they are within the scrotum.

Complications and Common Pitfalls

Dissection within the preperitoneal space can prove challenging and confusing. It is important to adequately visualize the entire myopectineal orifice and identify all hernias, as 15% of true hernias may actually be missed during laparoscopic repair, leading to "recurrence" [14].

Dissection at the pubic symphysis in the midline, in the prevesical space of Retzius, aims to sweep the bladder posteriorly to maximize the working space and avoid iatrogenic injury. Bladder injuries are typically identified upon sudden decompression of an earlier distended bladder or by the presence of urine in the field. Vesical injuries should be repaired in two layers with absorbable suture, using additional trocars if necessary. Complex urologic injuries and urethral injuries may require laparotomy and urologic repair. A Foley catheter should be kept in place postoperatively. Careful thought should be given to placing a Foley catheter preoperatively to avoid this complication when the hernia involves the bladder, is large, in the setting of prior preperitoneal surgery (including prior TEP), or when the surgeon or assistant is early in the TEP learning curve.

The medial dissection involves the space between the inferior epigastric vessels and Cooper's ligament. Bleeding during TEP inguinal hernia repair is a potentially life-threatening intraoperative event, and the inferior epigastric vessels are most commonly implicated. Injury may occur during any portion of the procedure. Inflation of the balloon dissector may lead to shearing of small branches of these vessels which will be noted upon insertion of the laparoscope and visualizing pooling blood in the field. In this situation, we recommend immediately placing the two additional trocars, irrigating the preperitoneal space, and evacuating any hematoma to identify the area of bleeding. Using a two-handed technique, one instrument can compress the epigastric bundle proximally so that the offending branch can be clipped, cauterized, or ligated. A similar strategy can be effective for bleeding from the epigastric vessels during the medial dissection.

The space between the vas deferens and the gonadal vessels houses the common iliac vessels and constitutes the so-called triangle of doom. The location of the vessels may be determined by observing for strong pulsations underneath the peritoneal layer. All dissection should avoid this area and be performed superior to it, as injury to the vessels engenders massive hemorrhage and can be fatal. Injury requires prompt laparotomy and repair.

Dissection and reduction of an indirect inguinal hernia sac involves separating it from the spermatic cord and the deep ring. Electrocautery should be avoided, with a predominant use of blunt dissection to accomplish this goal. Rough handling of the cord can lead to injury to the cremasteric or testicular vessels and/or hematoma formation, which can lead to testicular atrophy or orchitis. Transection of the vas deferens may occur as well and if identified should be repaired with an end-to-end anastomosis if feasible, particularly in young patients, even if the injury is unilateral. Conversion to an open procedure may be necessary. Bowel injuries are rare; however, should they occur, laparotomy and repair with or without resection are warranted.

Reduction of the hernia sac is also where inadvertent rents to the peritoneum may be introduced, leading to ramifications on cardiopulmonary physiology as well as loss of working domain in the preperitoneal space. A Veress needle or angiocatheter may be introduced at Palmer's point to allow for the pneumoperitoneum to be released and the preperitoneal space regained. Any peritoneal tears should be repaired with clips at the conclusion of the procedure to avoid future omental or visceral herniation and early small bowel obstruction.

Complications less likely to be noted intraoperatively include nerve injuries during mesh fixation. The lateral space of Bogros is created beyond the anterior superior iliac spine, thus exposing the triangle of pain and its nerves (ilioinguinal, iliohypogastric, and lateral femoral cutaneous nerves). Injury to these nerves, whether during dissection or during the deployment of tacks in mesh fixation, may lead to chronic groin pain. Tack placement in the lateral space is generally not recommended, to avoid this complication. The remedy includes removing the offending tack and infiltrating the injured nerve with local anesthetic. These interventions do not preclude chronic pain syndromes from developing postoperatively; the only effective management of nerve injuries is prevention, which involves careful dissection and judicious mesh fixation with laparoscopic tacking devices. There has been much work to develop self-adhering meshes and biologic glues to supplant tack fixation altogether to avoid nerve injury [15]. Early results of retrospective studies using such fixation with respect to recurrence, postoperative pain, and patient satisfaction appear promising [16, 17].

References

1. Kingsnorth A, Leblanc K. Hernias: inguinal and incisional. Lancet. 2003;362(9395):1561–71.
2. Scott NW, Mccormack K, Graham P, Go PM, Ross SJ, Grant AM. Open mesh versus non-mesh for repair of femoral and inguinal hernia. Cochrane Database Syst Rev. 2002;(4):CD002197.
3. Jacob BP, Ramshaw B. The SAGES manual of hernia repair. New York: Springer; 2012.
4. Ger R, Monroe K, Duvivier R, Mishrick A. Management of indirect inguinal hernias by laparoscopic closure of the neck of the sac. Am J Surg. 1990;159(4):370–3.
5. Schultz L, Graber J, Pietrafitta J, Hickok D. Laser laparoscopic herniorrhaphy: a clinical trial preliminary results. J Laparoendosc Surg. 1990;1(1):41–5.
6. McCormack K, Wake B, Perez J, Fraser C, Cook J, McIntosh E, Vale L, Grant A. Laparoscopic surgery for inguinal hernia repair: systematic review of effectiveness and economic evaluation. Health Technol Assess. 2005;9:1–203, iii–iv.
7. Dedemadi G, Sgourakis G, Karaliotas C, Christofides T, Kouraklis G, Karaliotas C. Comparison of laparoscopic and open tension-free repair of recurrent inguinal hernias: a prospective randomized study. Surg Endosc. 2006;20(7):1099–104.
8. Schrenk P, Woisetschläger R, Rieger R, Wayand W. Prospective randomized trial comparing postoperative pain and return to physical activity after transabdominal preperitoneal, total preperitoneal or Shouldice technique for inguinal hernia repair. Br J Surg. 1996;83(11):1563–6.
9. Wake BL, Mccormack K, Fraser C, Vale L, Perez J, Grant AM. Transabdominal pre-peritoneal (TAPP) vs totally extraperitoneal (TEP) laparoscopic techniques for inguinal hernia repair. Cochrane Database Syst Rev. 2005;(1):CD004703.
10. Krishna A, Misra MC, Bansal VK, et al. Laparoscopic inguinal hernia repair: transabdominal preperitoneal (TAPP) versus totally extraperitoneal (TEP) approach: a prospective randomized controlled trial. Surg Endosc. 2012;26(3):639–49.
11. Gong K, Zhang N, Lu Y, et al. Comparison of the open tension-free mesh-plug, transabdominal preperitoneal (TAPP), and totally extraperitoneal (TEP) laparoscopic techniques for primary unilateral inguinal hernia repair: a prospective randomized controlled trial. Surg Endosc. 2011;25(1):234–9.
12. Bringman S, Blomqvist P. Intestinal obstruction after inguinal and femoral hernia repair: a study of 33,275 operations during 1992-2000 in Sweden. Hernia. 2005;9(2):178–83.
13. Jones DB. Master techniques in surgery: hernia. Philadelphia, PA/London: Lippincott Williams & Wilkins; 2012.
14. Ryan EA. Recurrent hernias: an analysis of 369 consecutive cases of recurrent inguinal and femoral hernias. Surg Gynecol Obstet. 1953;96:343–54.
15. Lomanto D, Katara AN. Managing intra-operative complications during totally extraperitoneal repair of inguinal hernia. J Minim Access Surg. 2006;2(3):165–70.
16. Mangram A, Oguntodu OF, Rodriguez F, et al. Preperitoneal surgery using a self-adhesive mesh for inguinal hernia repair. JSLS. 2014;18(4):e2014.00229.
17. Berney CR, Yeo AE. Mesh fixation with fibrin sealant during endoscopic totally extraperitoneal inguinal hernia approach: a review of 640 repairs. Hernia. 2013;17(6):709–17.

Robotic Inguinal Hernia: The Why and the Hows

10

Gregory J. Mancini and Dennis R. Van Dorp

Minimally Invasive Inguinal Hernia

Within the minimally invasive surgery platform, laparoscopic inguinal hernia has remained a very controversial topic. Over the past 20 years, the battle lines have hardened between the open and laparoscopic inguinal hernia encampments. Few surgical procedures have received the volume of verbal debate, literary publication, and randomized clinical trial efforts without resolving the clinical debate. Inconsistent data regarding costs, operative times, outcomes, and chronic pain have all added to the controversy about the merit of minimally invasive hernia surgery. Within this ongoing debate enters the concept of robotic inguinal hernia repairs. For surgeons who favor the open approach, a robotic inguinal hernia repair is tantamount to surgical heresy. Surgeons who favor the laparoscopic approach argue that robotic surgery is a costly and redundant tool that offers little to the operation. Despite this, surgeons from each of these two encampments have found value in and have adopted the robotic platform for inguinal hernia surgery.

Data shows that only 17–22% of all inguinal hernia repairs in the USA are performed laparoscopically, utilizing either the totally extraperitoneal (TEP) or transabdominal preperitoneal (TAPP) techniques. This means that nearly 80% of all inguinal hernias are repaired using an open technique. Since introduced in the 1990s, the laparoscopic technique has seen an adoption rate of less than 1% per year, despite an increased case exposure during general surgical residency and the addition of over 100 minimally invasive surgery-trained fellows per year over the same time frame. Some argue that the outcomes data supporting laparoscopic inguinal hernia repair is negligible; however, similar soft outcomes data supports the use of laparoscopic appendectomy, yet over 80% of appendectomies are currently performed laparoscopically. The learning curve for TEP and TAPP has been estimated to be between 50 and 150 cases. Some argue this may be a contributing factor to its slow adoption; nevertheless, other technically complex operations such as laparoscopic gastric bypass have pushed the open technique to essentially be considered a complication. Others point out that the increased system cost and lower surgeon reimbursement are a disincentive to surgeon adoption. The robotic platform is generally considered to have a lower learning curve and may help to overcome some of the technical challenges of laparoscopic inguinal hernia repair. This system may demonstrate value if adopting surgeons can produce high-quality outcomes while lowering costs.

G. J. Mancini (✉) · D. R. Van Dorp
Department of Surgery, University of Tennessee,
Knoxville, TN, USA
e-mail: GMancini@utmck.edu; dvandorp@utmck.edu

© Springer International Publishing AG, part of Springer Nature 2018
M. P. LaPinska, J. A. Blatnik (eds.), *Surgical Principles in Inguinal Hernia Repair*,
https://doi.org/10.1007/978-3-319-92892-0_10

Current Published Data

An interest in robotic-assisted inguinal hernia repairs has arisen recently. Currently utilized primarily in gynecologic and urologic surgery, the robotic platform has been gaining popularity in general surgery, particularly in foregut, biliary, bariatric, and colorectal surgery [1]. Due to superior imaging, precision, accuracy, and articulating capabilities, there is interest in utilizing robotic technology among general surgeons to perform inguinal hernia repairs; however, this has been slow to develop, widely due to cost barriers [1]. Interestingly, the first reports of robot-assisted inguinal hernia repairs were performed by urologists at the time of robotic prostatectomy [2–6]. Since these initial descriptions, robot-assisted inguinal hernia repairs have been gaining popularity, with most surgeons performing the repairs in a transabdominal preperitoneal fashion, similar to the laparoscopic TAPP repair.

Due to this being a relatively new technique, there is little in the literature regarding outcomes. Early studies, with small population sizes, have demonstrated low complication rates [7–12]. One study followed a single surgeon's experience while transitioning from laparoscopic TEP to robotic TAPP (R-TAPP) repairs [12]. In this series, retrospective analysis compared 157 patients who underwent laparoscopic TEP to 118 patients who underwent R-TAPP. Operative times were higher in both groups at the beginning of the study and decreased as more cases were completed. During the study, no significant difference was noted in operative time between the two groups; this was true for both unilateral and bilateral hernia repairs. Mean surgical times were noted to be nearly identical, at approximately 69 min each. The study also demonstrated no significant difference in inguinodynia, seroma, or hernia recurrence at 1 year postop. This study did not, however, analyze cost or pain scores between the two groups. Two seromas were noted in each group [12].

In reviewing the literature, other studies have also demonstrated low complication rates for R-TAPP repairs. The most common complications are postoperative seroma and hematoma, which vary among studies from 0% to 20.5% identified in the first half of patients in the series, which was later reduced to 1.7% after modifying the operative technique [7, 10]. The vast majority of patients are discharged home on the same day of surgery, with overnight hospitalizations being due to comorbid conditions or social reasons [7, 10, 12]. Chronic pain was only reported in two patients [11, 12].

One series directly compared robotic versus laparoscopic TAPP repair over a series of 63 patients (24 laparoscopic, 39 robotic) in terms of cost and long-term outcomes [8]. This study utilized a tacking device for laparoscopic mesh placement and self-adhering mesh for the robotic group of patients. In their analysis, they found the direct cost for each group to be nearly identical, despite operative times being slightly longer for robotic repairs. The cost difference was attributed to a decreased time that the robotic group spent in the recovery room, and thus, were discharged home sooner. The study also noted that the robotic group experienced less pain than the laparoscopic group, with 7/39 patients reporting no pain at all after surgery. This difference was attributed to the avoidance of tacks in the robotic group as well as decreased trocar site trauma due to the fixed pivot point that the robotic platform offers. Final analysis showed no significant differences between the two groups, including an equal direct cost and contribution margin [8].

As surgeons gain experience performing robot-assisted transabdominal preperitoneal inguinal hernia repairs, operative times, docking times, and therefore costs will undoubtedly improve. With the introduction of the da Vinci Xi system, docking is generally considered easier. Early studies of robotic-assisted transabdominal preperitoneal hernia repair suggest that the cost may not be as prohibitive as once thought. With new self-adhering meshes, which eliminates the cost of a tacking device, combined with the elimination of a balloon dissector, costs may be reduced or net neutral when compared to laparoscopic methods [9, 13].

Who Should Have a Robotic Inguinal Hernia?

Patient Selection

When initiating a robotic inguinal hernia surgery program, it can be difficult to decide which patients will benefit from this technique. Though the learning curve for the R-TAPP is low, particularly if the surgeon is transitioning from an experienced laparoscopic practice, patient and case selection is an important consideration. Uncomplicated unilateral inguinal hernias are good learning cases; however, they may seem like a misapplication of the robotic platform, and some institutions may bar this type of utilization, despite the difficulty ascending the robotic inguinal hernia learning curve with complicated cases that involve issues of hernia multi-recurrence, high BMI, or prior mesh complications. Our foray into robotic inguinal hernia surgery began as an adjunct to other simultaneous robotic procedures. Performing a robotic inguinal hernia repair concurrently with a clean urologic or gynecologic robotic procedure may allow for skill acquisition on a simple inguinal hernia, and at the same time, utilize the robotic platform in a cost-effective manner.

Another patient cohort that may benefit from the robotic repair may be the complex hernia patient. Some joke that the robot may make a mediocre surgeon better; we believe the value that the robot should have is to make difficult cases easier for all surgeons. In the case of inguinal hernia, complex patients have worse outcomes. This includes the morbidly obese, the large scrotal hernia, and the multi-recurrent hernia. There is no data demonstrating that robotic outcomes are better in these patient groups compared to other surgical methods, but the current data shows that there is room for clinical improvement. Though starting a robotic practice on the hardest cases is not advisable, the true value of the system may be most apparent in the complex patient population.

Cost-Containment Strategy

Since cost continues to be the consistent barrier to robotic access, a cost-containment strategy can help surgeons and administrators maintain financial stewardship that can yield reasonable per-case costs. The robotic platform has built-in features of reusable instruments that help to reduce costs when compared to using the disposable instruments and accessories that can be cannibalized during laparoscopic surgery. Instruments such as balloon dissectors, tackers, and clip appliers are expensive and are usually not needed when performing a robotic inguinal hernia, thereby defraying overall robotic costs. Additionally, judicious use of the robotic instruments during the case can have a major impact on reducing the per-case cost. We typically limit the reusable instruments used during each case to just three: a grasper, a hook with cautery, and a needle driver. Limiting instrument use has the additional benefit of improving time and efficiency, since fewer instrument exchanges are done within each case.

TAPP Foundation

The robotic inguinal hernia repair is derived from the transabdominal preperitoneal (TAPP) laparoscopic technique. The trocar placement, planes of dissection, mesh positioning and fixation, and peritoneal lining closure are all similar to the TAPP. The largest migration of surgeons to the R-TAPP are those already proficient at TEP or TAPP. This differs from those moving to robotic ventral hernia, as both open and laparoscopic ventral hernia surgeons are equally represented.

The desire for laparoscopic surgeons to move to the robotic platform resides in the improved visualization provided by the 3-D optics, the enhanced ergonomics of both posture and arm positioning provided by the robotic console, and the ease of robotic suturing delivered by the 7 degrees of freedom of the robotic arms. When performing a laparoscopic TAPP, the camera is usually positioned in the center trocar with the surgeon standing at the side of and parallel to the patient, facing the foot of the bed, forcing the surgeon to extend both arms over the patient and operate in the extended "bullfighters" stance. Alternatively, the camera can be moved to the lateral port on the side of the hernia repair, allowing less arm extension and use of the umbilical port as an operating port. This strained posture of the TAPP has been cited as a major reason that many surgeons prefer the TEP technique. Additionally, the peritoneal closure to cover the mesh can be difficult, as laparoscopic sewing poses an ergonomic challenge and use of a tacker can increase both postoperative pain and the per-case cost.

Adaptations to the Robotic Platform

Patient Positioning

The room setup and patient position may depend on the version of the robot that the surgeon employs. For the S and Si versions of the robot, the patient can be either positioned in lithotomy, allowing docking between the legs, or in the supine position, if the parallel docking method is used. Docking between the legs permits optimal camera and robotic arm positioning within the designated "sweet spot," while parallel docking provides a simplified and safer patient setup. We prefer the parallel docking method because it saves approximately 30 min per case that is otherwise consumed by safe lithotomy positioning that is required at the beginning and end of the case. The Xi platform makes this efficiency adaptation debate moot, since the platform's side docking and rotating boom of the patient-side cart makes the lithotomy position unnecessary. The patient may be comfortably positioned and secured supine with the arms tucked and tilted in Trendelenburg (Fig. 10.1).

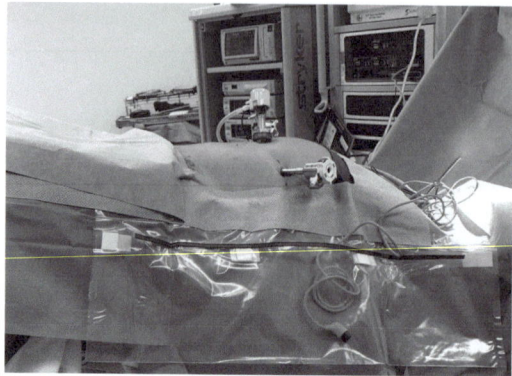

Fig. 10.1 Image demonstrates that the patient is positioned supine, with arms tucked, and in steep Trendelenburg

Trocar Placement

Trocar placement is similar to the TAPP trocar positioning. The inherent need of the robotic platform for greater distance from the target tissue (approximately 20 cm) means that the camera and arm trocars are most frequently placed in a parallel line located above the umbilicus (Fig. 10.2). In cases of patients with a short torso, we move the trocars further cephalad, toward the epigastric and subcostal locations. Trocar size depends on the robotic platform used. The S-series will typically use a supra-umbilical 12 mm trocar for the camera port and two 8 mm trocars placed parallel and 10 cm lateral to the camera port, bilaterally (Fig. 10.3). The Xi utilizes a uniform 8 mm instrument platform; thus, mesh and needle choice may impact ease of use. Larger mesh and needles may be more difficult to place into the abdomen. To facilitate their placement into the abdomen, we initially place a 12 mm trocar at the camera location, through which the mesh and needles are passed into the abdomen at the beginning of the case. We then telescope an 8 mm trocar through this 12 mm trocar to allow for docking of the robotic arm and subsequent placement of the 8 mm Xi camera (Fig. 10.4). Two additional 8 mm ports are then placed in parallel bilaterally.

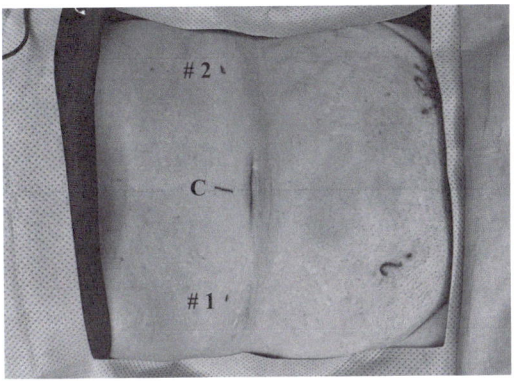

Fig. 10.2 Image shows the trocar placement for R-TAPP, with the skin markings in the pelvis for the laterality

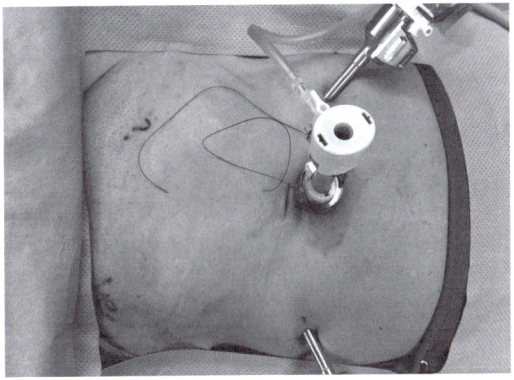

Fig. 10.3 Image shows the trocars placed prior to docking

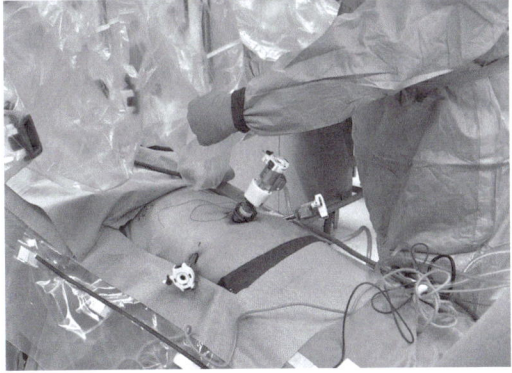

Fig. 10.4 Image demonstrates telescoping of the 8 mm trocar down the 12 mm Hasson trocar as an adaptation to the Xi platform

Instruments

As a surgeon begins to learn on the robotic platform, there is a tendency to employ multiple instruments with a variety of end effectors to accomplish the case. This tendency is due to a transfer of habits learned from both open and laparoscopic surgery, where all of the instruments are supplied in one tray (family-style) and all are re-sterilized after each case regardless of use. Conversely, the robotic instruments are individually processed and have a set number of uses ranging from 1 to 15 cases. This "à la carte" use of instruments has a significant impact on both cost and efficiency of a case. From the robotic surgeon's perspective, an instrument change during the case costs the system both time and money. We have worked to reduce the number of instruments used during an R-TAPP to just three. Typically, we use a grasper in the left arm and a hook with monopolar cautery in the right arm for the majority of the case, including mesh placement. Then the hook is replaced by the suture-cutting needle driver to sew the peritoneum closed. In difficult cases, we may exchange the hook for a second grasper.

Robotic Efficiency and Troubleshooting

Time and procedural efficiency are important considerations when employing the robotic platform to inguinal hernia disease. Most institutions have high utilization rates by multiple surgical specialties, so time and opportunities are often precious resources. We have found several procedural tips and tricks that have enhanced our robotic inguinal hernia efficiency.

Camera and instrument exchanges are the silent time killers in robotic surgery. Since mesh and suture are used in most cases and both require placement through the camera port, we have found that placing the mesh and suture into the abdomen at the beginning of the procedure speeds up the case. In and of itself, removing the camera to place mesh and suture mid-case is time-consuming, not to mention the extra lens cleaning and tip defogging that naturally follows each camera exchange. Placing the mesh and suture into the abdomen from the start of the case will not interfere with the hernia dissection.

Patient positioning and room setup are the next silent time thieves in robotic surgery. They do not add to the actual procedure time itself but rather the "white-space" time between cases. Simplifying room setup and patient positioning reduces time for both the setup and the breakdown of the case. The key to this concept is to place the patient in supine position with the arms tucked, avoiding the use of lithotomy position, which requires the use of leg stir-ups and bed reconfiguration, adding significant time to each case. With the Si platform, the supine position will require parallel side docking, as opposed to docking between the legs. The new Xi platform, with its rotating boom, has solved docking challenges and docks quite easily for this procedure.

Sewing the peritoneum closed at the completion of the hernia repair is one of the most advantageous aspects of using the robot for inguinal hernia repair. The quality and ease of the closure, due to the 7 degrees of freedom of the robotic arm, eliminate the most difficult parts of its laparoscopic counterpart. Due to its difficulty in laparoscopic surgery, many surgeons tack the peritoneum closed instead of sewing it, to save time and frustration, which adds cost to each case. To sew the peritoneum closed using the robot, we have found it is easier to sew in a medial to lateral direction because the posterior rectus sheath has integrity to hold the suture under tension. We use inexpensive 2–0 Vicryl suture on a SH or CT-2 needle. Some robotic surgeons prefer barbed sutures for peritoneal closure, but exposed barbed suture may adhere to the bowel and cause a postoperative obstruction [11].

Troubleshooting common problems encountered during robotic inguinal hernia surgery can have a major impact to saving time. A fogging camera can nag a surgeon throughout the case and often worsens with camera exchanges. Preheating, defogging, and minimizing camera exchanges can minimize camera fogging. Torn peritoneum is a frequent occurrence during the dissection of an R-TAPP, particularly early in a surgeon's experience. This may require additional suturing or a Z-plasty-type closure of the peritoneum to ensure mesh coverage. This is the moment you are glad that robotic suturing is easy. In cases in which the peritoneum cannot be repaired to cover mesh, a mesh with a microporous layer designed for intraperitoneal placement can be used. This can be encountered in cases of prior mesh repairs or open pelvic surgery. Overall, having a troubleshooting plan for common problems will keep your surgical pace on track and on time.

Si Versus Xi Platform Issues

In 2017, the *da Vinci* Surgical System (Intuitive Surgical, Inc., Sunnyvale, CA, USA) is the only FDA-approved robotic system on the market in the USA. This will likely change by late 2018 or 2019, as several competitors look to enter the surgical robot market. In 2014, the Xi version of the robot was launched. This platform provided several changes and upgrades to the S-series. The main focus of the new Xi platform was to increase the ease for surgeons to operate in multiple quadrants within the abdomen. Most general surgeons being trained today will likely train on the Xi platform, and only learn the S platform peripherally. For those surgeons who have been on the S platform, the Xi is a major change that should prompt simulation lab training before use. While the surgeon console is the same, the boomed patient-side cart has a total redesign that impacts trocar placement, bed positioning, and docking procedures.

In regard to the R-TAPP, the use of the Xi platform means rethinking how to place the mesh and suture into the abdomen, because it is based on all the cannulas being 8 mm in diameter. Our work-around for this issue is to place a 12 mm Hasson trocar in the supra-umbilical location and telescope the 8 mm cannula down it (Fig. 10.4). Additionally, the boomed patient-side cart and new positioning system solve the challenges of parallel docking of the Si platform. The integration of a bed control system with the robotic platform means that the patient position can be changed without undocking the robot on the Xi. Once docked and instruments are inserted, the surgeon has a familiar experience in the surgeon console on both Si and Xi platforms.

Summary

Robotic inguinal hernia based on the TAPP procedure is gaining popularity. Some of the migration comes from laparoscopic surgeons, but many are open inguinal hernia surgeons. This migration is occurring despite a lack of cost, outcomes, and value data proving equivalency. The R-TAPP may shorten the learning curve that has frustrated surgeons on the laparoscopic platform. The enhanced ergonomics, optics, and control provided by robotics may make the surgeons feel like they are performing better surgery. With inguinal hernia being one the most common general surgery operations, there will be plenty of data to collect to assess the value of robotics in inguinal hernia care. The greatest value may be in the complex hernia patient or in concomitant robotic procedures. The value proposition equation may change as competition enters the robotic market. Competition could drive both innovation and cost structures that may benefit the overall healthcare system. This would radically change the viewpoint of robotic surgery in the future.

References

1. Hussain A, Malik A, Halim MU, Ali AM. The use of robotics in surgery: a review. Int J Clin Pract. 2014;68(11):1376–82.

2. Collins JN, Britt RC, Britt LD. Concomitant robotic repair of inguinal hernia with robotic prostatectomy. Am Surg. 2011;77(2):238–9.

3. Joshi AR, Spivak J, Rubach E, Goldberg G, DeNoto G. Concurrent robotic trans-abdominal pre-peritoneal (TAP) herniorrhaphy during robotic-assisted radical prostatectomy. Int J Med Robot. 2010;6(3):311–4.

4. Lee DK, Montgomery DP, Porter JR. Concurrent transperitoneal repair for incidentally detected inguinal hernias during robotically assisted radical prostatectomy. Urology. 2013;82(6):1320–2.

5. Finley DS, Savatta D, Rodriguez E, Kopelan A, Ahlering TE. Transperitoneal robotic-assisted laparoscopic radical prostatectomy and inguinal herniorrhaphy. J Robot Surg. 2008;1(4):269–72.

6. Ito F, Jarrard D, Gould JC. Transabdominal preperitoneal robotic inguinal hernia repair. J Laparoendosc Adv Surg Tech A. 2008;18(3):397–9.

7. Engan C, Engan M, Bonilla V, Dyer DC, Randall BR. Description of robotically assisted single-site transabdominal preperitoneal (RASS-TAPP) inguinal hernia repair and presentation of clinical outcomes. Hernia. 2015;19(3):423–8.

8. Waite KE, Herman MA, Doyle PJ. Comparison of robotic versus laparoscopic transabdominal preperitoneal (TAPP) inguinal hernia repair. J Robot Surg. 2016;10(3):239–44.

9. Escobar Dominguez JE, Ramos MG, Seetharamaiah R, Donkor C, Rabaza J, Gonzalez A. Feasibility of robotic inguinal hernia repair, a single-institution experience. Surg Endosc. 2016;30(9):4042–8.

10. Arcerito M, Changchien E, Bernal O, Konkoly-Thege A, Moon J. Robotic inguinal hernia repair: technique and early experience. Am Surg. 2016;82(10):1014–7.

11. Iraniha A, Peloquin J. Long-term quality of life and outcomes following robotic assisted TAPP inguinal hernia repair. J Robot Surg. 2017. doi:https://doi.org/10.1007/s11701-017-0727-8.

12. Kudsi OY, McCarty JC, Paluvoi N, Mabardy AS. Transition from laparoscopic totally extraperitoneal inguinal hernia repair to robotic transabdominal preperitoneal inguinal hernia repair: a retrospective review of a single surgeon's experience. World J Surg. 2017;41(9):2251–7.

13. Escobar Dominguez JE, Gonzalez A, Donkor C. Robotic inguinal hernia repair. J Surg Oncol. 2015;112(3):310–4.

Laparoscopic Femoral Hernia Repair

11

Benjamin Carr and Dana Telem

Introduction

Laparoscopic repair of the femoral hernia (FH) is an essential skill for modern general surgeons. FH accounts for 3–5% of groin hernias, and up to 50,000 FH repairs are performed annually in the United States. Of these, approximately 65% are in women; though within the female population, inguinal hernia (IH) is still more common than FH (75% IH vs 25% FH). Femoral hernia accounts for only 1% of hernias in men. Risk factors for FH are similar those for IH – advanced age, smoking, chronic lung disease, family history, collagen vascular disease, peritoneal dialysis, and low BMI.

FH are less common than IH but are far more likely to become incarcerated. Up to 45% of FH become incarcerated within 2 years after diagnosis, and approximately 40% of FH are discovered when patients present with incarceration. In a Swedish study, more than one in five emergent femoral hernia repairs required bowel resection, with a tenfold mortality risk over non-emergent FH repairs. Thus, repair is indicated for any FH that is identified.

However, diagnosing a small FH by physical exam alone can be very challenging. FH involves the protrusion of the peritoneum and its contents into the femoral canal, passing under the inguinal ligament and medial to the femoral vessels. This can cause a bulge or discomfort in some patients, but many are asymptomatic until they present with obstruction or strangulation. FH may also be incidentally noted on cross-sectional imaging.

In clinical practice, FH is usually encountered in the operating room, either during treatment for incarceration or incidentally discovered during inguinal hernia repair (IHR). Even in patients undergoing repair of known IH, femoral hernias are often missed – in one Danish study, approximately 40% of women undergoing repair of "recurrent IH" were found to have a femoral hernia. It is therefore imperative that the surgeon performing an IHR thoroughly inspect all possible sites of herniation in the groin – the inguinal canal, the femoral canal, and the obturator canal (Fig. 11.1).

Even with an appropriate index of suspicion, FH can be difficult to identify, and care must be taken to adequately expose and inspect the myopectineal orifice.

The State of the Art

Before laparoscopic techniques were introduced, femoral hernias were challenging to identify because exposure of the femoral canal required either an infra-inguinal dissection or incision of

B. Carr · D. Telem (✉)
Department of Surgery, University of Michigan,
Ann Arbor, MI, USA
e-mail: dtelem@med.umich.edu

Fig. 11.1 Anterior view of indirect (A), direct (B), and femoral (C) hernia locations

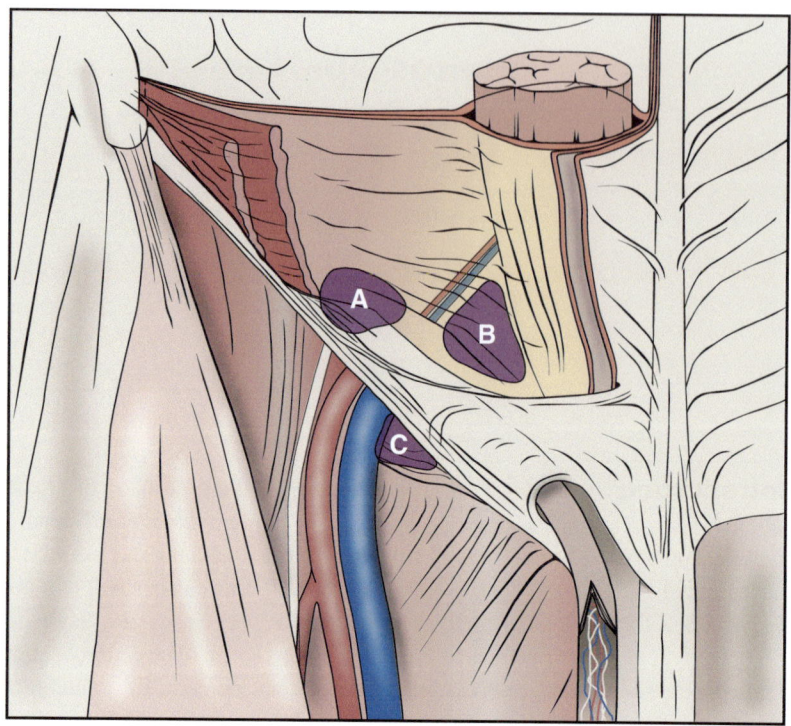

the inguinal ligament. Historically, open repairs used either a Cooper's ligament-based repair or a variety of mesh-based strategies (plug-and-patch, pre-peritoneal Kugel patch, or mesh bilayer).

Groin hernias are now preferentially repaired laparoscopically, either using a total extraperitoneal (TEP) approach or the transabdominal pre-peritoneal (TAPP) method. Laparoscopy provides excellent exposure of the femoral canal in addition to the inguinal canal (Fig. 11.2), and laparoscopic repair is the recommended operation for femoral hernias, whether diagnosed preoperatively or discovered incidentally during IHR.

For this reason, current trends in IHR have informed FH repair techniques to a large extent. Choice of mesh shape, materials, and method of securement all readily translate from IH to FH repairs.

A laparoscopic "critical view" of groin hernia anatomy has been recently defined and describes the benchmarks of an adequate dissection for mesh placement. An appropriate dissection should expose Hesselbach's triangle, the pubic tubercle, the space of Retzius, the Iliac vessels, the psoas muscle, and the antero-superior iliac spine (ASIS). The hernia sac should be completely freed from the canal and completely separated from the cord and vascular structures.

Management Strategy and Operative Technique

Because of their increased risk of incarceration, all FH should be repaired when identified.

Preoperative preparation, positioning, approach, and exposure for femoral hernia repair should follow established principles for repair of other groin hernias (see Chaps. 8, 9, and 10).

Femoral hernias are best approached by the laparoscopic technique with which the surgeon is most comfortable – either the TEP or TAPP exposure. If the operation is being undertaken for repair of IH, it is essential that the surgeon expose the femoral canal and rule out a femoral hernia in

Fig. 11.2 Laparoscopic view of indirect (A), direct (B), and femoral (C) hernia locations

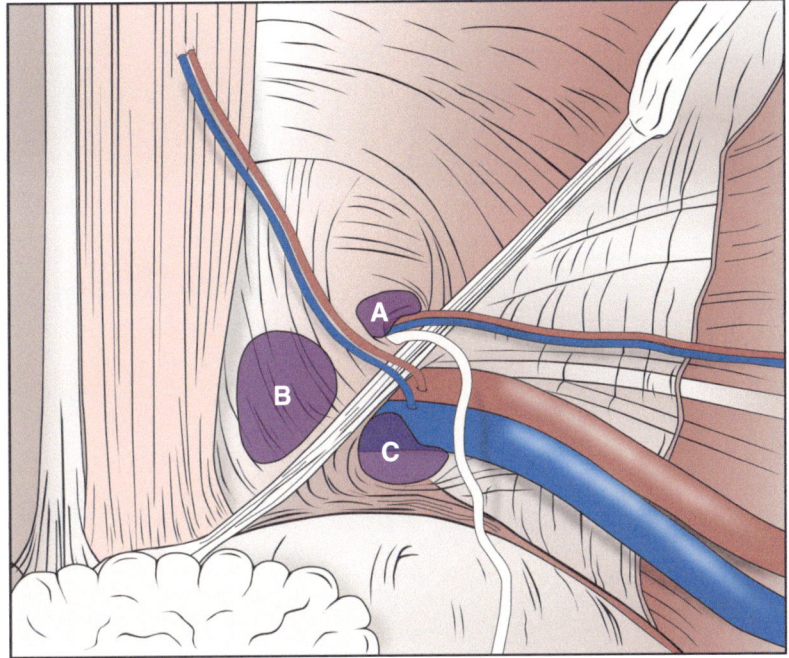

addition to the inguinal defect. Failure to perform an adequate dissection may lead to a missed femoral hernia, which carries a high risk of incarceration.

A thorough dissection should adhere to the principles of the critical view of the myopectineal orifice. In particular, the dissection should extend onto the pubic tubercle medially, extending inferiorly at least 2 cm into the space of Retzius to allow space for the mesh to lie anterior to the bladder. The lacunar ligament will be seen at the medial border of the femoral canal, and any corona mortis vessels should be identified and avoided. The inguinal ligament should be visualized coursing superior to the canal, with Cooper's ligament seen inferiorly and the wall of the femoral vein clearly visible laterally. An adequate dissection of the femoral ring will bring the inferior "gutter" of peritoneum well away from the femoral orifice, exposing the bladder fat medially and the femoral vessels laterally and proximally.

Once identified, a femoral hernia may be more difficult to reduce than an IH, due to the small diameter of the femoral ring. Occasionally, it may be necessary to carefully incise the lacunar ligament, iliopubic tract, or inguinal ligament to relax the femoral ring, or an infra-inguinal thigh incision may be required to lyse attachments of the sac.

Choice of mesh is a matter of surgeon preference. We favor pre-shaped concave polypropylene or polyester mesh, which is easy to place and provides excellent coverage of all possible hernia defects. Many surgeons anchor the mesh medially, usually with sutures or tacks to Cooper's ligament just over the pubis. However, recent studies in IHR have shown that using glue to secure the mesh is also sufficient, with no difference in recurrence compared to other anchoring methods and decreased postoperative pain. Similar results have been observed with self-gripping mesh. The essential point is to completely cover the inguinal, femoral, and obturator canals with a wide margin of mesh that lays out smoothly against the pelvic-abdominal wall (Fig. 11.3), with the medial edge snugged under the pubic tubercle anterior to the bladder and the lateral edge extending outward past the anterosuperior iliac spine.

Fig. 11.3 Laparoscopic view of indirect (A), direct (B), and femoral (C) hernia locations with mesh in place

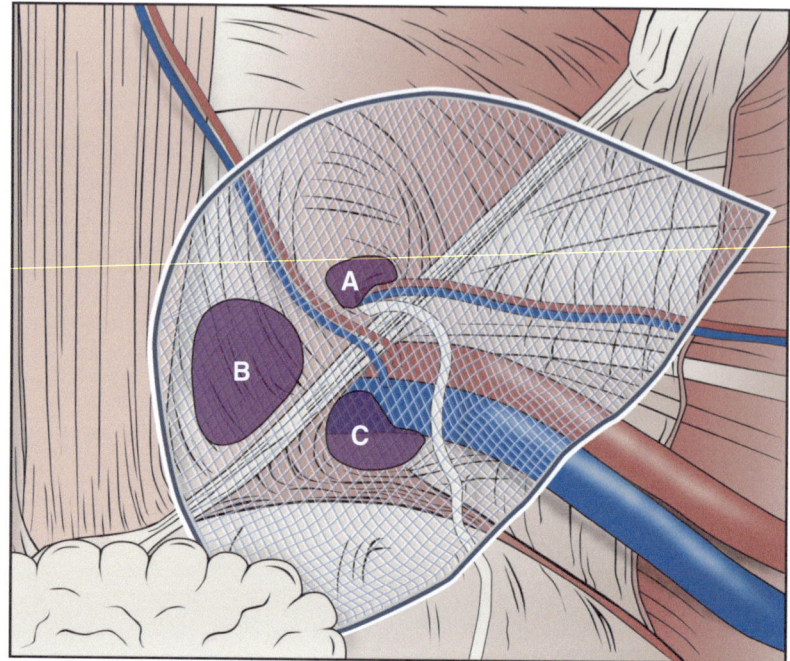

Conclusion

Femoral hernias may present incidentally during IHR, as a "recurrence" after previous IHR or as an independent problem either before or after becoming incarcerated. Fortunately, established principles of IHR can be readily applied to management of femoral hernias, with excellent exposure and coverage provided by laparoscopic techniques. Surgeons must maintain an appropriate index of suspicion for femoral hernia and take care to adequately inspect and cover all possible defects when repairing groin hernias.

Fixation in Laparoscopic Inguinal Hernia Repair

12

Nathaniel Stoikes, David Webb, and Guy Voeller

Fixation of mesh for laparoscopic preperitoneal hernia repair is an often debated and controversial topic. What we do laparoscopically has its origins in the work done by Jean Rives. He placed a unilateral piece of polyester mesh in the preperitoneal space through a lower midline incision. He fixated the mesh at multiple (>10) points with interrupted sutures. In a figure from his original description of the procedure, one can see he fixated the mesh in areas that we do not consider safe when using mechanical fixation through the laparoscope (Fig. 12.1).

In addition, Stoppa also recommended suture fixation of the mesh when used for unilateral preperitoneal inguinal hernia repair (Fig. 12.2). It was only with his giant prosthetic reinforcement of the visceral sac for multiple recurrent bilateral inguinal hernias that Stoppa advocated no fixation due to the large size of the mesh relative to the defect size. Many surgeons believe as did Rives and Stoppa that fixation for unilateral repair is mandatory to prevent mesh migration and displacement, while others have taken Stoppa's idea of nonfixation using a giant piece of mesh for bilateral recurrent repairs to the unilateral laparoscopic repair.

Regardless of technical laparoscopic approach of totally extraperitoneal (TEP) or transabdomi-nal preperitoneal (TAPP) repair, the confined space and contour of the preperitoneal space allows for an array of mesh fixation options. The three categories of fixation are no fixation, mechanical fixation, and adhesive or alternative fixation. They each have advantages and disadvantages depending on the clinical scenario.

No Fixation

There have been multiple studies evaluating no mesh fixation. Taylor et al. did a randomized prospective double-blinded trial comparing tack fixation versus no fixation in TEP inguinal hernia repair and found no differences in recurrence rates. Follow-up, however, was short at 8 months, and a majority of the hernias in the study were small (<2 cm in size). In their conclusions they cautioned against using no fixation in large inguinal hernias [1]. More recently, Golani et al. published a review of 538 patients undergoing TEP and no mesh fixation with over 6-year follow-up and recurrence rates of 1.5% and a 2.9% incidence of pain. In their series, they did use tacks in 11 patients that had direct hernia defects and were > 3 cm in size [2]. In general patients should be well selected for no mesh fixation in laparoscopic inguinal hernia repair. Specifically, patients with small indirect defects that maintain integrity of the inguinal floor may be considered candidates for no fixation.

N. Stoikes (✉) · D. Webb · G. Voeller
Division of Minimally Invasive Surgery,
University of Tennessee Health Science Center,
Memphis, TN, USA
e-mail: nstoikes@uthsc.edu

© Springer International Publishing AG, part of Springer Nature 2018
M. P. LaPinska, J. A. Blatnik (eds.), *Surgical Principles in Inguinal Hernia Repair*,
https://doi.org/10.1007/978-3-319-92892-0_12

Fig 12.1 Rives' open preperitoneal inguinal hernia repair. (Adapted from Hernia Healers 1998 page 116 chief editor Rene Stoppa, company is Arnette)

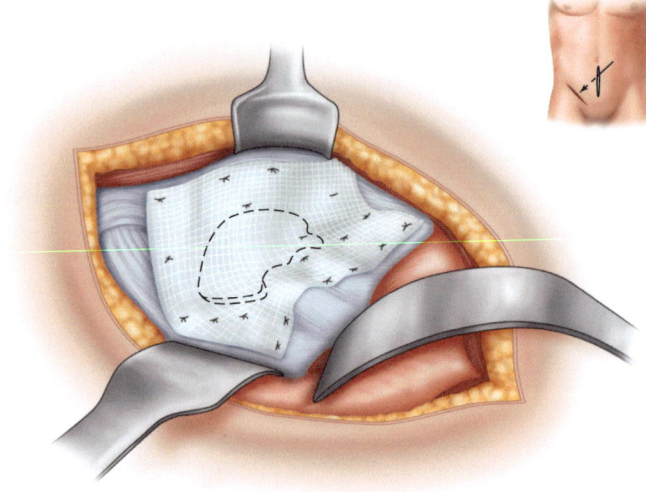

Fig. 12.2 Schematic anteromediolateral view of a unilateral prosthesis placed by the medial preperitoneal approach. The operator's left hand depressed; the peritoneal sac. The prosthesis split to let the cord pass through and is sewn to the parietal wall, the Cooper ligament, the femoral sheath, and the fascia iliaca. (Adapted from Hernia third edition (1989) chief editor Lloyd Nyhus. Lippincott. Chapter 10 page 208)

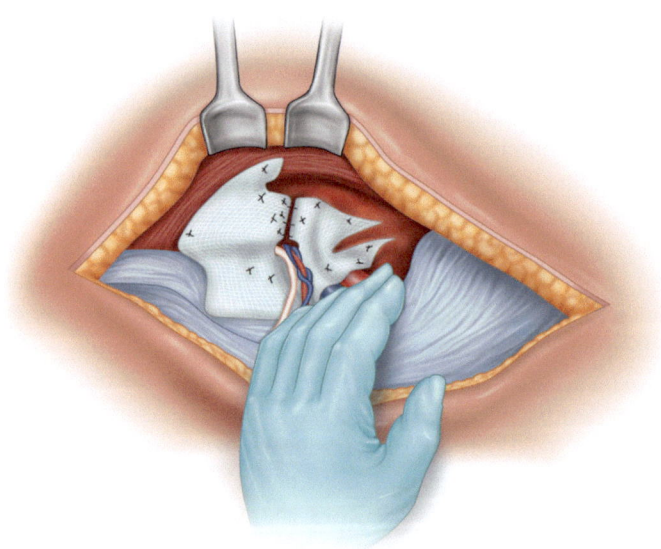

Mechanical Fixation

Tack fixation of mesh has been the mainstay since the inception of the procedure and has been the basis for comparison to all other forms of fixation. Biomechanically, mechanical fixation with a tack is stronger than other forms of fixation with the exception of suture fixation. Traditionally in the preperitoneal space suture fixation is technically difficult and cumbersome to perform making tack fixation the preferred method of mechanical fixation. One new caveat has been the introduction of robotic surgery, which has allowed for more degrees of articulation and made suturing possible.

Regardless of laparoscopic approach, tacking (when done properly) has been found to yield excellent results including low recurrence rates and low rates of chronic groin pain [3, 4].

Tacks are made both of absorbable and permanent materials. There have been few studies comparing these two types of fixation in the inguinal space. Most of the comparisons between absorbable and permanent mechanical fixation types have been done in laparoscopic ventral/incisional hernia. There is greater need for fixation strength in laparoscopic ventral hernia repair compared to laparoscopic inguinal hernia given the latter's confined space and contour. In terms of a pure biomechanical evaluation, Melman et al. evaluated acute fixation strength of permanent tacks vs absorbable tacks in a porcine model and found that tacks made of permanent materials were significantly stronger than tacks made of absorbable materials. In this study they also evaluated adhesive fixation utilizing fibrin glue and found absorbable tacks to have stronger fixation compared to fibrin glue [5].

Limitations of mechanical fixation are directly related to the anatomy of the preperitoneal space leading to point fixation in a few specific locations. Penetrating fixation is limited to medial placement on the rectus muscle, inferiorly on Cooper's ligament and laterally on the abdominal wall above the iliopubic tract. Below the iliopubic tract, there is the risk of vascular and nerve damage, and therefore the dissection itself and the orientation of the peritoneum as it rolls over the mesh serve as fixation in these areas.

Adhesive and Alternative Fixation

Adhesive fixation is principally different than mechanical fixation. Rather than point fixation in limited locations, adhesive fixation allows for non-penetrating fixation over a much larger surface area including the areas of the preperitoneal space that prohibit mechanical fixation due to the risk of injury to nerves, blood vessels, and other vital structures. As previously mentioned, the fixation is weaker per each point of fixation than a tack. It is not known if the larger surface area fixated increases fixation strength such that the two forms are biomechanically comparable in terms of strength. Clinically, adhesive fixation in laparoscopic inguinal hernia was originally described by Jourdan in the late 1990s using a cyanoacrylate. Due to dense inflammatory response, encapsulation, and oncogenic concerns, cyanoacrylates of the type used in this study are not commonly used [6]. In the early 2000s, original works by Kathkouhda and Schwab started the conversation about the feasibility of fibrin glue for mesh fixation in laparoscopic inguinal hernia repair. Katkhouda et al. established a porcine model for laparoscopic inguinal hernia comparing no fixation, tack fixation, and fibrin glue fixation of mesh. In their study they saw that there was significant migration with no fixation of the mesh but that tack and glue fixation were not

statistically different and both prevented mesh migration. In addition, the tensile strength of the repair was stronger when the mesh was fixated [7]. Schwab et al. found similar results when comparing suture fixation and fibrin glue using multiple different meshes. Mesh dislocation was consistently seen without fixation. Sutures and fibrin glue both prevented this dislocation. The highest stress resistance across the abdominal wall was seen with the fibrin glue. In addition, fibrin glue gave the best incorporation of the mesh and the best biomechanical stability of the mesh [8].

Multiple clinical studies comparing the use of fibrin glue and tacks for fixation of mesh in both TEP and TAPP inguinal hernia repair have shown clinical equivalency. Kaul et al. performed a meta-analysis of studies evaluating outcomes between fibrin glue fixation and tack fixation. Four studies that were evaluated included 662 repairs and showed that recurrence rates were similar between the two groups but that the incidence of chronic groin pain 3 months post-op was significantly higher in the tack group [9].

Self-gripping mesh is another alternative form of mesh fixation that has been available since 2009. The mesh itself contains absorbable barbs that allow the mesh to self-adhere to tissue. Only one clinical study comparing its use in laparoscopy to mechanical fixation has been done. Fumagalli et al. prospectively evaluated 96 patients undergoing TAPP inguinal hernia repair using self-gripping mesh versus mechanical fixation. Forty-nine patients had self-gripping mesh, and 46 patients had conventional mesh fixation with 4 permanent tacks. There was one recurrence in the series during follow-up at 13.8 months, which was conventional mesh fixation. The incidence of chronic pain trended to be lower with self-gripping mesh [10].

Biomechanics of Fixation

While the clinical results of each fixation modality have proven to be sound, there is no question that the biomechanics of fixation for each form is different. Fixation strength of the various modalities has been evaluated in animal studies. Stoikes et al. evaluated fibrin glue vs suture fixation of mesh in a porcine model. Fixation strength was evaluated at 24 h, 7 days, and 14 days. Shear strengths showed that suture was significantly stronger at 24 h (10.4 N/cm vs 4.9 N/cm), but by 7 days fixation strength was irrelevant because the mesh/fascia interface was stronger than the mesh or fascia itself leading to failure of either the mesh or fascia under shear stress testing. Conclusions were that while adhesive fixation was acutely less than suture fixation, the fixation provided by adhesives was adequate for mesh fixation [11].

Expounding on the concept of adequacy of fixation, Shahan et al. evaluated acute fixation of three alternative fixation methods including fibrin glue, self-gripping mesh, and a mesh coated with a synthetic adhesive. Shear strengths were evaluated acutely after application, and it was found that the coated mesh (8 N/cm) provided significantly stronger fixation than fibrin glue (2.6 N/cm) or self-gripping mesh (1.3 N/cm) [12].

Clinically, adhesive fixation has provided excellent results in laparoscopic inguinal hernia repair, which begs the question of how strong is strong enough? More studies are needed to evaluate the true mechanisms and behavior of the various technologies despite the proven clinical effectiveness. Understanding the details becomes very important and directly translates to decision-making in a clinical scenario. For example, Kes et al. evaluated protrusion of meshes through various-sized defects (3 cm, 4 cm, and 5 cm) with different meshes in a pressure chamber that simulated Valsalva. In general, it was found that as defect sizes increase there is more friction exerted on the edges of mesh and that the meshes collapse and deform into the defect more. This occurred at varying rates depending on the mesh used, but this phenomenon was seen uniformly [13].

Understanding this important study and the varying ways of fixating mesh can directly affect our decisions in the clinical arena. For example, in a patient with a small indirect defect less than 2 cm, a surgeon may choose to use no fixation or adhesive fixation only. In contrast, a patient presenting with a large direct defect >4 cm, a surgeon may choose to use both adhesive fixation and absorbable tacks medially on the rectus muscle. As more technologies become available, further study into the biomechanics of fixation is critical to our understanding of optimal fixation as it relates to recurrence and chronic pain in laparoscopic inguinal hernia repair.

References

1. Taylor C1, Layani L, Liew V, Ghusn M, Crampton N, White S. Laparoscopic inguinal hernia repair without mesh fixation, early results of a large randomised clinical trial. Surg Endosc. 2008;22(3):757–62. Epub 2007 Sep 21
2. Golani S1, Middleton P2. Long-term follow-up of laparoscopic total extraperitoneal (TEP) repair in inguinal hernia without mesh fixation. Hernia. 2017;21(1):37–43.
3. Fitzgibbons RJ Jr, Camps J, Cornet DA, Nguyen NX, Litke BS, Annibali R, Salerno GM. Laparoscopic inguinal herniorrhaphy. Results of a multicenter trial. Ann Surg. 1995;221(1):3–13.
4. Schwab JR1, Beaird DA, Ramshaw BJ, Franklin JS, Duncan TD, Wilson RA, Miller J, Mason EM. After 10 years and 1903 inguinal hernias, what is the outcome for the laparoscopic repair? Surg Endosc. 2002;16(8):1201–6. Epub 2002 May 3
5. Melman L, Jenkins ED, Deeken CR, Brodt MD, Brown SR, Brunt LM, Eagon JC, Frisella M, Matthews BD. Evaluation of acute fixation strength for mechanical tacking devices and fibrin sealant versus polypropylene suture for laparoscopic ventral hernia repair. Surg Innov. 2010;17(4):285–90.
6. Jourdan IC1, Bailey ME. Initial experience with the use of N-butyl 2-cyanoacrylate glue for the fixation of polypropylene mesh in laparoscopic hernia repair. Surg Laparosc Endosc. 1998;8(4):291–3.
7. Katkhouda N, Mavor E, Friedlander MH, Mason RJ, Kiyabu M, Grant SW, Achanta K, Kirkman EL, Narayanan K, Essani R. Use of fibrin sealant for prosthetic mesh fixation in laparoscopic extraperitoneal inguinal hernia repair. Ann Surg. 2001;233(1):18–25.
8. Schwab R, Schumacher O, Junge K, Binnebösel M, Klinge U, Becker HP, Schumpelick V. Biomechanical analyses of mesh fixation in TAPP and TEP hernia repair. Surg Endosc. 2008;22(3):731–8.
9. Kaul A, Hutfless S, Le H, Hamed SA, Tymitz K, Nguyen H, Marohn MR. Staple versus fibrin glue fixation in laparoscopic total extraperitoneal repair of inguinal hernia: a systematic review and meta-analysis. Surg Endosc. 2012;26(5):1269–78.
10. Fumagalli Romario U, Puccetti F, Elmore U, Massaron S, Rosati R. Self-gripping mesh versus staple fixation in laparoscopic inguinal hernia repair: a prospective comparison. Surg Endosc. 2013;27(5):1798–802.
11. Stoikes N, Sharpe J, Tasneem H, Roan E, Paulus E, Powell B, Webb D, Handorf C, Eckstein E, Fabian T, Voeller G. Biomechanical evaluation of fixation properties of fibrin glue for ventral incisional hernia repair. Hernia. 2015;19(1):161–6.
12. Shahan CP, Stoikes NF, Roan E, Tatum J, Webb DL, Voeller GR. Short-term strength of non-penetrating mesh fixation: LifeMesh™, Tisseel™, and ProGrip™. Surg Endosc. 2017;31(3):1350–3.
13. Kes E1, Lange J, Bonjer J, Stoeckart R, Mulder P, Snijders C, Kleinrensink G. Protrusion of prosthetic meshes in repair of inguinal hernias. Surgery. 2004;135(2):163–70.

Part IV

Postoperative Management

Postoperative Management

13

Steve R. Siegal and Sean B. Orenstein

Introduction

The surgical repair of inguinal hernias is a commonly performed general surgical procedure that has been practiced for generations. Though the postoperative management is not overly challenging, there is an ongoing trend in surgery toward quicker recovery and earlier return to activity, and these concepts are indeed evolving. In this chapter, postanesthesia care, discharge criteria, aftercare and activity restrictions, as well as short-term complications will be discussed.

Perioperative Care

After successful completion of inguinal hernia repair, patients will be awoken from anesthesia and taken to a postanesthesia care unit (PACU). The goal of "Post-Anesthesia Phase I" is to care for basic life-sustaining needs of the patient with constant vigilance to restore the patient to their preoperative state of function and alertness while minimizing postoperative pain, nausea, and adverse events. We advocate for a face-to-face

S. R. Siegal
Department of Surgery, Oregon Health & Science University, Portland, OR, USA

S. B. Orenstein (✉)
Oregon Health & Science University,
Portland, OR, USA
e-mail: orenstei@ohsu.edu

handoff to the PACU team with an appropriate "sign out" of the surgical and anesthesia course by the surgical team. This allows for transfer of important perioperative details and specific instructions for postoperative care to improve the safety of the patient and ensure a smooth transition out of the postoperative period.

Postoperative Analgesia

A mild to moderate amount of postoperative pain localized at the incision site(s) and/or the inguinal region(s) can be expected. For postoperative analgesia, we advocate for conservative use of parenteral opioid analgesics, if tolerated by the patient, to reduce postoperative urinary retention, nausea and vomiting, or ileus (discussed later). Oral nonsteroidal anti-inflammatory medications (NSAID) and acetaminophen may be used along with parenteral ketorolac as adjuncts to provide a synergistic effect of pain relief without the side effects of respiratory depression, altered mental status, or ileus. NSAIDs have been shown in prospective trials to provide effective pain control in inguinal hernia repairs without increased risk of bleeding [1]. Obvious contraindications to these medications exist, and careful use is warranted in patients with contraindications (e.g., renal dysfunction). Much discussion has been held with regard to the increased bleeding risk with perioperative use of ketorolac. A meta-analysis has shown no clinically increased risk of postoperative bleeding or adverse events in patients receiving perioperative ketorolac. This analysis also demonstrated improved pain control and decreased nausea and vomiting with ketorolac use [2]. As such, we favor the use of ketorolac in uncomplicated cases without underlying renal disease or a history of gastrointestinal ulcer disease or hemorrhage. Additionally, we apply ice packs to the surgical sites and inguinal region(s) during the postoperative period to provide local analgesia and reduced edema and inflammation. Patients are advised to continue ice pack application for the first 48 hours following surgery.

Postoperative Nausea Control

Mild postoperative nausea can be normal, and postoperative nausea with vomiting (PONV) is not uncommon. Nausea and vomiting is usually self-limited but may require medical intervention, delayed postoperative recovery, or even unanticipated hospital observation. Risk factors for PONV in adults include female gender, history of PONV or motion sickness, and age <50 years. The use of general anesthesia or volatile anesthetics, longer anesthetic time, and postoperative opioid administration can also increase the risk of PONV [3, 4].

The best strategy to avoid PONV is modification of anesthetic technique (if appropriate) and prophylaxis with multi-agent pain and nausea regimens with reduction or elimination of opioid use. Common antiemetic medications (such as ondansetron, diphenhydramine, and prochlorperazine) can reduce PONV by approximately 25% [5]. Close consideration should be given to side effect profiles and contraindications in patients with comorbidities (i.e., prolonged QT interval for ondansetron). A scoring system for PONV has been developed and can help guide perioperative management based on risk stratification of those predisposed to PONV [6]. For refractory PONV, alternative regimens are available and should be discussed with participation of the anesthesiology team.

Fluid Management

Conservative use of perioperative intravenous crystalloid infusions is recommended to prevent hypervolemia, increased bladder volume leading to urinary retention, and potential pulmonary sequelae in select patients. If a patient has normal or acceptable vital signs (normotension without tachycardia) in the PACU, their IV fluids are turned off or minimized to a "keep-vein-open" (KVO) rate to maintain IV patency. Ongoing fluid administration may be appropriate or even required for vital sign abnormalities, nausea/vomiting, per oral intolerance, or at the discretion of the anesthesiologist.

Urinary Retention

Postoperative urinary retention (POUR) most commonly follows anorectal, spine, and pelvic surgery. POUR can be quite common following laparoscopic inguinal hernia repair, with incidences as high as 22–25% [7, 8]. This can prevent same-day discharge in some patients and requires others to perform self-catheterization at home, both of which elevate medical costs and reduce patient satisfaction. While high rates of POUR have been described, a laparoscopic series including over 1000 inguinal repair patients demonstrated the occurrence of POUR in 0.2–3.1% of cases [9–11]. Retention is diagnosed as an inability to void with an overfilled bladder (often imaged with bladder sonography). Though normal bladder volume capacity is 400–500 ml, volumes greater than 270 ml are a risk factor for POUR. Bladder volume can be estimated by catheterization or ultrasonography, though there is decreased accuracy in obese patients [12].

A number of risk factors have been identified for urinary retention [12]. Patient-specific factors include neurologic disorders, male gender, older than 50 years, and benign prostatic hypertrophy. Several drugs used in the perioperative period can predispose patients to POUR, including anticholinergics, beta-blockers, and sympathomimetics. The incidence of POUR does vary based on anesthetic technique, occurring in 0.37% of local anesthetic cases, 2.42% of regional cases, and in 3% of cases using general anesthesia [13]. Similarly, over 1200 ml of intravenous fluids used perioperatively has been shown to increase the risk of POUR [14]. In our practice, we commonly restrict intraoperative fluid to less than 1,000 ml, and prefer closer to 500 ml.

Because of a potential high rate of POUR following inguinal hernia repair, it is standard that patients void after repair, and those who spontaneously void may discharge home. There is variation among surgeons for treatment of POUR, with some surgeons discharging patients regardless of voiding status, while others prefer a more aggressive approach to retention. We prefer to actively monitor the ability to spontaneously void and to ensure there is adequate emptying prior to discharge. Patients unable to void by the time of discharge receive an ultrasonography of the bladder (aka bladder scan). Patients with bladder volumes less than approximately 500 ml are given additional time to spontaneously void. Continued failure to void necessitates straight catheterization to empty the bladder. An indwelling Foley catheter is commonly placed for patients that fail a second voiding trial as well as patients with >500 ml upon bladder scanning or with a strong history of urinary retention (e.g., BPH). These patients receive specific discharge instructions on catheter removal with voiding trial at home 12–24 h after catheterization or to come back to clinic in for catheter removal and voiding trial. Those unable to spontaneously void, or who require repeat catheterization, are referred for urologic consultation.

Discharge Criteria

The goal of "Post-Anesthesia Phase II" of care is preparing the patient for discharge and care at home. We routinely discuss the outcomes of our surgery with the patient (and caregivers) and send a copy of the operative report to the referring physician (if able). A patient should now be fully awake and able to answer questions appropri-ately. Oxygen supplementation should be weaned to room air or preoperative oxygen requirements, and the patient should have normal respiratory/ventilation parameters. Systolic blood pressure should be within 20 mmHg of the pre-anesthesia level with the same variation in heart rate. The patient's pain should be adequately controlled, thus allowing for transfer out of the hospital bed and ambulation without overwhelming discomfort. Patients are routinely given standard dosing of oral analgesics prior to discharge to assist with their travel comfort as well as to evaluate their response to the prescribed analgesics. Patients not meeting these criteria may require longer postanesthesia observation or alterations in their management depending on the clinical scenario and should be determined on a case-by-case basis. If adjustments in postanesthesia care and longer observation fail to improve lingering discharge criteria or if other concerning features are present, inpatient admission and further workup are strongly considered. Rare, but not unforeseen, circumstances that may necessitate admission include persistent oxygen requirement; vital sign aberrances including hypotension, tachycardia, and tachypnea; pain unrelieved with an oral medication regimen; and altered mental status. Obvious signs of ongoing bleeding (e.g., expanding hematoma) or neurologic sequelae warrant further evaluation and possibly return to the operating room for exploration.

Aftercare

The cornerstones of postoperative recovery and home care after inguinal hernia surgery include pain relief with tapering and cessation of narcotics, early mobilization and ambulation, resumption of diet and bowel habits, and adherence to activity instructions.

Pain Management

Specific pain medication choice, dosage, and amount prescribed vary widely across practices and from surgeon to surgeon. A recent single institution study analyzed postoperative opiate use in opiate-naïve patients after 165 laparoscopic and open inguinal hernia repairs [15]. Among the hernia patients who completed their surveys, the average amount of 5 mg oxycodone equivalents prescribed was 33 pills. Interestingly, 45% of laparoscopic patients and 22% of open patients did not take any opiate pills. The authors calculated the "ideal" number of pills to be prescribed based on criteria that would satisfy 80% of patients' postoperative opiate use and determined a hernia repair patient's ideal prescription is 15 pills of 5 mg oxycodone equivalents. This data should be interpreted as suggestive, rather than guidelines, though it parallels our approach to narcotic prescriptions.

Patients taking chronic preoperative narcotics may resume their prescription. Our practice is to strongly emphasize "staggered" dosing of NSAID medication and/or acetaminophen to achieve synergistic pain control and encourage prompt opiate cessation.

Activity Level and Restriction

One of the most important and beneficial aspects of postoperative care at home is early mobilization and ambulation. Early ambulation improves pulmonary toileting, reduces postoperative ileus risk, and prevents postoperative deconditioning. After discharge, we encourage our patients to achieve adequate pain control to allow for low-speed, low-impact ambulation two to three times a day starting on the first postoperative day.

Postoperative activity and weight lifting restriction is a frequently recommended discharge instruction for patients after inguinal hernia repair. The duration and amount of this restriction is quite varied from practice to practice, and restriction is often quite protracted [16]. Recommendations for prolonged convalescence likely stem from a fear of recurrence. This fear, however, is unfounded and based on data that fail to attribute activity with recurrence. A 2-year prospective multicenter Danish Hernia Collaboration study of Lichtenstein repair of inguinal hernia evaluated patients who were instructed to resume usual work and daily activities the day after surgery. The median time off work was 7 days; those employed in sedentary work returned in a median of 4.5 days, and those with a strenuous job returned in 14 days. Patients resumed their most strenuous activity at a median of 14 days. There was no difference in reoperation rate for recurrence compared to controls that were not asked to resume activity the day after surgery, indicating that the recommendation for short convalescence does not increase risk of recurrence [17]. Similarly, there is no clear evidence that postoperative activity instructions should vary by surgical approach. One trial comparing Shouldice repair, TAPP, and TEP allowed patients to resume activity as tolerated, rather than a predefined time, and found no difference in return to walking, running, sexual intercourse, sports, or resumption of work between groups [16].

There have been concerted efforts to best compile evidence to support postoperative activity instructions. In 2009 the European Hernia Society published their guidelines on inguinal hernia management in adults. This group found Level 3 evidence negating the imposition of lifting bans after inguinal surgery and gave a Grade C recommendation to not place limitations. Rather, they offer a "Do what you feel you can do" approach, though state that heavy weight lifting "probably" necessitates a 2–3-week limitation [13]. A separate set of guidelines was published in 2015 addressing management of TAPP and TEP repairs of inguinal hernias. This study presented Level 1B evidence showing no increased risk for recurrence due to physical strain and Level 3 evidence supporting return to work and resumption of daily activity within 1–3 days assuming pain is controlled [18]. As such, it is our belief that the surgeon should keenly emphasize to the patient that postoperative physical activity does not increase the risk of recurrence and resumption of normal activity and return to work should be considered as early as postoperative day 1 as long as adequate pain control is achieved. In general, our patients are allowed to proceed with most physical activity as long as they are comfortable enough and not "fighting" through pain. Two exceptions to this are patients that perform heavy manual labor (e.g., lifting 50–100+ pounds as a part of their employment) and patients that perform heavy weight lifting in the gym. These cohorts of patients are typically advised to hold off on heavy work or exercise for 4–6 weeks, though they can return to "lighter duty" (e.g., <50 lbs) when comfortable enough for the activity without excessive groin pain.

Postoperative Diet and Bowel Function

After inguinal hernia surgery, a regular diet is resumed in the immediate postoperative period during the PACU phase of care. If the patient's nausea is minimal without emesis, they are allowed to resume normal diet as tolerated once discharged. Opioid-induced constipation (OIC) is a recognized issue in the era of high narcotic use. For patients with chronic opioid use and those discharged with short-term opioid prescriptions, we recommend increased fluid and fiber intake as well as daily use of a laxative or stool softener (such as polyethylene glycol or docusate) to reduce constipation. Milk of magnesia (two tablespoons, twice daily) is added as a second-line therapy for constipation, and a bisacodyl suppository may also be used for refractory constipation. A bowel regimen is continued until normal, consistent bowel function returns.

Resumption of Held Medications

Anticoagulation is a topic of interest as many patients take anticoagulants for atrial fibrillation, venous thromboembolism, and/or stroke prophylaxis. Coumadin requires at least 48 h for its anticoagulation properties to take effect. If a normalized INR is obtained preoperatively and non-coagulopathic bleeding is observed during the procedure, we ask patients to resume their medication 24 h

postoperatively. For patients at increased bleeding risk, resumption of anticoagulation is initiated 48–72 h after surgery. Special cases of anticoagulation "bridging" with unfractionated or low-molecular-weight heparin should be considered on a case-by-case basis and discussed with the patient's primary care physician or anticoagulation team.

For those patients whose antiplatelet therapy (e.g., aspirin, clopidogrel, etc.) is held for surgery, we typically allow resumption of these medications 24–48 h after surgery. For patients with coagulopathic bleeding or who are at increased bleeding risk, we delay reinitiation of antiplatelet therapy until 48–72 h after surgery. If stroke or cardiac risk is elevated, same day resumption can be considered in cases with minimal intraoperative hemorrhage or coagulopathy.

Patients taking chronic angiotensin-converting enzyme inhibitors (ACE-I) or angiotensin receptor blockers (ARB) are allowed to resume these medications after 24 h postoperative since fluid shifts are minimal and intravascular volume should approximate normal by this time.

Follow-Up and Wound Care

Patients generally return to clinic 2–3 weeks following hernia repair to assess wound/trocar site healing as well as for a thorough groin examination. For men, examination of the entire groin region and scrotum allow for assessment for early hernia recurrence as well as to ensure proper testicular health. Specific attention to postoperative seromas and hematomas should be made. It is common to have some degree of dependent (soft) ecchymosis of the groin crease and scrotum. Any firm masses should be further evaluated for hematoma, seroma, or early recurrence (discussed below). Any questionable finding prompts a return visit in 2–4 weeks to evaluate for improvement or resolution. While not mandatory, we routinely ask patients to return to clinic at 1 year postop for reassessment of overall healing, degree of activity level achieved since surgery, and symptoms of pain or discomfort, as well as assessment for hernia recurrence.

Short-term Complications

Both open and minimally invasive approaches to inguinal hernia repair result in low morbidity. Many immediate postoperative complications such as seromas and hematomas are monitored without the need for intervention. For questionable findings at time of postoperative evaluation, a groin/scrotal duplex ultrasound is commonly obtained as a noninvasive diagnostic tool to assess for testicular blood flow and fluid collections such as seromas/hematomas, as well as to assess for hernia recurrence.

Seroma

A seroma is a collection of benign serous fluid that can occur in a dead space created during a surgical procedure. Seromas are one of the more frequent early complications following inguinal hernia repair with an incidence ranging from 0.5% to 12.2%. Some evidence points toward an increased risk following laparoscopic, rather than open, repairs [13]. Additionally, direct inguinal defects may increase the risk of seromas given the inability to close the dead space within the direct space, though more recently surgeons are exploring the option of closing direct defects to reduce seroma formation. If a large direct defect is seen at time of repair, we typically counsel patients and family to expect a medial bulge from seroma accumulation in the postop period. In general, the body should reabsorb the serous fluid in 1 to 2 months following surgical repair, and thus initial management includes close observation without routine drainage. If, however, the seroma persists for an extended period of time, or if the seroma is so large as to cause pain/pressure or overlying changes to the skin, sterile aspiration is appropriate. No evidence points to routine need for culture of aspirated fluid, though seromas can become infected. As such, if seroma fluid appears purulent or turbid or the patient has signs of infection (fevers, cellulitis, leukocytosis), culture is recommended and appropriate antibiotics are given.

Hematoma

Similar to a seroma, a hematoma is a localized collection of blood outside of a source vessel that presents as scrotal swelling and ecchymosis. The risk of hematomas in open surgery is similar to seromas, 5.6–16%. Laparoscopic repairs have a mildly reduced risk [13]. Management of hematomas parallels that of seromas. For small, asymptomatic hematomas, we employ conservative management. Cold packs can be applied to the hematoma, though more importantly patients must be educated that hematomas can take many weeks or even months to resolve completely. Hematomas that are large and painful or necessitate blood transfusion are rare though require special attention. These hematomas should be operatively drained with close attention to hemostasis and consideration of drain placement after evacuation.

Wound Infection

Wound infections after both laparoscopic and open inguinal hernia repairs are rare, often reported to be less than 5% in the literature with even less occurrence in laparoscopic repairs [13]. Additionally, there is not an increased risk of infection in mesh versus non-mesh repairs. Deep surgical site infections (SSIs) are even less common. If a deep SSI is identified, drainage and antibiotics are the mainstay of therapy and are usually sufficient. Rarely, removal of a permanent synthetic mesh is required to attain source control of the infectious nidus if chronic or recurrent.

Testicular Complications

Spermatic cord and testicular complications such as ischemic orchitis, testicular atrophy, and vas deferens ligation are rare in both open and laparoscopic repairs. Ischemic orchitis after inguinal hernia repair presents within the first few days after surgery and may result in atrophy or even necrosis. Injury to the cremasteric vessels or pampiniform plexus or tight closure of the internal ring can lead to thrombosis of testicular veins with resultant outflow obstruction and testicular complications. Ischemic orchitis is an inflammation of the testicle usually presenting the first few days after surgery as a painful, indurated, and edematous testicle. Patients may also experience a fever. Testicular duplex ultrasound should be used to elucidate blood flow and determine if the testicle is ischemic or necrotic. For an ischemic testicle, treatment is conservative with NSAIDS and reassurance that the orchitis should resolve in 4–6 weeks as blood flow is restored. Routine antibiotics are not required. Testicular necrosis, with a complete lack of blood flow, is an urgent surgical complication that necessitates prompt urology consultation for detorsion versus orchiectomy.

Vas Deferens Injury

Transection or obstruction of the vas deferens is a rare event, though more pronounced in open repairs due to maneuvers that isolate it from other cord structures. There is increased risk of injury during recurrent operations as well. If complete transection is recognized early, the vas deferens can be reanastomosed over a stent with monofilament suture. Urology consultation is highly recommended for proper evaluation and treatment. Obstruction of the vas deferens can occur from scarring or crushing of the anatomical structure leading to fibrosis which points to the need for gentle and minimal handling of the tissue. This complication can lead to infertility and dysejaculation (groin pain during ejaculation). Symptoms often self-resolve, though ongoing pain should prompt urology referral.

Long-term Complications

Inguinodynia

Chronic postoperative groin pain after inguinal hernia repair (inguinodynia) remains a topic of interest and can be quite concerning and bothersome for patients. The reported incidence in the literature of inguinodynia after inguinal hernia repair ranges from 0% to 60%, but approximately

only 2–4% of patients find the pain adversely affects their daily life [19]. Though this incidence is small, the volume of inguinal hernia repairs preformed worldwide allows for a large amount of patients left with inguinodynia. As such, this topic necessitates specific mention. Please see Chaps. 14 and 15 for further information regarding diagnosis and management of chronic groin pain.

Hernia Recurrence

Hernia recurrence after initial repair also deserves special mention. A large series from the Danish Hernia Database reported a hernia recurrence of 3% after inguinal hernia repair [20]. Recurrent hernias can be debilitating to a patient and a challenge for the surgeon and deserve further discussion. Please see Chap. 21 for further information regarding evaluation and management of recurrent hernias.

> **Conclusion**
> Following the principles discussed in this chapter, the postoperative and post-discharge care of inguinal hernia repairs can be straightforward and uncomplicated. Certain complications require strict attention and further workup, but they are rare in inguinal surgery. Most patients recover quickly and return to their full baseline functional capacity and activities of daily living without a prolonged rehabilitation course.

References

1. Mixter CG 3rd, Meeker LD, Gavin TJ. Preemptive pain control in patients having laparoscopic hernia repair: a comparison of ketorolac and ibuprofen. Arch Surg. 1998;133(4):432–7.
2. Gobble RM, et al. Ketorolac does not increase perioperative bleeding: a meta-analysis of randomized controlled trials. Plast Reconstr Surg. 2014;133(3):741–55.
3. Apfel CC, et al. Evidence-based analysis of risk factors for postoperative nausea and vomiting. Br J Anaesth. 2012;109(5):742–53.
4. Apfel CC, et al. Volatile anaesthetics may be the main cause of early but not delayed postoperative vomiting:

a randomized controlled trial of factorial design. Br J Anaesth. 2002;88(5):659–68.

5. Apfel CC, et al. A factorial trial of six interventions for the prevention of postoperative nausea and vomiting. N Engl J Med. 2004;350(24):2441–51.

6. Apfel CC, et al. A simplified risk score for predicting postoperative nausea and vomiting: conclusions from cross-validations between two centers. Anesthesiology. 1999;91(3):693–700.

7. Gonullu NN, et al. Prevention of postherniorrhaphy urinary retention with prazosin. Am Surg. 1999;65(1):55–8.

8. Koch CA, Grinberg GG, Farley DR. Incidence and risk factors for urinary retention after endoscopic hernia repair. Am J Surg. 2006;191(3):381–5.

9. Aeberhard P, et al. Prospective audit of laparoscopic totally extraperitoneal inguinal hernia repair: a multicenter study of the Swiss Association for Laparoscopic and Thoracoscopic Surgery (SALTC). Surg Endosc. 1999;13(11):1115–20.

10. Dulucq JL, Wintringer P, Mahajna A. Laparoscopic totally extraperitoneal inguinal hernia repair: lessons learned from 3,100 hernia repairs over 15 years. Surg Endosc. 2009;23(3):482–6.

11. Swadia ND. Laparoscopic totally extra-peritoneal inguinal hernia repair: 9 year's experience. Hernia. 2011;15(3):273–9.

12. Baldini G, et al. Postoperative urinary retention: anesthetic and perioperative considerations. Anesthesiology. 2009;110(5):1139–57.

13. Simons MP, et al. European hernia society guidelines on the treatment of inguinal hernia in adult patients. Hernia. 2009;13(4):343–403.

14. Petros JG, et al. Factors influencing postoperative urinary retention in patients undergoing elective inguinal herniorrhaphy. Am J Surg. 1991;161(4):431–3; discussion 434.

15. Hill MV, et al. Wide variation and excessive dosage of opioid prescriptions for common general surgical procedures. Ann Surg. 2016;

16. Schrenk P, et al. Prospective randomized trial comparing postoperative pain and return to physical activity after transabdominal preperitoneal, total preperitoneal or Shouldice technique for inguinal hernia repair. Br J Surg. 1996;83(11):1563–6.

17. Bay-Nielsen M, et al. Convalescence after inguinal herniorrhaphy. Br J Surg. 2004;91(3):362–7.

18. Bittner R, et al. Update of guidelines on laparoscopic (TAPP) and endoscopic (TEP) treatment of inguinal hernia (international Endohernia Society). Surg Endosc. 2015;29(2):289–321.

19. Hakeem A, Shanmugam V. Inguinodynia following Lichtenstein tension-free hernia repair: a review. World J Gastroenterol. 2011;17(14):1791–6.

20. Bisgaard T, Bay-Nielsen M, Kehlet H. Re-recurrence after operation for recurrent inguinal hernia. A nationwide 8-year follow-up study on the role of type of repair. Ann Surg. 2008;247(4):707–11.

Inguinodynia: Nonoperative Management

14

Janavi Rao and Michael Bottros

Introduction

Persistent postsurgical pain (all cause) has been described by Macrae et al. as pain which persists for more than 2 months after surgery, after other etiologies and pre-existing conditions have been explored and excluded [1]. Others define it as pain which persists for 3–6 months after surgery [2].

The reported incidence of inguinodynia after mesh inguinal hernia surgical repair varies among studies and is estimated to be 11–54% [3, 4] and is responsible for significant morbidity after surgery, affecting the quality of life of patients and limiting their daily activities.

Anatomy (Fig. 14.1)

The nerves involved are the ilioinguinal nerve (IIN), the iliohypogastric nerve (IHN), the genital branch of the genitofemoral nerve (GFN), and, rarely, the lateral femoral cutaneous nerve (LFN) [4, 5]. The ilioinguinal nerve arises from the anterior ramus of L1. It accompanies the spermatic cord through the superficial inguinal ring and provides sensation to the skin in the upper medial part of the thigh, the root of the penis, the superior portion of the scrotum (referred to as the anterior scrotal nerve) in males, and the skin covering the mons pubis and labia majora in females. It does not pass through the deep inguinal ring.

The iliohypogastric nerve also arises from the anterior ramus of L1 and has two branches:

- The lateral cutaneous branch (iliac branch) pierces the internal and external oblique muscles just above the iliac crest and provides sensation to the skin of the gluteal region. It is prone to damage during bone harvesting for spinal fusion operations and is unlikely to be damaged during hernia repair.
- The anterior cutaneous branch (hypogastric branch) runs through the internal oblique and then pierces the aponeurosis of the external oblique muscle to become superficial about 2.5 cm above the superficial inguinal ring. It does not pass through the inguinal canal. It provides sensation to the skin of the lower part of the abdomen overlying the rectus abdominis (hypogastric region) as well as the pubic region.

The genitofemoral nerve originates from L1 to L2 nerve roots. The genital branch enters the deep inguinal ring and enters the inguinal canal. It provides sensation to the majority of the skin of the scrotum and also supplies the cremaster muscle in men. In women, it innervates the labia majora and mons pubis along with the ilioinguinal nerve. The femoral branch passes deep to the

J. Rao · M. Bottros (✉)
Department of Anesthesiology, Washington
University School of Medicine, St. Louis, MO, USA
e-mail: bottrosm@anest.wustl.edu

© Springer International Publishing AG, part of Springer Nature 2018
M. P. LaPinska, J. A. Blatnik (eds.), *Surgical Principles in Inguinal Hernia Repair*,
https://doi.org/10.1007/978-3-319-92892-0_14

Fig. 14.1 Landmarks for the different nerve blocks: ilioinguinal, iliohypogastric, and genital branch of genitofemoral nerves. (From: Medscape-Testicle and epididymis anesthesia- Meda Raghavendra (Raghu), MD; Chief Editor: Alex Macario, MD, MBA)

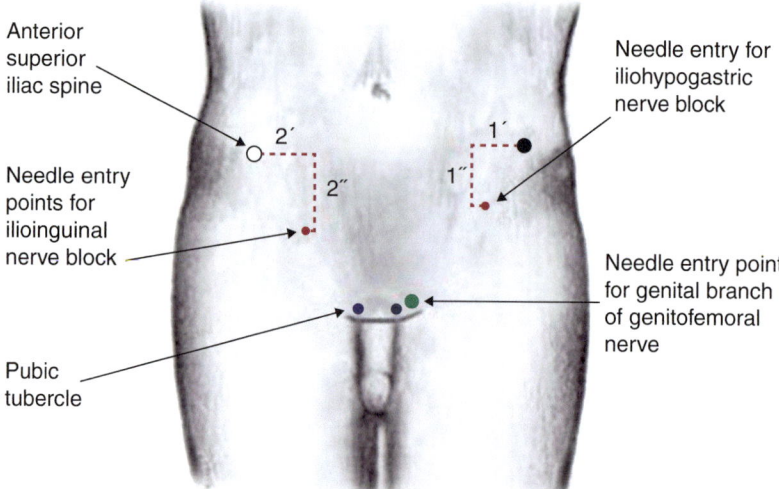

inguinal ligament and then enters the femoral canal. Hence, it is unlikely to be damaged during inguinal hernia repair. It supplies the skin of the superomedial portion of the thigh. Together, the two branches are responsible for the cremasteric reflex – stroking of the superomedial portion of the thigh (femoral branch – sensory) causing contraction of the cremasteric muscle resulting in upward movement of the scrotal sac (genital branch – motor).

The lateral femoral cutaneous nerve arises from the dorsal horns of L2 to L3. It passes under the inguinal ligament and into the lateral compartment of the thigh to run over the sartorius muscle. It divides into anterior and posterior branches in the thigh. The anterior branch becomes cutaneous about 10 cm below the inguinal ligament and supplies the skin over the lateral and anterior thigh, up to the knee. The posterior branch pierces the fascia lata and supplies the skin from the greater trochanter to the middle of the thigh. Entrapment of this nerve is called meralgia paresthetica.

Etiology and Pathophysiology

Damage to the abovementioned nerves can occur intraoperatively or postoperatively. Intraoperative damage occurs by stretching, crushing, cautery, tacking sutures, staples, or direct transection.

Postoperatively, the nerves can get entrapped in a "meshoma," or they can be damaged by excessive fibrosis or granuloma formation [4]. Inguinodynia is classified into neuropathic vs nociceptive types.

A. *Neuropathic pain*

Neuropathic pain is either due to direct damage to the nerves or inflammation adjacent to the nerves (e.g., granuloma formation). Mechanisms for direct damage include complete or partial transection, crush injury, injury from electrocauterization, stretching during retraction, entrapment in suture material, or mesh tacks.

Based on the location of the nerves around the inguinal ring – the ilioinguinal nerve being lateral and the genital branch being medial to the ring – these nerves can be damaged by handling during surgery. The iliohypogastric nerve is most vulnerable to damage caused by staples or tacks placed during laparoscopic repair [6].

Once a peripheral nerve is damaged, the main mechanisms that lead to the development of neuropathic pain are:

(i) Ectopic activity: Stimulus-independent paresthesias are likely due to hyperexcitability of the afferent neurons. Increased action potentials in voltage-gated sodium (e.g., Nav1.3, Nav1.6, and

Nav1.9) channels, voltage-gated potassium (e.g., KCNQ Kv7) channels, and hyperpolarization-activated cyclic nucleotide-gated (e.g., HCN2) channels are responsible for stimulus-independent paresthesias [7].

(ii) Central sensitization: Peripheral nerve damage triggers central neuroplastic changes leading to neuronal hyperexcitability and increased efficacy – this is termed central sensitization [8]. The typical symptoms arising from central sensitization include allodynia (perceived pain from non-painful stimulus), hyperalgesia (exaggerated response to painful stimulus), exaggerated temporal summation (repeated stimuli causing increasing pain), and secondary hyperalgesia (perception of pain beyond the dermatome of the damaged nerve) [8]. Mechanisms responsible for this include increased N-methyl-D-aspartate (NMDA) activity as well as increased production of neuropeptides, namely, calcitonin gene-related peptide and substance P [9]. Other mechanisms include post-injury activation and modification of glial cells, also termed "gliopathy." This occurs by release of glial cytokines and growth factors, phosphorylation of mitogen-activated protein kinase, and chemokine receptor upregulation. There is also hypertrophy and proliferation of glial networks [10].

Impaired central inhibitory modulation from post-injury apoptosis of GABAergic inhibitory neurons may also contribute to the hypersensitivity experienced after nerve injury [11].

(iii) Peripheral sensitization: This is the main mechanism for inflammatory mediated pain; however it plays an important role in neuropathic pain. Changes in transient receptor potential TRPV1 ion channel have led to the development of the TRPV1 agonist, capsaicin, used topically in various concentrations to treat neuropathic pain [12].

B. *Nociceptive pain*

Nociceptive pain is further subdivided into the following:

(i) Inflammatory nociceptive pain: Due to mesh-related inflammation and subsequent excessive fibrosis or "meshoma" [13]. Inflammatory mediators like fibrinogen, C-reactive protein, alpha-1-antitrypsin, and interleukin-6 have been shown to be increased in patients who have a Lichtenstein mesh hernioplasty compared to the conventional Bassini (no mesh) repair [14]. Lightweight mesh causes considerably less chronic groin pain compared to heavyweight mesh. The lightweight mesh is more elastic and causes less of an inflammatory response, thus reducing foreign body sensation and stiffness [15]. A "meshoma" is a radiological entity where the mesh rolls up into a ball due to inadequate fixation or insufficient room for the mesh due to inadequate dissection [16].

(ii) Somatic nociceptive pain: Periostitis pubis is an important entity which occurs due to anchoring of the mesh to the pubic tubercle [4].

(iii) Visceral nociceptive pain occurs when there is intestinal (residual or recurrent hernias) or spermatic cord involvement within the mesh. Funiculodynia (pain related to the spermatic cord) can be due to strictures in the spermatic duct, twisting of the spermatic cord, venous congestion, disturbance in the coordination of ejaculatory muscles, or encasement of the spermatic cord within scar tissue [4, 17] (Table 14.1).

Risk Factors

A. *Preoperative risk factors*: Numerous studies have shown that young age, female gender, the presence of preoperative inguinal pain [18–21], lower preoperative optimism [22], as well as patients having repeat surgery for recurrent hernia [21] or having a history of

Table 14.1 Classification of inguinodynia

Etiology	Percentage
A. Neuropathic causes	46.5
Inguinal nerves	45.8
Meralgia paresthetica	0.6
B. Non-neuropathic causes	25.8
Periostitis pubis	11.6
Recurrent inguinal hernia	8.4
Referred lumbosacral pain	1.9
Urological problems	1.3
Femoral hernia	0.6
Iliopectineal bursitis	0.6
Adductor tendinitis	0.6
Hip osteoarthritis	0.6
C. Tender spermatic cord/tight feeling	27.7

Adapted from: Loos et al. [17].

Table 14.2 Risk factors for chronic postherniorrhaphy inguinodynia

Preoperative factors
  (a) Young age
  (b) Female sex
  (c) High preoperative pain score
  (d) Lower preoperative optimism
  (e) Impairment of daily activities
  (f) Recurrent hernia surgery
  (g) Genetic predisposition (*DQBI*03:02 HLA* haplotype)
Perioperative factors
  (a) Less experienced surgeon
  (b) Open repair technique
  (c) Heavyweight mesh
  (d) Mesh fixation: Suture (open), staple (laparoscopic)
  (e) Ilioinguinal nerve neurolysis in Lichtenstein repair
Postoperative factors
  (a) Postoperative complications: Hematoma, infection
  (b) High early postoperative pain score
  (c) Lower perceived pain control
  (d) Sensory dysfunction in the groin

Adapted from: Bjurstrom et al. [6]

chronic pain in other areas [23] are predisposed to the development of chronic postherniorrhaphy inguinal pain. Psychosocial factors like depression, psychological vulnerability, stress, and duration of disability are good predictors of all-cause persistent postsurgical pain [24] and can likely be extrapolated to chronic postherniorrhaphy pain; however, specific studies regarding psychosocial factors in the development of chronic postherniorrhaphy pain are lacking.

B. *Operative risk factors:* Hernia repairs performed by inexperienced surgeons or outside of a dedicated hernia facility put patients at an increased risk of developing chronic pain [21]. Intraoperative factors include open hernia repair vs laparoscopic repair [20, 21], use of mesh, in particular, heavyweight mesh [15] and fixation of mesh (by suture in open repair and staples in laparoscopic repair) [25–27].

C. *Postoperative risk factors:* Postoperative complications like hematoma and infection [20] as well as higher early postoperative pain intensity [21] and lower perceived pain control at 1 week [22] are implicated in the development of chronic inguinal pain (Table 14.2).

Symptoms

The location of pain depends on which nerve is affected; however, due to overlapping sensory areas covered by the three nerves as well as

mesh-related fibrosis and scarring, the diagnosis is often challenging [5, 28].The pain may radiate to the scrotum, upper leg, or back.

Symptoms of pain include hyperesthesia (heightened response to painful stimulus), hypoesthesia (partial loss of sensation to sensory stimulation), paresthesia (tingling or burning with lack of a specific stimulation), or allodynia (painful response to non-painful stimulation).

Depending on whether the pain is neuropathic or non-neuropathic, the symptomatology may differ. Neuropathic pain is typically described as episodic sharp, shooting, or burning pain, worse with activity/changes in position, having a specific trigger point [29]. Non-neuropathic pain is typically a diffuse dull ache over the groin lacking a specific trigger point described as gnawing, pulling, or pounding sensation [13].

The ilioinguinal nerve is the likely etiology if the pain is mainly in the upper medial part of the thigh and the root of the penis radiating to the superior portion of the scrotum. Pain in the lower part of the abdomen overlying the rectus abdominis muscle is likely due to involvement of the iliohypogastric nerve. Pain localized scrotum is often attributed to the genital branch of the genitofemoral nerve. If the pain is localized to the lateral thigh, then the lateral femoral cutaneous nerve is the likely offender.

Patients with periostitis pubis complain of tenderness over the pubic symphysis [17].

Other symptoms include pain at the pubic tubercle, ejaculatory pain, labial pain, numbness over the thigh, sexual dysfunction, mood swings, reduction in activity tolerance, and depression.

Diagnosis

An individualized approach including a sound history and physical examination with good knowledge of the anatomy of the inguinal region is essential to tease out which nerve is the root cause of inguinodynia.

Due to overlapping sensory areas covered by the three nerves, nerve regeneration after injury, and intertwining of nerve endings in addition to mesh-related fibrosis and scarring, the diagnosis is often challenging, and the region of pain is not clearly demarcated unlike if normal nerve anatomy persisted [5, 28].

Tinel's test (tapping the skin medial to the anterosuperior iliac spine or over an area of local tenderness with reproduction of pain) may aid in the diagnosis [5].

In the case of neuropathic pain, diagnostic nerve blocks can be helpful in determining which nerves are involved. However, evidence is controversial. The presence of a mesh along with postsurgical fibrosis distorts the anatomy and local anesthetic medications injected, while performing these blocks may not be able to spread along the injected nerve, thus confusing the picture.

For non-neuropathic pain, imaging modalities like CT scan or MRI will highlight pathologies like granulomas, neuromas, mesh-related pathologies, or recurrent hernias [30]. Ultrasonography is usually the first test to be performed to detect occult hernias [31]. MRI is considered to be the most validated diagnostic tool for detecting hernias [32]; however in patients with persistent postherniorrhaphy pain, interpretation is radiologist dependent. Findings like "contrast enhance-

ment in groin," "edema," and "spermatic cord caliber increased" were consistently seen more often in patients with persistent pain compared to those who were pain-free [33].

Nonsurgical Treatment Options

Persistent postherniorrhaphy pain is difficult to treat due to multiple factors like vague symptoms, difficulty in correctly identifying the nerves involved, central sensitization of pain, and psychological comorbidities. A multimodal, multidisciplinary treatment approach is prudent to obtain maximal benefit from the available treatment options.

A. *Non-pharmacological modalities*

Postherniorrhaphy pain is typically exacerbated on bending, walking, and lifting. Lifestyle changes to avoid these exacerbating factors make patients sedentary and adversely affect quality of life; hence most clinicians do not advocate this as a treatment option [19]; in fact, it is important to avoid harmful inactivity [6].

Physiotherapy, acupuncture, massages, and stretching can be helpful in temporarily abating the pain, but as the sole treatment option, they do not cure or prevent the recurrence of pain [29]. Physiotherapy, in particular, is important in collaboration with other treatment modalities.

Transcutaneous electrical nerve stimulation (TENS) works via the gate control theory where cortical transmission of a nociceptive stimulus is blocked by a non-nociceptive stimulus, which in the case of TENS is an electrical stimulation to the skin. There is evidence supporting the efficacy of TENS in the acute postoperative period following hernia repair [34]; however, no studies have been performed in patients with chronic inguinal pain.

Given the psychosocial aspect of chronic pain, it is prudent to ensure treatment of other associated conditions like depression, anxiety, and/or substance abuse. Prompt referral to a psychologist, psychiatrist, or tertiary care pain management clinic is important to assess and treat these coexisting conditions [35].

B. *Pharmacological modalities* (Table 14.3)
Neuropathic pain is challenging to treat. The International Association for the Study of Pain (IASP) guidelines are based on studies conducted on postherpetic neuralgia and diabetic neuropathy. There have been no well-conducted trials for medication management in patients with inguinodynia, and in our practice, we

Table 14.3 Mechanisms of action and dosing of the first-line drugs and opioids for neuropathic pain

Medication	Mechanism of action	Starting dose	Titration	Maximum recommended dose	Major adverse effects	Contraindications
TCAs						
Nortriptyline and desipramine	Serotonin and noradrenalin reuptake inhibition, sodium channel block, N-methyl-D-aspartate receptor antagonist	10–25 mg at bedtime	Increase by 10–25 mg every 3–7 d as tolerated	150 mg/d; further titration guided by blood concentration of the drug and its active metabolite	Cardiac conduction block, sedation, confusion anticholinergic effects (dry mouth, constipation urinary retention, blurred vision), orthostatic hypotension, weight gain	Recovery phase after myocardial infarction, arrhythmias (particularly heart block) concomitant use of MAO inhibitors, porphyria
SNRIs						
Duloxetine	Serotonin and noradrenalin reuptake inhibition	30 mg once daily	Increase to 60 mg once daily after 1 week	120 mg/d	Nausea, loss of appetite constipation, sedation, dry mouth, hyperhidrosis, anxiety	Concomitant use of MAO inhibitors; uncontrolled hypertension
Venlafaxine		37.5 mg once or twice daily	Increase by 75 mg each week	225 mg/d		
Gabapentinoids						
Gabapentin	Calcium channel alpha-2-delta ligand which reduces release of presynaptic transmitters	100–300 mg at bedtime	Increase by 100–300 mg 3 times daily every 1–7 d as tolerated	3600 mg/d (divided into 3 doses)	Sedation, dizziness, weight gain, edema, blurred vision	None
Pregabalin		75 mg twice daily	Increase to 300 mg/d after 3–7 d, then by 150 mg/d every 3–7 d as tolerated	600 mg/d (divided into 2–3 doses)		
Topical lidocaine (5% lidocaine patch)	Block of peripheral sodium channels and thus of ectopic discharges	Maximum 3 patches daily for a maximum of 12 h	None	Maximum 3 patches daily for a maximum of 12 h	Local erythema, rash; no systemic adverse effect	Known history of sensitivity to amide local anesthetics

Legend: *TCA* tricyclic antidepressant, *SNRI* selective noradrenergic reuptake inhibitor
From: Haanpaa et al. [55]

extrapolate the IASP guidelines for neuropathic pain to chronic postherniorrhaphy pain.

(i) Antidepressants: Antidepressants reduce pain in patients with and without depression, suggesting a separate mechanism of action for analgesia-increased supraspinal availability of norepinephrine leading to an enhancement of descending inhibitory bulbospinal control, activation of endogenous opioid receptors, sodium channel blockade, and NMDA receptor inhibition [36]. The analgesic doses of antidepressants are lower than the antidepressant doses. The classes of antidepressants are:

    (a) Tricyclic antidepressants (TCAs)

    (b) Selective serotonin reuptake inhibitors (SSRIs)

    (c) Serotonin-norepinephrine reuptake inhibitors (SNRIs)

(ii) Anticonvulsants: Gabapentin and pregabalin are alpha-2-delta calcium channel blockers which were first developed to treat seizures but have been found more effective in treating neuropathic pain and are recommended as first-line agents.

(iii) Topical agents:

    (a) Lidocaine patches: These are generally safe and well tolerated and have low systemic absorption.

    (b) Capsaicin cream: Capsaicin is an agonist of the transient receptor potential vanilloid receptor (TRPV1) and activates TRPV1 ligand-gated channels on nociceptive fibers which then depolarizes, generates an action potential, and transmits pain signals to the spinal cord. Application of capsaicin cream for several days leads to desensitization of the TRPV1 receptor and reduced transmission of pain signals [37].

(iv) Opioid medications: These are often prescribed; however they have limited benefit, and patients are prone to developing tolerance, requiring dose escalation with inadequate pain relief.

(v) Botulinum toxin A: Botox is a potent neurotoxin used for the treatment of focal muscle hyperactivity but has been shown to be effective in treating neuropathic pain independent of muscle relaxation. This is likely due to its ability to reduce neurogenic inflammation and inhibit neurotransmitter release from sensory neurons thus reducing peripheral sensitization indirectly leading a reduction in central sensitization [38]. The drug has an excellent safety profile with no systemic side effects and mild discomfort during injection.

Nociceptive pain can be treated with anti-inflammatory drugs, the first line being NSAIDS. Short courses of oral steroids have been tried, but evidence on the efficacy are inconclusive.

Unfortunately, medications alone are seldom adequate and recurrences common. Most patients require further interventions.

C. *Interventional pain management*

(i) Ultrasound/fluoroscopy-guided nerve blocks:

Nerve blocks of the IIN, IHN, and/or GFN serve both diagnostic and therapeutic purposes. Historically, these nerve blocks were performed using anatomic landmarks to guide needle placement. Prior to the advancement in ultrasound technology, these nerve blocks were performed with nerve stimulator guidance. With the development of ultrasound technology and its use in regional anesthesia, these nerve blocks are now performed successfully under direct visualization, which reduces the risk of intraperitoneal injection, nerve damage, and allows for a smaller volume of injectate due to improved accuracy [6]. A study by Thomassen et al. showed that for a median follow-up time of 21 months, 55% of patients no longer reported neuropathic pain, and 32% of patients no longer reported moderate to severe neuropathic pain. A combination of a local anesthetic solution and a corticosteroid is used for these nerve blocks [39] (Figs. 14.2 and 14.3).

(ii) Neuroablation:

If nerve blocks provide significant temporary analgesia but not long-term

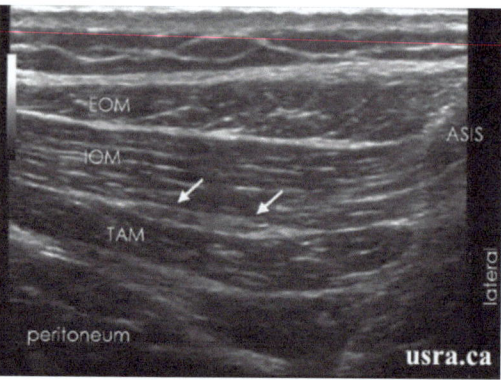

Fig. 14.2 Ultrasound image of ilioinguinal and iliohypogastric nerves. Arrows ilioinguinal/iliohypogastric nerves, ASIS anterior superior iliac spine, EOM external oblique muscle, IOM internal oblique muscle, TAM transverse abdominis muscle. (From: usra.ca)

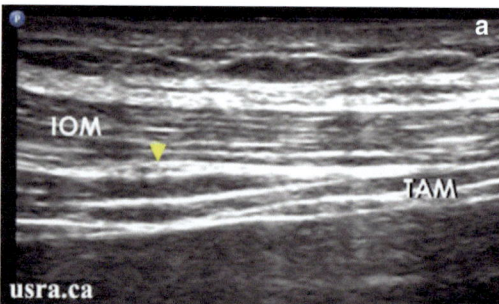

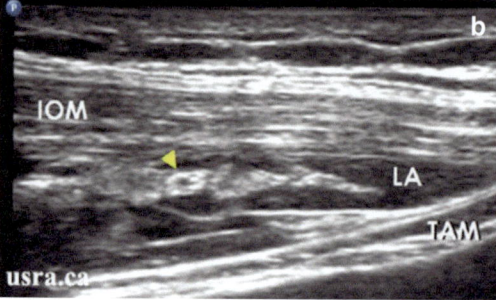

Fig. 14.3 Ultrasound images of the ilioinguinal and iliohypogastric nerves. (**a**) Shows hypoechoic nerves within the plane between the internal oblique muscle (IOM) and the transverse abdominis muscle (TAM). (**b**) Shows the II/IH nerves completely surrounded by local anesthetic (LA). IOM internal oblique muscle, TAM transverse abdominis muscle. (From: usra.ca)

relief, neuroablative techniques such as chemical neurolysis, cryoablation, and pulsed radiofrequency (PRF) may be considered for longer-lasting pain relief. Studies using chemical neurolysis with phenol [40] and cryoablation [41, 42] are few, and sample sizes are small; however there are multiple case studies for PRF at T12, L1, and L2 nerve roots [43, 44] as well as directly to the affected nerves in the groin [45, 46].

A systematic review published by Werner et al. found both neuraxial and peripheral PRF techniques gave 63–100% relief [n = 8] in a 3–9-month follow-up period. They conclude that the evidence base is fairly limited and suggests improved research into this modality [47].

PRF delivers high-intensity currents in pulses, allowing heat (typically 42 °C) to dissipate, thus preventing neurodestructive temperatures from being attained, which lowers the risk of complications like neuroma formation, neuritis-type reaction, and deafferentation pain. The mechanism of action for analgesia is thought to be temporary inhibition of nerve conduction; however, the exact mechanism is unclear [6].

(iii) Neuromodulation:

Neuromodulation techniques such as peripheral nerve field stimulation or spinal cord stimulation may be considered for use in a select group of patients with intractable groin pain who are refractory to conventional methods including pharmacological, interventional, and even surgical treatment options. Case reports for peripheral nerve stimulators [48–50], spinal cord stimulators [51, 52], nerve root simulators [53], as well as combined spinal-peripheral neurostimulators [54] have shown to provide significant relief from pain. These implantable devices provide pain relief by producing gentle paresthesias in the concordant areas of pain. The success rate of these techniques is improved by a rigorous screening process, psychiatric clearance, documentation of conventional treatment failure, and a stimulator trial of 3–7 days [48].

Conclusion

Chronic postherniorrhaphy pain is a significant burden on society, and prevention by meticulous hernia repair is essential to reduce this burden. Preoperative identification of patients who are likely to suffer from chronic pain is possible by identifying risk factors. A detailed history and targeted physical examination is required to identify the cause of pain, and diagnostic tests like CT scan or MRI can help rule out treatable causes of pain. Once the diagnosis of chronic postherniorrhaphy pain has been made, a multimodal, multidisciplinary approach to treatment is necessary. Referral to a dedicated pain management facility may be warranted. Identification and treatment of comorbidities is important in the management of all types of chronic pain. Patients should be pharmacologically optimized with antidepressants, antiepileptics, NSAIDs, and topical medications. Patients who have pain in classical nerve distributions should undergo diagnostic and potentially therapeutic nerve blocks. Neuroablation and neuromodulation are promising techniques that may help avoid repeat surgery.

References

1. Crombie IK, Davies HT, Macrae WA. Cut and thrust: antecedent surgery and trauma among patients attending a chronic pain clinic. Pain. 1998;76(1–2):167–71.
2. Kehlet H, Jensen TS, Woolf CJ. Persistent postsurgical pain: risk factors and prevention. Lancet. 2006;367(9522):1618–25.
3. Nienhuijs S, et al. Chronic pain after mesh repair of inguinal hernia: a systematic review. Am J Surg. 2007;194(3):394–400.
4. Poobalan AS, et al. A review of chronic pain after inguinal herniorrhaphy. Clin J Pain. 2003;19(1):48–54.
5. Hakeem A, Shanmugam V. Current trends in the diagnosis and management of post-herniorraphy chronic groin pain. World J Gastrointest Surg. 2011;3(6):73–81.

6. Bjurstrom MF, et al. Pain control following inguinal herniorrhaphy: current perspectives. J Pain Res. 2014;7:277–90.
7. Chaplan SR, et al. Neuronal hyperpolarization-activated pacemaker channels drive neuropathic pain. J Neurosci. 2003;23(4):1169–78.
8. Woolf CJ. Central sensitization: implications for the diagnosis and treatment of pain. Pain. 2011;152(3 Suppl):S2–15.
9. Nitzan-Luques A, Devor M, Tal M. Genotype-selective phenotypic switch in primary afferent neurons contributes to neuropathic pain. Pain. 2011;152(10):2413–26.
10. Ji RR, Berta T, Nedergaard M. Glia and pain: is chronic pain a gliopathy? Pain. 2013;154(Suppl 1):S10–28.
11. Scholz J, et al. Blocking caspase activity prevents transsynaptic neuronal apoptosis and the loss of inhibition in lamina II of the dorsal horn after peripheral nerve injury. J Neurosci. 2005;25(32):7317–23.
12. Simpson DM, et al. Controlled trial of high-concentration capsaicin patch for treatment of painful HIV neuropathy. Neurology. 2008;70(24):2305–13.
13. Heise CP, Starling JR. Mesh inguinodynia: a new clinical syndrome after inguinal herniorrhaphy? J Am Coll Surg. 1998;187(5):514–8.
14. Di Vita G, et al. Tension-free hernia repair is associated with an increase in inflammatory response markers against the mesh. Am J Surg. 2000;180(3):203–7.
15. Sajid MS, et al. A systematic review and meta-analysis evaluating the effectiveness of lightweight mesh against heavyweight mesh in influencing the incidence of chronic groin pain following laparoscopic inguinal hernia repair. Am J Surg. 2013;205(6):726–36.
16. Amid PK, Hiatt JR. New understanding of the causes and surgical treatment of postherniorrhaphy inguinodynia and orchalgia. J Am Coll Surg. 2007;205(2):381–5.
17. Loos MJ, Roumen RM, Scheltinga MR. Classifying post-herniorrhaphy pain syndromes following elective inguinal hernia repair. World J Surg. 2007;31(9):1760–5. discussion 1766-7
18. Bay-Nielsen M, et al. Pain and functional impairment 1 year after inguinal herniorrhaphy: a nationwide questionnaire study. Ann Surg. 2001;233(1):1–7.
19. Courtney CA, et al. Outcome of patients with severe chronic pain following repair of groin hernia. Br J Surg. 2002;89(10):1310–4.
20. Franneby U, et al. Risk factors for long-term pain after hernia surgery. Ann Surg. 2006;244(2):212–9.
21. Aasvang E, Kehlet H. Chronic postoperative pain: the case of inguinal herniorrhaphy. Br J Anaesth. 2005;95(1):69–76.
22. Powell R, et al. Psychological risk factors for chronic post-surgical pain after inguinal hernia repair surgery: a prospective cohort study. Eur J Pain. 2012;16(4):600–10.
23. Dennis R, O'Riordan D. Risk factors for chronic pain after inguinal hernia repair. Ann R Coll Surg Engl. 2007;89(3):218–20.

24. Hinrichs-Rocker A, et al. Psychosocial predictors and correlates for chronic post-surgical pain (CPSP) - a systematic review. Eur J Pain. 2009;13(7):719–30.

25. de Goede B, et al. Meta-analysis of glue versus sutured mesh fixation for Lichtenstein inguinal hernia repair. Br J Surg. 2013;100(6):735–42.

26. Colvin HS, et al. Glue versus suture fixation of mesh during open repair of inguinal hernias: a systematic review and meta-analysis. World J Surg. 2013;37(10):2282–92.

27. Kaul A, et al. Staple versus fibrin glue fixation in laparoscopic total extraperitoneal repair of inguinal hernia: a systematic review and meta-analysis. Surg Endosc. 2012;26(5):1269–78.

28. Rab M, Ebmer J, Dellon AL. Anatomic variability of the ilioinguinal and genitofemoral nerve: implications for the treatment of groin pain. Plast Reconstr Surg. 2001;108(6):1618–23.

29. Vuilleumier H, Hubner M, Demartines N. Neuropathy after herniorrhaphy: indication for surgical treatment and outcome. World J Surg. 2009;33(4):841–5.

30. Amid PK. Radiologic images of meshoma: a new phenomenon causing chronic pain after prosthetic repair of abdominal wall hernias. Arch Surg. 2004;139(12):1297–8.

31. Bradley M, et al. The groin hernia - an ultrasound diagnosis? Ann R Coll Surg Engl. 2003;85(3):178–80.

32. van den Berg JC, et al. Detection of groin hernia with physical examination, ultrasound, and MRI compared with laparoscopic findings. Investig Radiol. 1999;34(12):739–43.

33. Aasvang EK, et al. MRI and pathology in persistent postherniotomy pain. J Am Coll Surg. 2009;208(6):1023–8; discussion 1028–9

34. DeSantana JM, et al. Hypoalgesic effect of the transcutaneous electrical nerve stimulation following inguinal herniorrhaphy: a randomized, controlled trial. J Pain. 2008;9(7):623–9.

35. Gilron I, Baron R, Jensen T. Neuropathic pain: principles of diagnosis and treatment. Mayo Clin Proc. 2015;90(4):532–45.

36. Mico JA, et al. Antidepressants and pain. Trends Pharmacol Sci. 2006;27(7):348–54.

37. Wong GY, Gavva NR. Therapeutic potential of vanilloid receptor TRPV1 agonists and antagonists as analgesics: recent advances and setbacks. Brain Res Rev. 2009;60(1):267–77.

38. Aoki KR. Review of a proposed mechanism for the antinociceptive action of botulinum toxin type A. Neurotoxicology. 2005;26(5):785–93.

39. Thomassen I, et al. Ultrasound-guided ilioinguinal/ iliohypogastric nerve blocks for chronic pain after inguinal hernia repair. Hernia. 2013;17(3):329–32.

40. Parris D, et al. A novel CT-guided transpsoas approach to diagnostic genitofemoral nerve block and ablation. Pain Med. 2010;11(5):785–9.

41. Fanelli RD, et al. Cryoanalgesic ablation for the treatment of chronic postherniorrhaphy neuropathic pain. Surg Endosc. 2003;17(2):196–200.

42. Campos NA, Chiles JH, Plunkett AR. Ultrasound-guided cryoablation of genitofemoral nerve for chronic inguinal pain. Pain Physician. 2009;12(6):997–1000.

43. Rozen D, Ahn J. Pulsed radiofrequency for the treatment of ilioinguinal neuralgia after inguinal herniorrhaphy. Mt Sinai J Med. 2006;73(4):716–8.

44. Rozen D, Parvez U. Pulsed radiofrequency of lumbar nerve roots for treatment of chronic inguinal herniorrhaphy pain. Pain Physician. 2006;9(2):153–6.

45. Mitra R, Zeighami A, Mackey S. Pulsed radiofrequency for the treatment of chronic ilioinguinal neuropathy. Hernia. 2007;11(4):369–71.

46. Cohen SP, Foster A. Pulsed radiofrequency as a treatment for groin pain and orchialgia. Urology. 2003;61(3):645.

47. Werner MU, et al. Pulsed radiofrequency in the treatment of persistent pain after inguinal herniotomy: a systematic review. Reg Anesth Pain Med. 2012;37(3):340–3.

48. Banh DP, et al. Permanent implantation of peripheral nerve stimulator for combat injury-related ilioinguinal neuralgia. Pain Physician. 2013;16(6):E789–91.

49. Rosendal F, et al. Successful treatment of testicular pain with peripheral nerve stimulation of the cutaneous branch of the ilioinguinal and genital branch of the genitofemoral nerves. Neuromodulation. 2013;16(2):121–4.

50. Carayannopoulos A, Beasley R, Sites B. Facilitation of percutaneous trial lead placement with ultrasound guidance for peripheral nerve stimulation trial of ilioinguinal neuralgia: a technical note. Neuromodulation. 2009;12(4):296–301.

51. Elias M. Spinal cord stimulation for post-herniorrhaphy pain. Neuromodulation. 2000; 3(3):155–7.

52. Yakovlev AE, et al. Spinal cord stimulation as alternative treatment for chronic post-herniorrhaphy pain. Neuromodulation. 2010;13(4):288–90; discussion 291

53. Alo KM, et al. Lumbar and sacral nerve root stimulation (NRS) in the treatment of chronic pain: a novel anatomic approach and neuro stimulation technique. Neuromodulation. 1999;2(1):23–31.

54. Mironer YE, Monroe TR. Spinal-peripheral neurostimulation (SPN) for bilateral postherniorrhaphy pain: a case report. Neuromodulation. 2013;16(6):603–6.

55. Haanpaa ML, et al. Treatment considerations for patients with neuropathic pain and other medical comorbidities. Mayo Clin Proc. 2010;85(3 Suppl):S15–25.

Operative Management of Inguinodynia

15

Michael W. Robinson and David C. Chen

Introduction

Inguinodynia following inguinal hernia repair is unfortunately a significant cause of postoperative morbidity and arguably the most important patient-centered clinical outcome affecting patient satisfaction, physical activity, productivity, employment, and quality of life. Throughout the last few decades, techniques for hernia repair have advanced, resulting in lower recurrence rates. However, chronic postherniorrhaphy inguinal pain remains an infrequent but significant condition. The rate of chronic pain after hernia repair varies according to the literature and the definition used to identify this condition but has been reported as high as 60% [1]. The Swedish Hernia Registry reports severe postherniorrhaphy pain between 5% and 7% with a subset of these patients experiencing debilitating complications [2].

The majority of patients with postoperative inguinodynia experience improvement of their symptoms with time, requiring only expectant management and conservative measures. Postoperative pain, however, should not be ignored as chronic pain develops from persistence of acute pain, and longer durations may lead to centralization which may not be fixable. Initial management should include analgesics, rest, and diagnostic evaluation to rule out recurrence or other remediable causes. Neuropathic pain may respond to neuropathic medications such as gabapentin or pregabalin as well as atypical antidepressants. Physical therapy, cognitive behavioral therapy, acupuncture, and biofeedback are all useful adjuncts to manage chronic pain. Chronic pain specialists and a multidisciplinary approach are helpful to manage complex patients that are refractory to standard therapy. Interventions such as nerve blocks and trigger point injections with a local anesthetic with or without steroids may serve a diagnostic and therapeutic role helping to delineate neuropathic pain.

Operative management of postherniorrhaphy chronic pain should be considered in patients refractory to conservative treatment with potentially remediable causes of pain: recurrence, neuropathic pain, "meshoma," foreign body sensation, and orchialgia. In order to pursue operative treatment, one must have a full understanding of many potential contributing factors, which include but are not limited to groin neuroanatomy, likely causative mechanisms of pain, onset and timing of symptoms, prior operations, character and intensity of pain, and the response to interventions and nerve blocks [3, 4].

The diagnostic evaluation must also discriminate specific types of pain including nociceptive, neuropathic, somatic, and visceral pain. Nociceptive pain is a result of tissue injury and

M. W. Robinson · D. C. Chen (✉)
Lichtenstein Amid Hernia Clinic, David Geffen
School of Medicine at UCLA,
Los Angeles, CA, USA
e-mail: dcchen@mednet.ucla.edu

© Springer International Publishing AG, part of Springer Nature 2018
M. P. LaPinska, J. A. Blatnik (eds.), *Surgical Principles in Inguinal Hernia Repair*,
https://doi.org/10.1007/978-3-319-92892-0_15

inflammation and is typically characterized as deep, aching, squeezing, stabbing, or throbbing. This type of pain may also be directly related to the implantation of mesh. Wrinkling, folding, contraction, and mesh scarring can progress to "meshoma" pain or foreign body sensation, and excision may benefit the patient [4]. Neuropathic pain is generally related to direct nerve injury, entrapment, or perineural scarring causing symptoms of hyperalgesia, paresthesia, hyperesthesia, hypoesthesia, and/or allodynia [5]. This pain generally radiates down to the scrotum or to the femoral triangle and follows the dermatomal distributions corresponding to the course of these nerves. There is considerable neuroanatomic variation, cross-innervation, and dermatomal overlap between the inguinal nerves making selective neurectomy of the exact involved nerve(s) a challenge. As simple as the etiology of post-inguinal hernia pain seems, the diagnosis and treatment are both complex, due to the multifactorial aspect that affects the patient's subjective experience of pain (i.e., social, psychological, genetic) and the overlapping types of pain.

In consideration of timing and patient selection for operative management of chronic post-inguinal hernia repair pain, failure of conservative measures, in of itself, is not an indication for further surgery. Successful outcomes are entirely dependent upon choosing patients with correctable causes of inguinodynia. In general, operative intervention of chronic post-inguinal hernia repair pain should be reserved for pain lasting greater than 3 months – the accepted definition for chronic pain. In mesh hernia repairs, this is often extended to 6 months as mesh integration and remodeling continue and the symptoms may still improve with expectant management. The preoperative evaluation must include review of the prior operative report for technique (type of repair, type of mesh used, position of the mesh, method of fixation), imaging to assess for "meshoma" or other anatomic abnormalities, and response to prior interventions.

Hernia recurrence either overt or occult may cause or contribute to pain and should be addressed. Neuropathic pain that developed after the initial operation, follows a definable dermatomal pattern with a reasonable mechanism of injury, improves with neuropathic medications, and responds to nerve blocks, ablation, or ne uromodulation suggests that there are reasonable targets for remedial surgery. "Meshoma" when identified clinically and radiographically may improve with meshectomy to address foreign body sensation and compression or entrapment of inguinal structures. Coexisting orchialgia is a complex problem that may also be neuropathic or nociceptive in origin. Neurectomy of the autonomic nerves investing the vas deferens (paravasal nerves) at the time of remedial surgery may be beneficial.

Anatomy

Experience, familiarity, and mindfulness of the neuroanatomy of the inguinal region are essential to avoid nerve injury and to operatively address neuropathic pain. The distribution and variations of the inguinal nerves must be considered for both anterior and posterior repairs. The inguinal nerves originate from the lumbar plexus in the retroperitoneum and exit through the inguinal canal [6]. In the anterior plane above the transversalis fascia, the ilioinguinal nerve, iliohypogastric nerve, and the genital branch of the genitofemoral nerve pass through the operative field and are susceptible to injury.

In an open transinguinal repair, the ilioinguinal nerve typically enters the canal medial to the anterior superior iliac spine. It then travels parallel to the spermatic cord most often residing on the anterior surface of the cord and exits through the external ring. It is covered by an investing fascia derived as it passes through the transversalis and internal oblique muscle. Unnecessary mobilization or dissection of this layer should be avoided in order to protect the nerve from direct contact and perineural scarring with mesh.

The iliohypogastric nerve typically enters the inguinal canal medial to the ilioinguinal nerve and travels between the internal and external oblique muscle layers of the abdominal wall. The investing fascia similarly protects this nerve from contacting the mesh. The iliohypogastric nerve reliably exits at the cleavage plane between the external and internal oblique at the conjoint tendon. Ten to 15% of patients do not have a visible iliohypogastric nerve in the inguinal canal as it may run a subaponeurotic course below the internal oblique aponeurosis which can lead to potential injury during medial suturing and fixation of mesh. In these cases, identification is performed by opening the anatomic cleavage plane to expose the exit and course of this nerve. There is an additional intramuscular segment of the nerve that lies within the internal oblique muscle cephalad and lateral to its visible entry into the canal. This portion of the nerve may be injured because it is not usually seen during herniorrhaphy. Suturing the internal oblique muscle above the level of the internal ring during open repair can potentially result in nerve injury.

The genital branch of the genitofemoral nerve enters the deep inguinal ring and traverses the inguinal canal within the spermatic cord covered by the deep cremasteric fascia. Its location is most easily identified by its close proximity to the external spermatic vein. The nerve is usually protected from entrapment by the cremasteric fascia, and disruption may result in direct injury or scarring due to exposure and direct contact with mesh.

In a posterior open preperitoneal repair through the inguinal canal, in addition to the anterior nerves, the femoral branch of the genitofemoral nerve and the lateral femoral cutaneous nerve may also be implicated. In a posterior laparoscopic preperitoneal approach, the genital and femoral branches of the genitofemoral nerve and the lateral femoral cutaneous nerve are found in the operative field and must be considered. The genitofemoral trunk exits from the lumbar plexus typically from the nerve roots of L1. The nerve reliably exits the psoas in the retroperitoneum and travels on its anterior surface. As it courses to the preperitoneal plane, its course becomes more variable. It will typically divide into a genital and femoral branch with the genital coursing medial adjacent to the iliac vessels toward the internal ring and the femoral passing lateral under the iliopubic tract toward the anterior thigh. The ilioinguinal and iliohypogastric nerves are not visible in the preperitoneal field but are at risk of injury with penetrating fixation through the transversalis fascia (i.e., suture, tacks) as they traverse the inguinal canal superficial to the operative field. The femoral nerve trunk traverses in the retroperitoneal space posterolateral to the psoas and infrequently may be injured with fixation, energy, thermal injury, or overdissection presenting with motor deficits. Understanding the potential location of sensory and motor nerve injury based upon subjective symptoms, mechanism of prior repair, physical exam findings, somatosensory evaluation with dermatome mapping, and imaging is crucial to successful operative intervention [7].

Surgical Management of Neuropathic Pain

Operative management for chronic pain after inguinal hernia repair refractory to conservative measures requires tailoring based upon an optimal approach to the likely pathology. The goal of remedial surgery is to simultaneously address all likely causes to prevent subsequent risk and difficulty of reoperation while balancing this against the potential morbidity of surgery. In general, selective neurolysis or neurectomy, removal of mesh, or repair/revision of prior herniorrhaphy alone is a less effective strategy for treatment due to overlapping nerve distribution, coexisting causes of pain, and intrinsic disruption of nerves, mesh, and native anatomy with remedial surgery. Neurolysis has limited efficacy and is not recommended considering it does not address the overall structural changes to the inflamed and potentially entrapped nerves. Removal of entrapping sutures or fixating devices while leaving the injured nerves behind will also not necessarily alleviate inguinodynia.

For most anterior inguinal hernia repairs and posterior approaches utilizing fixation, multiple inguinal nerves may be involved or will be placed at risk with reoperation. Triple neurectomy is more effective but results in greater numbness and potential for deafferentation hypersensitivity. Selective neurectomy may be considered when the likely mechanism of injury, prior operation, physical examination, and dermatome mapping isolate to a discrete nerve without likely overlap (i.e., isolated genitofemoral neurectomy after lap repair with no fixation, isolated pain in lateral femoral cutaneous distribution, isolated scrotal pain with plug repair) [8, 9]. In these cases, neurectomy should be tailored to minimize collateral damage from the repair.

Operating in the scarred reoperative field also contributes to the complexity of this operation. Bischoff et al. described their experience with selective neurectomy in 54 patients with chronic pain after open mesh repair. The ilioinguinal, iliohypogastric, and genitofemoral nerves were identified in 40 (74%), 20 (37%), and 13 (24%) patients, respectively, illustrating the challenge of reoperative nerve identification even in experienced hands [10]. In the reoperative field, it is difficult to precisely isolate the inguinal nerves involved, and frequently there is more than one nerve implicated in postherniorrhaphy chronic neuropathic pain.

Triple neurectomy is an accepted surgical treatment for neuropathic pain refractory to conservative measures and, in most cases, is arguably the most effective option [8, 9]. In our experience with over 800 patients using an open approach and over 90 selected cases using a laparoscopic retroperitoneal approach, we are able to achieve an 85% and 90% success rate, respectively [11]. Figures for efficacy rates of these operations should be interpreted in the context of rigorous and experienced patient selection which is by far the most important factor with regard to predicting successful intervention. When combined with "meshoma" excision and removal, open triple neurectomy provides effective relief in a majority of carefully selected patients with refractory neuropathic and nociceptive inguinodynia. Those most likely to benefit from operative neurectomy are those with neuropathic pain that was not present prior to the original operation, that is isolated to the inguinal distribution, and that experienced improvement with therapeutic nerve blocks.

Risks of Surgery

Open triple neurectomy and groin re-exploration is not a benign operation. It does carry risk of complications including novel and ongoing pain, deafferentation hypersensitivity, and anticipated permanent numbness. In female patents, this may include ipsilateral labial numbness and potential associated sexual dysfunction. Risks related to reoperation in the scarred field include bleeding, disruption of the prior hernia repair, recurrence, vascular injury, and testicular atrophy or loss. These risks should be discussed and documented prior to proceeding to surgery. In general, patients should be counseled to pursue operative intervention for higher intensity or debilitating pain as the anticipated outcome of surgery is not a normal, pain-free existence. Rather, successful intervention is defined as improvement or alleviation of high-intensity pain and suffering and improvement of functionality.

Technique

Triple neurectomy involves resecting segments of the ilioinguinal nerve, the genital branch of the genital femoral nerve, and the iliohypogastric nerve from a point proximal to the original surgical field to the most distal accessible point. Exposure for open triple neurectomy typically utilizes the same incision as the original anterior repair. If the original repair was done laparoscopically, a standard inguinal incision is used. Extending the incision more cephalad and lateral than typical for a hernia repair facilitates the exposure of the proximal portions of the ilioinguinal and iliohypogastric nerves in a less scarred location.

The ilioinguinal nerve is typically identified lateral to the deep inguinal ring and divided as proximally as possible (Fig. 15.1). The iliohypogastric nerve is identified in the plane between the internal and external oblique aponeurosis (Fig. 15.2). It is traced proximally to its intramuscular segment and divided proximal to the field of the original repair. As mentioned prior, care must be taken to resect this segment of the nerve for a complete neurectomy. If the iliohypogastric nerve is noted to be one of the subaponeurotic variants, the internal oblique aponeurosis is split proximal to the point where the nerve traverses both internal and external oblique aponeurosis, and the nerve is found and transected.

The genital branch of the genitofemoral nerve is identified adjacent to the external spermatic

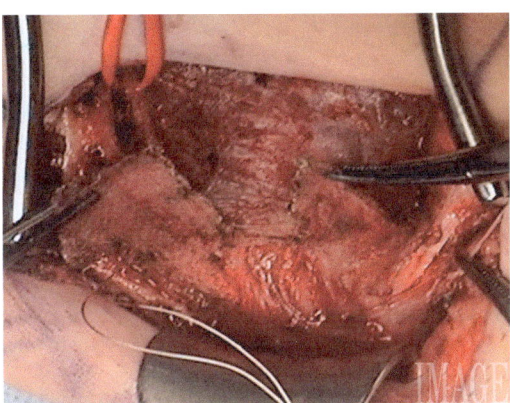

Fig. 15.1 Open anterior mesh removal and neurectomy. Red vessel loop around ilioinguinal nerve. Mesh split to internal ring

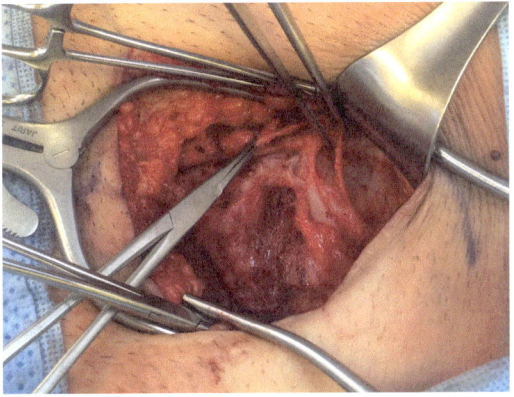

Fig. 15.2 Open anterior neurectomy. Iliohypogastric nerve (in forceps) identified at conjoined tendon

vein under the cord or through the lateral crus of the internal ring. During the neurectomy, this nerve is ligated and divided at the internal ring. We generally perform ligation of the cut nerves, which may reduce nerve sprouting and neuroma formation. Our standard practice includes burying the proximal nerve stump into surrounding muscle to protect it from the inflammation and scarring of the operative field.

Chronic Pain After Preperitoneal Hernia Repair

With widespread adoption of preperitoneal open and minimally invasive (laparoscopic and robotic) inguinal hernia repairs, chronic inguino-

dynia after posterior repairs has increased in frequency and poses different challenges for operative remediation. The preperitoneal nerves and posteriorly placed mesh are less accessible and more technically challenging to remove. After posterior repair, the most commonly implicated nerves are the main trunk, femoral branch, and the preperitoneal segment of the genital branch of the genitofemoral nerve. These nerves do not possess a separate fascial covering and are therefore at increased risk of injury if they are placed in contact with mesh. With the wider lateral dissection of the myopectineal orifice in laparoscopic and robotic repairs, injury to the lateral femoral cutaneous nerve must also be considered. Nerve injury after posterior repair can be addressed by laparoscopic triple neurectomy or an open extended triple neurectomy, which includes segmental resection of the main genitofemoral trunk in the retroperitoneum [12].

For open extended triple neurectomy, a standard anterior approach is used to address the ilioinguinal and iliohypogastric nerves. The field is then extended to expose the retroperitoneum dividing the inguinal floor utilizing the same split made in the internal oblique muscle during resection of the intramuscular segment of the iliohypogastric nerve. The underlying transversus abdominis muscle is split, which exposes the parietal peritoneum. This is then swept medially and cephalad to expose the psoas muscle and the main trunk of the genitofemoral nerve as it courses over the body of the muscle (Fig. 15.3). This approach treats neuropathic pain due to injury of the main trunk, the femoral branch, or the preperitoneal segment of the genital branch, which is inaccessible during standard triple neurectomy.

Alternatively, minimally invasive laparoscopic and robotic approaches to inguinal neurectomy improve access and identification of the retroperitoneal and preperitoneal nerves while avoiding the scarred reoperative field. If the presentation is primarily neuropathic pain without meshoma or mesh-related problems, laparoscopic neurectomy can be performed with limited operative morbidity (i.e., no risk to the testicle, cord structures, recurrence with disruption of the prior repair, or vascular injury with

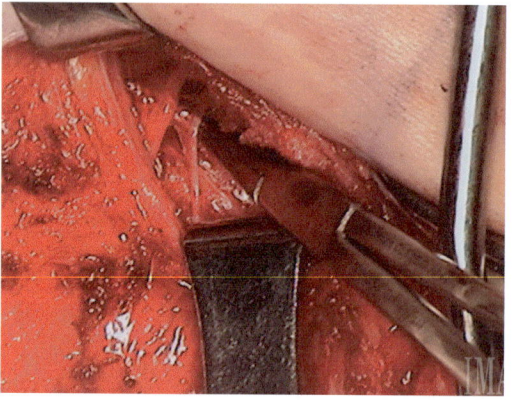

Fig. 15.3 Open extended anterior neurectomy preformed through inguinal floor. Genital branch of genitofemoral nerve identified over the psoas muscle

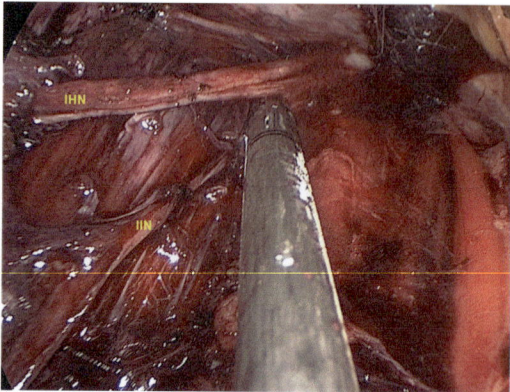

Fig. 15.5 Endoscopic retroperitoneal exposure with ilio-hypogastric and ilioinguinal nerve trunks over quadratus muscle

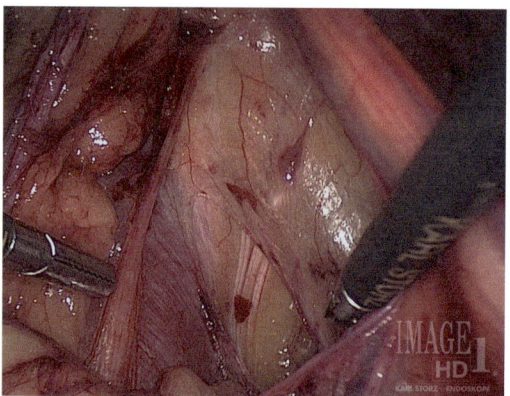

Fig. 15.4 Laparoscopic preperitoneal neurectomy. Genital branch of genitofemoral nerve identified over the psoas muscle (indicated by left grasper). Femoral branch of genitofemoral nerve with three branches lateral to the psoas

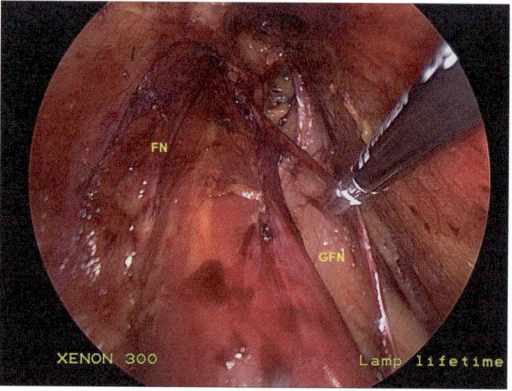

Fig. 15.6 Endoscopic retroperitoneal exposure with genitofemoral nerve trunk over the psoas muscle

mesh removal). Isolated access to the genitofemoral or lateral femoral cutaneous nerve can be achieved using the same approach as a laparoscopic transabdominal or total extraperitoneal inguinal hernia repair to identify and isolate these nerves in the preperitoneal plane (Fig. 15.4). This can also be combined with an open approach as a hybrid operation if anterior mesh removal and iliohypogastric or ilioinguinal neurectomy are indicated.

For patients that present with isolated or predominant neuropathic pain after a prior laparoscopic repair, after multiple prior open anterior inguinal interventions, after prior infection with extensive inguinal scarring, or after failed attempted anterior inguinal neurectomy, laparoscopic retroperitoneal triple neurectomy is the best option to definitively access and address these nerves. The iliohypogastric and ilioinguinal nerves are found in the retroperitoneum as they exit the L1 nerve root and travel over the quadratus lumborum muscle (Fig. 15.5). While neuroanatomic variation still exists, the course of these nerves is much more constant and reliable along its proximal extent in the lumbar plexus. The genitofemoral nerve trunk may be found over the psoas muscle exiting from the L1 level (Fig. 15.6). Separate genital and femoral branches are noted over 30% of the time, and the distal course of the genital nerve passing toward the internal ring should be confirmed prior to neurectomy. The lateral femoral cutaneous nerve exits from L3 and then travels below the iliac crest over the iliacus muscle exiting to the lateral thigh and may be addressed along its proximal course if needed.

Neurectomy at this proximal level is highly reliable and effective but does not address recurrence, nociceptive pain, or mesh-related etiologies. It may be used alone or in conjunction with a hybrid approach with open mesh removal or repair. However, the same factors that make proximal neurectomy successful for neuropathic pain lead to its morbidities. Special consideration of the anticipated side effects and complications of proximal neurectomy must be considered, understood, and explained to the patient in the consent process. The resultant area of anticipated numbness is larger after proximal neurectomy. The entire field of the nerve is affected along with the proximal branches that are preserved in open neurectomy. The iliohypogastric nerve typically has a posterior branch that extends toward the lower back and upper gluteal region. Neurectomy of a common genitofemoral trunk will sacrifice sensation to the anterior upper thigh innervated by the femoral branch of the nerve. Larger areas of denervation may increase the risk for deafferentation hypersensitivity. Proximal iliohypogastric neurectomy will also result in loss of the motor innervation to the lower oblique muscles which may result in lateral bulging and abdominal wall laxity. This typically improves with time due to cross-innervation and compensation but is a known result of proximal denervation. In general, it is preferable to perform a neurectomy as distal as reasonably possible where it is proximal to the likely site of injury with less unwanted side consequences.

Mesh-related Pain

Mesh-related pain and meshoma may exist independently or in conjunction with neuropathic pain. The type, configuration, and location of the prosthetic and resultant symptoms determine options for remediation. Anterior flat mesh may fold, extrude, or dislodge leading to pain and foreign body sensation. Plug and patch and bilayer meshes may migrate, contract, or fold, or the three-dimensional configuration of the mesh may lead to foreign body sensation. Posterior flat meshes placed through an open or laparoscopic approach may fold, clamshell, migrate, or lead to foreign body sensation. Removal of mesh is challenging, and the approach depends on the logistics of the prior operation, location, and coexisting symptoms. The greatest operative morbidities with regard to vascular injury, testicular atrophy or loss, disruption of the repair, and visceral injury are associated with mesh removal. If neuropathic pain is present, simultaneous neurectomy of the involved nerves should be performed. Mesh removal may also require pragmatic neurectomy as inguinal nerves adjacent to the mesh are at risk and should be sacrificed to prevent the development of neuropathic pain.

Anterior flat mesh, plug, and bilayer mesh may be removed through an anterior approach (Fig. 15.1). Specific care to preserve the cord structures and spermatic vessels should be taken. Complete mesh removal is not mandatory, and removing the bulk of the mesh may be adequate to improve symptoms. If separation is difficult, leaving a small rim of mesh adjacent to the cord or on vessels is prudent to minimize risk and complications. Meshes that cross the anterior and posterior plane (i.e., plug and patch, bilayer mesh, ONSTEP) may be approached through an anterior inguinal operation or may be combined with a hybrid laparoscopic and open approach. Posterior mesh placed at the time of open or laparoscopic surgery may be removed through an anterior operation, but removal is often morbid given the challenges of exposure. Laparoscopic and robotic mesh removal may be performed typically through a transabdominal approach following the same principles of protecting the vascular, visceral, and cord structures (Fig. 15.7). These remedial minimally invasive surgeries require a high degree of technical skill, experience, and most importantly clinical and operative judgment and are best reserved for experienced specialists.

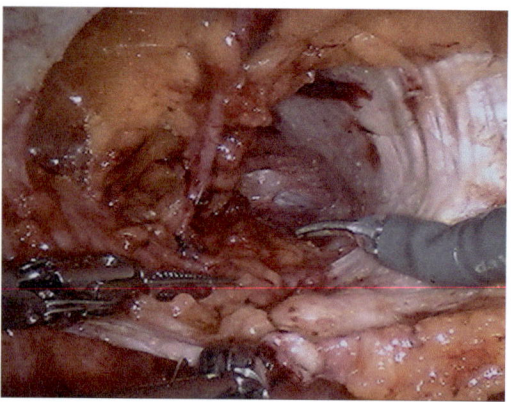

Fig. 15.7 Robotic transabdominal preperitoneal mesh removal

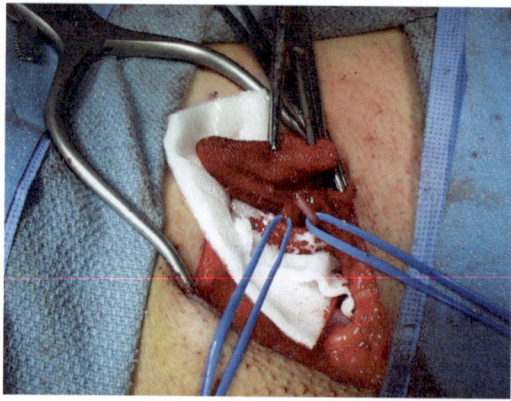

Fig. 15.8 Open anterior paravasal neurectomy. Vas adherent to plug

Postherniorrhaphy Orchialgia

In a subset of patients, orchialgia accompanies inguinodynia following inguinal hernia repair. It is important to distinguish testicular pain from the scrotal pain often associated with genital neuralgia. If this presents, triple neurectomy alone will not alleviate the pain. As with inguinodynia, postherniorrhaphy orchialgia may be caused by different overlapping etiologies. Nociceptive testicular pain may be due to direct injury to the testicular parenchyma or ischemia from vascular compromised from arterial infarction or venous obstruction. This type of pain is difficult to address and may be refractory to conservative measures as well as interventions including orchiectomy. Neuropathic testicular pain secondary to hernia repair may be caused by neuropathy of the paravasal nerve fibers, the autonomic nerve fibers that run with the cord structures, and coalesce at the level of the internal ring to envelop the vas deferens. In patients identified with neuropathic orchialgia, paravasal neurectomy may be performed at the time of triple neurectomy or mesh removal. After an anterior repair with a flat mesh, plug and patch, or bilayer mesh, this can be performed just proximal to the internal ring and mesh (Fig. 15.8). In orchialgia after laparoscopic mesh repair, anterior vas neurolysis is unlikely to be effective due to the injury being proximal to cord structures. Accessing the paravasal autonomic nerve plexus proximal to the mesh may be

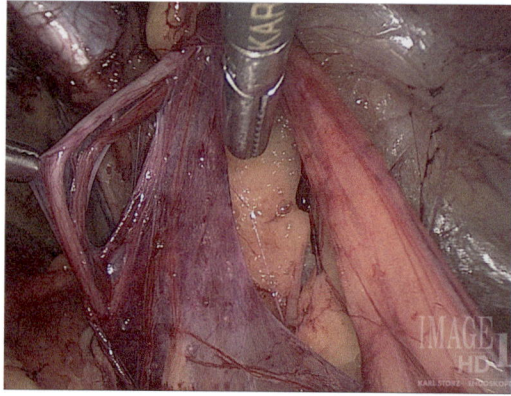

Fig. 15.9 Laparoscopic preperitoneal paravasal neurectomy. Nerves enveloping the vas deferens (left)

accomplished laparoscopically or robotically in these cases of preperitoneal repair (Fig. 15.9).

Results

Our experience includes over 800 patients that have undergone open triple neurectomy. In patients whose original repair did not enter the preperitoneal space, we achieve satisfactory improvement or resolution of postherniorrhaphy inguinodynia in 95% of patients. These results represent patients whose triple neurectomy included resection of the intramuscular segment of the iliohypogastric nerve. Prior to this modification, only the inguinal portion of the iliohypogastric nerve was resected, with a lower associated success rate of 85% [4].

Open extended triple neurectomy including the main trunk of the genitofemoral nerve has been performed in patients with chronic inguinodynia following preperitoneal mesh inguinal hernia repair with over 90% of these patients experiencing significant improvement of their pain. Laparoscopic triple neurectomy of the inguinal nerves in the retroperitoneal lumbar plexus is an effective option for patients that have pain after a posterior repair and those that have failed multiple prior anterior open interventions. In carefully selected cases where the pain is primarily neuropathic, this operative technique improves neuropathic complaints in over 90%. We have additionally combined both open and minimally invasive paravasal neurectomy with triple neurectomy for patients with posthernior-rhaphy groin pain and coexisting neuropathic orchialgia. In our original description, orchialgia was eliminated in 83% of patients [11]. Other overlapping etiologies for orchialgia make successful intervention less defined. These limited series suggest that these procedures are safe and successful, and future studies should be completed to determine a standardized clinical effectiveness.

Conclusion

Chronic post-inguinal herniorrhaphy pain is a challenging complication and may occur with all methods of inguinal hernia repair – open, laparoscopic, robotic, mesh, and tissue. It is a function of several factors including complex and variable neuroanatomy, inguinal floor dynamics, operative technique, mesh configuration and integration, individual patient predisposition, and psychosocial factors that modulate the subjective experience of pain. While the majority can be managed with conservative measures, a small subset of patients is significantly debilitated with implications on daily life, physical activity, employment, relationships, socialization, sexual activity, sleep, and overall quality of life. In refractory cases, operative management may help to improve symptoms and restore function.

Neuropathic inguinodynia may improve with neurectomy of the involved inguinal nerves. Mesh removal may ameliorate symptoms associated with "meshoma," displacement, migration, and foreign body sensation. Recurrence should be addressed at the time of any remedial operation. Associated orchialgia that arises after inguinal repair may respond to paravasal neurectomy of the autonomic nerve fibers surrounding the vas deferens. Outcomes and prevention of further complications are contingent upon knowledge of likely mechanisms of injury and neuroanatomy, meticulous operative technique, operative decision making, and judicious patient selection. For patients with severe symptoms, disability, and unrelenting pain, operative remediation may restore some degree of function, quality of life, and hope.

References

1. Hakeem A, Shanmugam V. Inguinodynia following Lichtenstein tension-free hernia repair: a review. World J Gastroenterol. 2011;17(14):1791–6.
2. Franneby U, Sandblom G, Nordin O, Nyren O, Gunnarsson U. Risk factors for long-term pain after hernia surgery. Ann Surg. 2006;244(2):212–9.
3. Lichtenstein IL, Shulman AG, Amid PK, Montllor MM. Cause and prevention of postherniorrhaphy neuralgia: a proposed protocol for treatment. Am J Surg. 1988;155(6):786–90.
4. Amid PK, Hiatt JR. New understanding of the causes and surgical treatment of postherniorrhaphy inguinodynia and orchalgia. J Am Coll Surg. 2007;205(2):381–5.
5. Aavsang E, Kehlet H. Surgical management of chronic pain after inguinal hernia repair. Br J Surg. 2005;92(7):795–801.
6. Klaassen Z, Marshall E, Tubbs RS, Louis RG Jr, Wartmann CT, Loukas M. Anatomy of the ilioinguinal and iliohypogastric nerves with observations of their spinal nerve contributions. Clin Anat. 2011;24(4):454–61.
7. Klaassen Z, Marshall E, Tubbs RS, Louis RG Jr, Wartmann CT, Loukas M. Anatomy of the ilioinguinal and iliohypogastric nerves with observations of their spinal nerve contributions. Clin Anat (New York, NY). 2011;24(4):454–61.
8. Aavsang E, Kehlet H. The effect of mesh removal and selective neurectomy on persistent postherniotomy pain. Ann Surg. 2009;249(2):327–34.

9. Loos MJ, Scheltinga MR, Roumen RM. Tailored neurectomy for treatment of postherniorrhaphy inguinal neuralgia. Surgery. 2010;147(2):275–81.

10. Bischoff JM, Enghuus C, Werner MU, Kehlet H. Long-term follow-up after mesh removal and selective neurectomy for persistent inguinal postherniorrhaphy pain. Hernia. 2013;17(3):339–45.

11. Lange JF, Kaufmann R, Wijsmuller AR, Pierie JP, Ploeg RJ, Chen DC, et al. An international consensus algorithm for management of chronic postoperative inguinal pain. Hernia. 2014;19(1):33–43. https://doi.org/10.1007/s10029-014-1292-y.

12. Chen DC, Hiatt JR, Amid PK. Operative management of refractory neuropathic inguinodynia by a laparoscopic retroperitoneal approach. JAMA Surg. 2013;148(10):962–7.

Surgical Outcomes: The Importance of Surgeon-Kept Data in Hernia Care

Nicholas H. Carter and Richard A. Pierce

Perhaps the most apt example of the power of surgeon-kept data to advance hernia care can be found in the contributions of Drs. Irving Lichtenstein and Parviz Amid. In a remarkable effort of long-term surveillance of outcomes, Drs. Lichtenstein and Amid followed their 4000 patients with primary inguinal hernias repaired from 1984 to 1995 with annual physical exams. The surgeons achieved an 87% follow-up rate with mean time of 5 years. By collecting and reviewing assiduous data, these surgeons identified four recurrences attributed to technical errors and subsequently modified their technique. The combined rate of infection, seroma, and hematoma was less than 1%. Their findings helped establish the Lichtenstein technique as a safe and effective option for inguinal hernia repair and spur the transition from tissue-based to mesh closures [1, 2].

Repair of the primary inguinal hernia is considered an essential skill of every general surgeon, but operative technique varies widely. Recent decades have seen considerable innovation in inguinal hernia repair, and large data cohorts with adequate long-term follow-up are crucial for validating new approaches. In addition, the diversity of techniques for umbilical, incisional, and parastomal hernia repair continues to grow. In this chapter, we present a brief review of some of the landmark recent studies in hernia surgery with a focus on methods for approaching major questions in this field. We describe persistent challenges in collecting meaningful data to guide surgeons toward achieving improved outcomes. Finally, we outline the various national and international collaborative hernia databases designed to assist surgeons by generating standardized metrics to identify areas for improvement.

Brief Review of Methods in Landmark Studies

In the United States, surgeon-researchers conducting most major hernia studies have had to collect their own prospective data. Maintaining long-term follow-up for large cohorts of patients has been a principal challenge in hernia research. With support from federal entities such as the Agency for Healthcare Research and Quality and the Veteran Affairs Cooperative Studies Program, several key papers have addressed crucial questions including whether open or laparoscopic inguinal hernia approaches should be favored and which inguinal hernia patients may be safely observed. In recent years, focus has shifted to measuring and preventing chronic pain following hernia surgery as data drives increased awareness of the grave morbidity associated with this complication.

N. H. Carter · R. A. Pierce (✉)
Department of Surgery, Vanderbilt University
Medical Center, Nashville, TN, USA
e-mail: Richard.pierce@vanderbilt.edu

© Springer International Publishing AG, part of Springer Nature 2018
M. P. LaPinska, J. A. Blatnik (eds.), *Surgical Principles in Inguinal Hernia Repair*,
https://doi.org/10.1007/978-3-319-92892-0_16

The Veterans Affairs system has provided infrastructure for several of the oft-cited American studies, including a randomized trial of open versus laparoscopic mesh inguinal repairs published in the *New England Journal of Medicine* in 2004 [3]. In this study, patients were examined at 2 weeks, 3 months, and yearly thereafter by a surgeon who had not been involved in the index operation with a primary endpoint of recurrence at 2 years. Recurrence was identified by physical examination by the independent surgeon, by ultrasound, or during reoperation. This study assigned 1087 patients to open Lichtenstein repair and 1077 patients to laparoscopic repair and achieved a high rate of follow-up with overall 90% of eligible patients evaluated at 2 years. The authors reported a higher rate of recurrence for laparoscopic repair compared to open Lichtenstein repairs. In subsequent studies, however, laparoscopic and open repairs were shown to have comparable recurrence rates when performed by surgeons with adequate experience in each procedure [4–6].

Another key study in hernia management is the randomized trial of watchful waiting for asymptomatic inguinal hernia published in the *Journal of the American Medical Association* in 2006 [7]. In this study, 724 patients with asymptomatic or minimally symptomatic inguinal hernias were enrolled from five North American community and academic centers and randomized to watchful waiting versus immediate Lichtenstein repair. Primary outcomes included pain and discomfort interfering with usual activities 2 years after enrollment. Patients were examined at 2 weeks, 6 months, and annually. The median time of follow-up was 3.2 years. This study found similar rates of pain interfering with activities in the watchful waiting versus operative groups. The rate of acute incarceration for patients randomized to watchful waiting was negligible although the rate of crossover to operative intervention was 27.9% with median time to crossover of 24 months. The authors concluded that watchful waiting is a reasonable option for management of healthy patients with minimally symptomatic inguinal hernias.

Given that recurrence rates are now consistently low with mesh-based repairs, the focus of

hernia research has shifted to methods for preventing and treating chronic pain associated with hernia repair [8–10]. This shift has been spurred by increasing evidence that pain, rather than recurrence, represents the more common and often more debilitating long-term complication of hernia surgery [11, 12]. This area of research, while crucial, has faced challenges in achieving long-term, standardized measurements [13]. Even a recent meta-analysis that included only five studies that examined surgeons using similar operative techniques with similar study design and primary outcomes found rates of chronic pain ranging from 0 to 24% [14]. Consensus regarding the best techniques for preventing chronic pain following hernia surgery is fleeting, with leading voices variously calling for routine identification and preservation of nerves, prophylactic neurectomy, or even abandonment of mesh repairs [15–17].

These studies, among the most widely cited trials among hernia surgeons, also reveal considerable limitations of hernia research to date. They are designed to address the big questions of management and technique and employ considerable resources to collect data that follows patients for only 2 years. In the United States, both longer-term and individualized data are rarely available. Few surgeons can truthfully cite their own basic outcomes such as rates of recurrence or chronic pain following hernia repairs.

Persistent Challenges in Collecting Meaningful Data

The appropriate methods for long-term follow-up of hernia patients are controversial. For example, recurrences have historically been evaluated by physical examination by a surgeon with or without adjunct imaging [18, 19]. Modalities for imaging have included CT scanning, standard ultrasound, or Dynamic Abdominal Sonography for Hernia (DASH) [20]. There is early evidence that complications including recurrence may be elicited by simply asking patients if they have felt pain or a bulge at the site of their prior repair [21]. This strategy of using patient-reported outcomes (PROs) to screen for late complications of hernia operations promises to assist overburdened surgeons in following larger cohorts of postoperative patients and may help generate more reliable data regarding late complications of these operations.

Data collection regarding hernia outcomes is made even more complex by a growing evidence that rates of complications for specific surgical techniques are not static but rather vary notably *among individual surgeons* and even *within* an individual surgeon's practice at various points in his or her own learning curve. The existence of a learning curve, however, is well-documented in both open and laparoscopic hernia repairs. Involvement of junior surgical residents in open inguinal hernia repairs has been shown to be associated with increased recurrence rates compared to more senior surgical residents [22]. The learning curve in laparoscopic hernia techniques has been even more clearly demonstrated [23–26]. Overall, recurrence rates for individual surgeons can vary from 0.2 to 10% [27]. In the absence of routinely collected individualized hernia outcome data in the United States, the specific technical causes of this individual variation are perhaps the least understood factors in hernia surgery and the most under-explored field for quality improvement.

In an age of increasing demands for clinical productivity, many surgeons find routine data collection regarding hernia outcomes unfeasible. To date, rigorous tracking of individual outcomes has been the purview of exceptional efforts such as demonstrated by Drs. Lichtenstein and Amid. Most practicing surgeons simply are unable or unwilling to follow all of their postoperative hernia patients year after year. Patients who suffer a late postoperative complication often seek the care of a different surgeon, and infrastructure to provide feedback to the original surgeon is usually informal or nonexistent. Yet our current healthcare financing environment mandates a transition from sheer productivity, as measured by number of operations performed, to value-based metrics set to patient-oriented outcomes. This requires far better tracking of individual surgical results. Quality improvement collaboratives offer opportunities to standardize metrics

for measuring complications such as recurrence or chronic pain [28]. To make surgeon-kept data feasible and useful, individual surgeons need support from database-driven collaboratives.

Collaborative Hernia Databases

In recent decades, collaborative data collection has become a favored approach for comparing methods for hernia repair as well as individualized outcomes. Europe has led the way with several large collaborative databases. Surgeons in Sweden and Denmark pioneered national data collection and public reporting of outcomes. Since 1992, the Swedish Hernia Register has collected voluntary data on hernia repairs in patients of ages 15 and older [29]. Starting with 8 participating hospitals, the Swedish registry grew to include 19 facilities by 1995 and 29 by 1997, ultimately capturing an estimated 98% of hernia operations performed nationally [30, 31]. Between 2002 and 2011, the registry included more than 143,000 patients who underwent inguinal hernia operations. This large cohort of patients has permitted analysis of lesser studied aspects of hernia repair such as operative time and frequency of cardiovascular complications [31, 32].

In Denmark, the Danish Hernia Database has collected prospective information on recurrence, surgical technique, chronic pain, sexual dysfunction, and recovery time since 1998 [33]. Data is reviewed by a scientific steering committee and presented at two annual national conferences. In the early years, surgeon participation was voluntary. The national surgical society played an important role in promoting surgeon participation and achieved 95% participation rates. In 2005, a national law mandated that surgeons report all hernia repairs to the registry. Nationwide and individual surgeon outcomes are publicly reported twice yearly [34]. Since the inception of the Danish registry, national recurrence rates have dropped from more than 10% to 2–3% [35]. Danish and Swedish surgeons have pooled their databases to study specific topics ranging from technical causes of recurrence following Lichtenstein repair to chronic pain following mesh vs. tissue-based repairs [36, 37].

The success of Scandinavian national registries in documenting improved outcomes following hernia operations spurred efforts to collect pooled hernia data across Europe. In 2009, a network of hospitals and private practice surgeons in Germany, Austria, and Switzerland launched Herniamed, an Internet-based registry of hernia operations [38]. In less than 10 years, Herniamed has grown to include 460 participating institutions and generated analyses of diverse topics including the need for prophylactic antibiotics, self-adhesive mesh, and the effect of surgeon volume on outcomes in laparoscopic inguinal hernia repairs [39–41]. In 2012, the European Hernia Society launched EuraHS, the European Registry for Abdominal Wall Hernias [42]. This registry has validated key metrics for quality of life reporting following hernia repair [43].

In the United States, prospective databases have been slower to develop. Large studies of hernia outcomes have required retrospective review of the Veteran Affairs Surgical Quality Improvement Database (VASQIP) or American College of Surgeons National Surgical Quality Improvement Database (ACS NSQIP) to identify hernia patients by CPT codes [44, 45]. Many of these studies, while notable in their findings, have relied heavily on ICD-9 coding or laborious retrospective data abstraction from operative reports [46, 47]. These databases capture postoperative complications up to 30 days after an operation and are therefore limited in their ability to identify several of the primary adverse events related to hernia operations including chronic pain and recurrence [45, 48].

The Americas Hernia Society Quality Collaborative (AHSQC) was formed in 2013 with the mission to "provide health care professionals real-time information for maximizing value in hernia care" [49]. In an effort to focus on types of hernias with particularly wide variations in practice and poor pre-existing data, the AHSQC was limited initially to incisional or parastomal hernias, and the following year was expanded to include ventral hernias of any kind, including epigastric, umbilical, Spigelian, or lumbar. From the beginning, the AHSQC emphasized the importance of consistent data collection. Surgeons alone are permitted to enter operative information although designated support staff and data entry personnel may enter other patient data. To improve long-term follow-up rates, the database includes phone and email surveys administered yearly to supplement standard postoperative clinical visits. Recurrence may be assessed using clinical, radiographic, and patient-reported outcomes. In February 2017, the AHSQC began collecting data on inguinal hernias in addition to those mentioned above. To date, over 4,000 inguinal cases have been entered into the database.

Quality collaboratives like the AHSQC promise to help shift the burden of long-term data collection away from individual surgeons while providing a mechanism for pooling of detailed, relevant outcomes information. Since these registries are designed by surgeon-researchers with expertise in hernia care, they can be crafted to capture precise data points relevant to clinical decisions. With the assistance of patient-reported outcomes, hernia registries may achieve long-term follow-up that extends far beyond the 30-day postoperative period reported to NSQIP and VASQIP databases. In fact, at the time of this publication, since its inception 5 years ago, the AHS-QC has already accrued over 35,000 patients and resulted in 8 unique publications with several more soon to come [49, 50].

In conclusion, US hernia research to date has largely relied on individual surgeons or study groups to collect detailed, long-term data on hernia patients. This process is burdensome for surgeons and lends itself to wide variability in metrics. European national and regional databases have demonstrated the use of collaborative data collection to assist surgeons in reviewing and improving their outcomes. The AHSQC represents a new effort to harness the power of surgeon-kept data in the Americas to provide readily available information for quality improvement.

References

1. Amid PK, Shulman AG, Lichtenstein IL. Open "tension-free" repair of inguinal hernias: the Lichtenstein technique. Europ J Surg = Acta chirurgica. 1996;162(6):447–53.
2. Scott NW, McCormack K, Graham P, Go PM, Ross SJ, Grant AM. Open mesh versus non-mesh for repair of femoral and inguinal hernia. Cochrane Database Syst Rev. 2002(4):Cd002197.
3. Neumayer L, Giobbie-Hurder A, Jonasson O, Fitzgibbons R Jr, Dunlop D, Gibbs J, et al. Open mesh versus laparoscopic mesh repair of inguinal hernia. N Engl J Med. 2004;350(18):1819–27.
4. Eklund A, Carlsson P, Rosenblad A, Montgomery A, Bergkvist L, Rudberg C. Long-term cost-minimization analysis comparing laparoscopic with open (Lichtenstein) inguinal hernia repair. Br J Surg. 2010;97(5):765–71.
5. Karthikesalingam A, Markar SR, Holt PJ, Praseedom RK. Meta-analysis of randomized controlled trials comparing laparoscopic with open mesh repair of recurrent inguinal hernia. Br J Surg. 2010;97(1):4–11.
6. Cavazzola LT, Rosen MJ. Laparoscopic versus open inguinal hernia repair. Surg Clin North Am. 2013;93(5):1269–79.
7. Fitzgibbons RJ Jr, Giobbie-Hurder A, Gibbs JO, Dunlop DD, Reda DJ, McCarthy M Jr, et al. Watchful waiting vs repair of inguinal hernia in minimally symptomatic men: a randomized clinical trial. JAMA. 2006;295(3):285–92.
8. Johner A, Faulds J, Wiseman SM. Planned ilioinguinal nerve excision for prevention of chronic pain after inguinal hernia repair: a meta-analysis. Surgery. 2011;150(3):534–41.
9. Amid PK, Hiatt JR. New understanding of the causes and surgical treatment of postherniorrhaphy inguinodynia and orchalgia. J Am Coll Surg. 2007;205(2):381–5.
10. Amid PK, Chen DC. Surgical treatment of chronic groin and testicular pain after laparoscopic and open preperitoneal inguinal hernia repair. J Am Coll Surg. 2011;213(4):531–6.
11. Poobalan AS, Bruce J, King PM, Chambers WA, Krukowski ZH, Smith WC. Chronic pain and quality of life following open inguinal hernia repair. Br J Surg. 2001;88(8):1122–6.
12. Courtney CA, Duffy K, Serpell MG, O'Dwyer PJ. Outcome of patients with severe chronic pain following repair of groin hernia. Br J Surg. 2002;89(10):1310–4.
13. Chen DC, Amid PK. Prevention of inguinodynia: the need for continuous refinement and quality improvement in inguinal hernia repair. World J Surg. 2014;38(10):2571–3.
14. Shah NS, Fullwood C, Siriwardena AK, Sheen AJ. Mesh fixation at laparoscopic inguinal hernia repair: a meta-analysis comparing tissue glue and tack fixation. World J Surg. 2014;38(10):2558–70.
15. Alfieri S, Rotondi F, Di Giorgio A, Fumagalli U, Salzano A, Di Miceli D, et al. Influence of preservation versus division of ilioinguinal, iliohypogastric, and genital nerves during open mesh herniorrhaphy: prospective multicentric study of chronic pain. Ann Surg. 2006;243(4):553–8.
16. Mui WL, Ng CS, Fung TM, Cheung FK, Wong CM, Ma TH, et al. Prophylactic ilioinguinal neurectomy in open inguinal hernia repair: a double-blind randomized controlled trial. Ann Surg. 2006;244(1):27–33.
17. Fischer JE. Hernia repair: why do we continue to perform mesh repair in the face of the human toll of inguinodynia? Am J Surg. 2013;206(4):619–23.
18. Burger JW, Luijendijk RW, Hop WC, Halm JA, Verdaasdonk EG, Jeekel J. Long-term follow-up of a randomized controlled trial of suture versus mesh repair of incisional hernia. Ann Surg. 2004;240(4):578–83. discussion 83–5
19. Heniford BT, Park A, Ramshaw BJ, Voeller G. Laparoscopic ventral and incisional hernia repair in 407 patients. J Am Coll Surg. 2000;190(6):645–50.
20. Baucom RB, Beck WC, Phillips SE, Holzman MD, Sharp KW, Nealon WH, et al. Comparative evaluation of dynamic abdominal sonography for hernia and computed tomography for characterization of incisional hernia. JAMA Surg. 2014;149(6):591–6.
21. Baucom RB, Ousley J, Feurer ID, Beveridge GB, Pierce RA, Holzman MD, et al. Patient reported outcomes after incisional hernia repair-establishing the ventral hernia recurrence inventory. Am J Surg. 2016;212(1):81–8.
22. Wilkiemeyer M, Pappas TN, Giobbie-Hurder A, Itani KM, Jonasson O, Neumayer LA. Does resident post graduate year influence the outcomes of inguinal hernia repair? Ann Surg. 2005;241(6):879–82. discussion 82–4
23. Lal P, Kajla RK, Chander J, Ramteke VK. Laparoscopic total extraperitoneal (TEP) inguinal hernia repair: overcoming the learning curve. Surg Endosc. 2004;18(4):642–5.
24. Schouten N, Elshof JW, Simmermacher RK, van Dalen T, de Meer SG, Clevers GJ, et al. Selecting patients during the "learning curve" of endoscopic totally Extraperitoneal (TEP) hernia repair. Hernia : J Hernias Abdominal Wall Surg. 2013;17(6):737–43.
25. Schouten N, Simmermacher RK, van Dalen T, Smakman N, Clevers GJ, Davids PH, et al. Is there an end of the "learning curve" of endoscopic totally extraperitoneal (TEP) hernia repair? Surg Endosc. 2013;27(3):789–94.
26. Neumayer LA, Gawande AA, Wang J, Giobbie-Hurder A, Itani KM, Fitzgibbons RJ Jr, et al. Proficiency of surgeons in inguinal hernia repair: effect of experience and age. Ann Surg. 2005;242(3):344–8; discussion 8–52
27. Gawande AA. The bell curve: what happens when patients find out how good their doctors really are? The New Yorker. 2004.
28. Muysoms FE, Deerenberg EB, Peeters E, Agresta F, Berrevoet F, Campanelli G, et al. Recommendations

for reporting outcome results in abdominal wall repair: results of a consensus meeting in Palermo, Italy, 28-30 June 2012. Hernia : J Hernias Abdom Wall Surg. 2013;17(4):423–33.

29. Nilsson H, Angeras U, Sandblom G, Nordin P. Serious adverse events within 30 days of groin hernia surgery. Hernia : J Hernias Abdominal Wall Surg. 2016;20(3):377–85.

30. Nilsson E. Outcomes. In: Kark AE, Kurzer MN, Wantz GE, editors. Surgical Management of Abdominal Wall Hernias. Malden, MA: Blackwell Science Inc; 1999. p. 11–8.

31. Lundstrom KJ, Sandblom G, Smedberg S, Nordin P. Risk factors for complications in groin hernia surgery: a national register study. Ann Surg. 2012;255(4):784–8.

32. van der Linden W, Warg A, Nordin P. National register study of operating time and outcome in hernia repair. Arch Surg (Chicago, Ill : 1960). 2011;146(10):1198–203.

33. Bay-Nielsen M, Kehlet H, Strand L, Malmstrom J, Andersen FH, Wara P, et al. Quality assessment of 26,304 herniorrhaphies in Denmark: a prospective nationwide study. Lancet (London, England). 2001;358(9288):1124–8.

34. Kehlet H, Bay-Nielsen M. Nationwide quality improvement of groin hernia repair from the Danish Hernia Database of 87,840 patients from 1998 to 2005. Hernia : J Hernias Abdominal Wall Surg. 2008;12(1):1–7.

35. Friis-Andersen H, Bisgaard T. The Danish inguinal hernia database. Clin Epidemiol. 2016;8:521–4.

36. Bay-Nielsen M, Nordin P, Nilsson E, Kehlet H. Operative findings in recurrent hernia after a Lichtenstein procedure. Am J Surg. 2001;182(2):134–6.

37. Bay-Nielsen M, Nilsson E, Nordin P, Kehlet H. Chronic pain after open mesh and sutured repair of indirect inguinal hernia in young males. Br J Surg. 2004;91(10):1372–6.

38. Stechemesser B, Jacob DA, Schug-Pass C, Kockerling F. Herniamed: an internet-based registry for outcome research in hernia surgery. Hernia : J Hernias Abdominal Wall Surg. 2012;16(3):269–76.

39. Kockerling F, Bittner R, Jacob D, Schug-Pass C, Laurenz C, Adolf D, et al. Do we need antibiotic prophylaxis in endoscopic inguinal hernia repair? Results of the Herniamed registry. Surg Endosc. 2015;29(12):3741–9.

40. Klobusicky P, Feyerherd P. Usage of a self-adhesive mesh in TAPP hernia repair: a prospective study based on Herniamed register. J minim Access Surg. 2016;12(3):226–34.

41. Kockerling F, Bittner R, Kraft B, Hukauf M, Kuthe A, Schug-Pass C. Does surgeon volume matter in the outcome of endoscopic inguinal hernia repair? Surg Endosc. 2016.

42. Muysoms F, Campanelli G, Champault GG, DeBeaux AC, Dietz UA, Jeekel J, et al. EuraHS: the development of an international online platform for registration and outcome measurement of ventral abdominal wall hernia repair. Hernia : J Hernias Abdominal Wall Surg. 2012;16(3):239–50.

43. Muysoms FE, Vanlander A, Ceulemans R, Kyle-Leinhase I, Michiels M, Jacobs I, et al. A prospective, multicenter, observational study on quality of life after laparoscopic inguinal hernia repair with ProGrip laparoscopic, self-fixating mesh according to the European registry for Abdominal Wall hernias quality of life instrument. Surgery. 2016;160(5):1344–57.

44. Snyder CW, Graham LA, Gray SH, Vick CC, Hawn MT. Effect of mesh type and position on subsequent abdominal operations after incisional hernia repair. J Am Coll Surg. 2011;212(4):496–502; discussion −4

45. Froylich D, Haskins IN, Aminian A, O'Rourke CP, Khorgami Z, Boules M, et al. Laparoscopic versus open inguinal hernia repair in patients with obesity: an American College of Surgeons NSQIP clinical outcomes analysis. Surg Endosc. 2016.

46. Hawn MT, Snyder CW, Graham LA, Gray SH, Finan KR, Vick CC. Hospital-level variability in incisional hernia repair technique affects patient outcomes. Surgery. 2011;149(2):185–91.

47. Mason RJ, Moazzez A, Sohn HJ, Berne TV, Katkhouda N. Laparoscopic versus open anterior abdominal wall hernia repair: 30-day morbidity and mortality using the ACS-NSQIP database. Ann Surg. 2011;254(4):641–52.

48. Chung PJ, Lee JS, Tam S, Schwartzman A, Bernstein MO, Dresner L, et al. Predicting 30-day postoperative mortality for emergent anterior abdominal wall hernia repairs using the American College of Surgeons National Surgical Quality Improvement Program database. Hernia: J Hernias Abdominal Wall Surg. 2016.

49. Poulose BK, Roll S, Murphy JW, Matthews BD, Todd Heniford B, Voeller G, et al. Design and implementation of the Americas hernia society quality collaborative (AHSQC): improving value in hernia care. Hernia : J Hernias Abdominal Wall Surg. 2016;20(2):177–89.

50. Krpata DM, Haskins IN, Phillips S, Prabhu AS, Rosenblatt S, Poulose BK, et al. Does preoperative bowel preparation reduce surgical site infections during elective ventral hernia repair? J Am Coll Surg. 2016.

Part V

Special Situations in Inguinal Hernia Repair

Sports Hernia and Athletic Pubalgia

17

Arghavan Salles and L. Michael Brunt

Background

Athletes, both professional and recreational, are at risk for groin injuries. This is particularly true for those who play sports that require cutting, kicking, or other rapid acceleration and deceleration movements that rely on pelvic stability. [1] Consequently, these types of injuries tend to occur in soccer, hockey, and football players more often than in baseball players, cyclists, and swimmers. By some estimates, up to 18% of all hip/groin injuries occur in elite soccer players [2], and up to 58% of soccer players report symptoms consistent with groin injuries [3]. In a small series of 15 patients in the United Kingdom who had surgery for groin injuries, Tansey et al. noted that 67% of them were injured playing either rugby or soccer [4].

In another study of 998 sub-elite male soccer players over the course of a 10-month season, the most common groin injuries were adductor-related followed by iliopsoas-related and abdominal-related. Major risk factors for injury were age and a history of prior groin injury. A total of 447 groin injuries were recorded for an overall incidence of 3.41 injuries per 1000 h of training or competition [5].

Terminology

A number of terms are used to describe groin injuries: athletic pubalgia, sports hernia, sportsman's groin, inguinal disruption, abdominal core injury, Gilmore's groin, and hockey groin syndrome, among others. Two recent consensus conferences have come to different conclusions about appropriate terminology. The British Hernia Society guidelines from 2014 suggest that the term hernia should be avoided as there is usually no true hernia [6]. Rather, they recommend using the term "inguinal disruption" instead of sports hernia. They define this as "pain, either of an insidious or acute onset, which occurs predominantly in the groin area near the pubic tubercle where no obvious other pathology, such as a hernia, exists to explain the symptoms" [6]. The First World Conference on Groin Pain, which was held in Doha, Qatar, in 2014, developed four categories of groin pain: (1) adductor-related groin pain, (2) iliopsoas-related groin pain, (3) inguinal-related groin pain, and (4) pubic-related groin pain [7]. Thus, there is no agreement currently on what terminology to use. However, both consensus meetings favored descriptive anatomical terms rather than athletic pubalgia and sports hernia. Nonetheless, these are the most commonly used

A. Salles · L. M. Brunt (✉)
Department of Surgery and Section of Minimally Invasive Surgery, Washington University School of Medicine, St. Louis, MO, USA
e-mail: arghavan@wustl.edu; bruntm@wustl.edu

© Springer International Publishing AG, part of Springer Nature 2018
M. P. LaPinska, J. A. Blatnik (eds.), *Surgical Principles in Inguinal Hernia Repair*,
https://doi.org/10.1007/978-3-319-92892-0_17

terms in the field and are both firmly ingrained in the popular and surgical literature. Thus, throughout this chapter we will use the terms athletic pubalgia and sports hernia interchangeably to refer to pathology related to the abdominal rectus or inguinal floor with or without associated adductor pathology.

Pathophysiology

Groin injuries occur due to the high degree of strain placed across the pubis in the region of the insertion of the rectus abdominis, inguinal ligament, and adductor longus tendon. Such injuries may be acute from a sudden force applied with one or more muscle groups eccentrically contracted or can result from a more gradual process due to an imbalance in forces. Most commonly this results from the force of the powerful thigh muscles (mainly the adductor group) across the pubis which is transmitted to the distal rectus and inguinal floor [8]. The three major categories of anatomical findings in these athletes are (1) rectus tendon injury [8, 9], (2) posterior abdominal wall/inguinal floor defect [10], and (3) adductor-related groin injury. Rectus abdominis insertion injuries typically occur at the attachment of the rectus aponeurosis to the pubis (Fig. 17.1). Similarly, there can be a tear or tendinopathy in the adductor longus leading to pain at the tendinous insertion into the pubis with any adduction-related movements. The second type of injury, related to weakness of the posterior abdominal wall or inguinal disruption, (Fig. 17.2) may be a more gradual result from an imbalance in forces across the pubis, particularly if the adductors are much stronger than the rectus and associated lower abdominal muscles. A common associated finding in this setting is an attenuated external oblique aponeurosis, although it is unclear to what extent this contributes to symptoms (Fig.17.3). It is also not uncommon for these different injuries to coexist in one athlete.

Pathology of the inguinal or genital nerves has been postulated to contribute to athletic groin pain in some cases, but this is rarely the

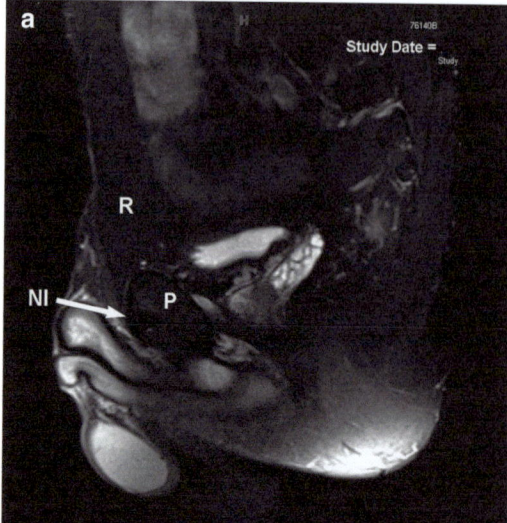

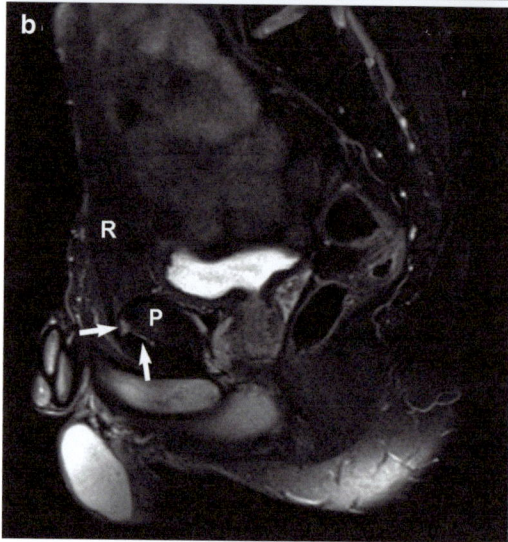

Fig. 17.1 Pelvic MRI that shows a rectus abdominal tear. (**a**) Normal side. (**b**) Rectus aponeurosis tear at pubis (*arrow*). P pubis, R rectus

sole source of pain [11]. However, this theory is countered by the fact that most authorities have good outcomes, regardless of approach, without resecting either the ilioinguinal or genital nerves. The role of neurectomy in the treatment of athletic groin injuries is, therefore, controversial. It should also be stated that athletic pubalgia is not just one isolated condition but rather comprises a spectrum of pathology that mandates an individualized approach to the evaluation and assessment of a given athlete.

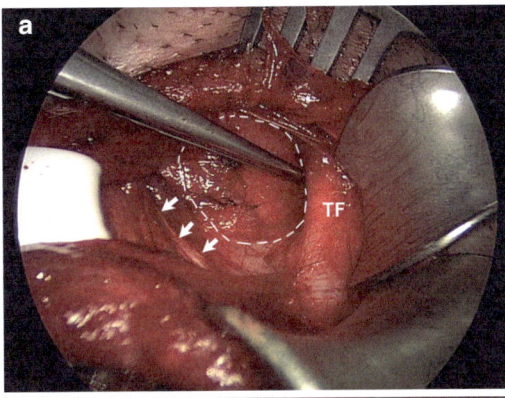

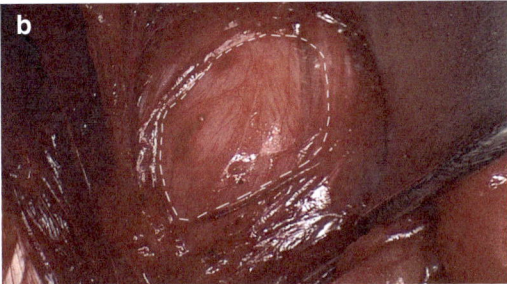

Fig. 17.2 Operative photo of a weakened posterior inguinal floor. (**a**) The dotted circle outlines the area of weakness in the inguinal floor. Also seen is the healthy transversalis fascia (TF) medially and the inguinal ligament laterally (*arrows*). (**b**) Magnified view of the bulging posterior floor

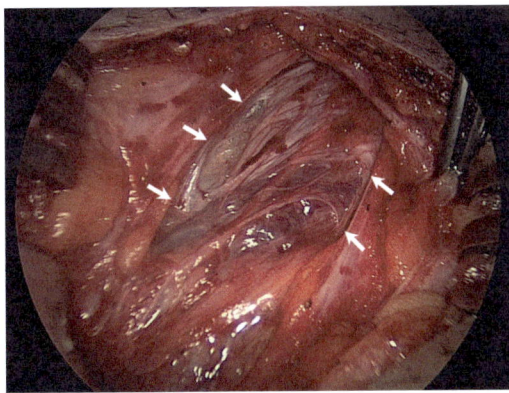

Fig. 17.3 Operative view of a markedly attenuated external oblique aponeurosis (*arrows*)

Differential Diagnosis

Groin anatomy is complex, and there are a number of other conditions that need to be considered when evaluating a patient for sports-related

Table 17.1 Differential diagnosis for groin pain

General
Abdominal muscle strain/tear of rectus abdominis or obliques
Osteitis pubis
Pubic rami stress fracture
Adductor strain
Hip flexor strain
Inguinal hernia
Nerve entrapment
Hip-related
Labral tear
Femoroacetabular impingement
Osteoarthritis
Femoral neck stress fracture
Avascular necrosis
In women
Endometriosis
Ovarian pathology
Other gynecologic abnormalities
In men
Prostatitis

groin injuries. Among the causes of groin pain are abdominal muscle strains, osteitis pubis, pubic rami stress fractures, adductor strain, hip flexor strains, inguinal hernias, and nerve entrapment (Table 17.1). Hip-related etiologies of groin pain include labral tears, femoroacetabular impingement, osteoarthritis, femoral neck stress fractures, and avascular necrosis. In women, gynecologic etiologies of groin pain, such as endometriosis and ovarian pathology, may enter into the differential diagnosis as does prostatitis in men. In 1 recent systematic literature review of 73 articles on the treatment of athletic groin injuries, the 5 most common entities that required surgical intervention were femoroacetabular impingement (32%), athletic pubalgia (24%), adductor-related pathology (12%), inguinal-related pathology (10%), and labral pathology (5%) [12].

Some of these problems may coexist in the same athlete. For example, Hammoud et al. noted significant overlap in symptoms between athletes with athletic pubalgia, as defined by lower abdominal or adductor pain, and femoroacetabular impingement (FAI) [13]. In their series, 32% of patients had persistent symptoms after surgery for athletic pubalgia which did not resolve until arthroscopic management of FAI was undertaken. These findings highlight the difficulty of making the correct diagnosis and the importance of a thorough history and physical exam as well as multidisciplinary evaluation.

A diagnosis of inguinal disruption or inguinal-related groin injury should be suspected when an athlete presents with exertional pain in the lower abdomen or groin, in the absence of an inguinal hernia, which does not improve with non-operative treatments. Adductor injuries typically present with pain in the adductor longus tendon region which is exacerbated with resisted adduction.

Clinical Evaluation

History

While groin injuries are common, their evaluation is nuanced and requires a thorough history and physical exam. Initial evaluation is often multidisciplinary, involving orthopedic surgeons or sports medicine physicians, athletic trainers, and physical therapists with referral to a general surgeon after failure of conservative management.

During the history, one should ask about the onset and duration of symptoms as well as the precise location and quality of pain. An effort should be made to determine if the symptoms originate from the inguinal region, abdominal muscles, the hip, adductors, or a combination thereof. A history of a bulge in the groin that would suggest a true inguinal hernia is rarely present. Typically, the pain from a groin injury does not occur at rest or sitting but may be aggravated with activities such as running, skating, cutting, coughing, sneezing, and getting in and out of bed. Since one of the risk factors for a groin injury is previous groin injury [7], this should be inquired about as well.

Physical Exam

A careful physical exam is essential to reach the correct diagnosis. A complete exam will include both standing and supine assessment of the patient.

With the patient standing, it is important to evaluate for inguinal hernias or testicular pathology which could be contributing to pain. The external inguinal ring should be examined for laxity or tenderness. With the patient supine, one should begin by palpation over the pubic symphysis to elicit tenderness there which could suggest osteitis pubis. Both inguinal floors should be palpated to assess for weakness or asymmetry (Fig. 17.4a). Pelvic stability should be assessed by pressing down on the iliac wings bilaterally. Resisted sit-ups and trunk rotation may reveal pain related to the rectus abdominis insertion or the oblique muscles. A thorough hip exam is recommended to rule out hip pathology and should include flexion/adduction/internal rotation (FADIR) as well as flexion/abduction/external rotation (FABER) which may indicate a labral inury [12]. The thigh exam should include testing of strength and pain with straight leg raising, resisted hip flexion, and passive and resisted adduction and abduction. Any other sites of pain should be examined as well. Finally, the adductor insertion site should be palpated to identify tightness or tenderness.

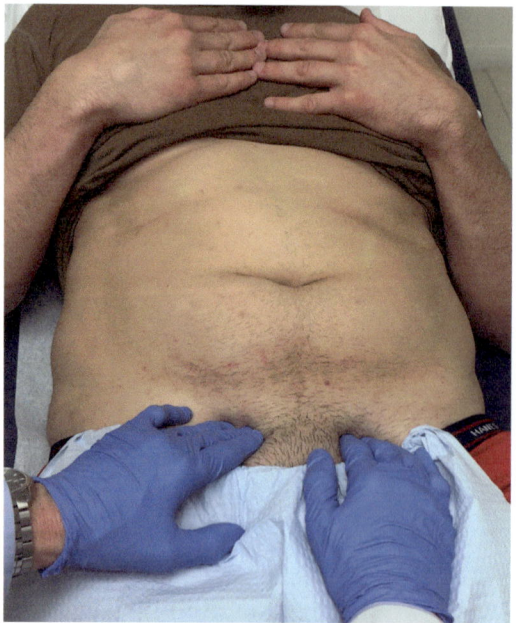

Fig. 17.4 Inguinal floor exam with palpation of inguinal floors and distal rectus insertion at rest and during a sit-up

Imaging

There is no clear consensus on the use of imaging to evaluate groin injuries. Plain x-rays [4], ultrasound [14], and MRI [4, 6] have been used and advocated by different groups. Plain x-rays are effective for ruling out avulsion of bony fragments but are rarely informative in this population of athletes. Dynamic ultrasound can be helpful in identifying inguinal hernias or posterior weakness in the inguinal floor but does not typically identify rectus injuries or adductor pathology. Ultrasound is also operator dependent and does not allow assessment of pubis-, adductor-, or hip-related pathology. In the authors' experience, a pelvic MRI is the most useful imaging modality for the evaluation of acute and chronic athletic groin injuries. Findings that may be seen on MRI include bone marrow edema (Fig. 17.5), stress fractures, rectus or adductor aponeurosis tears (Fig. 17.6), and hip pathology. MRI, combined with a careful history and physical exam, should allow a precise diagnosis of sports-related groin injury in the vast majority of cases.

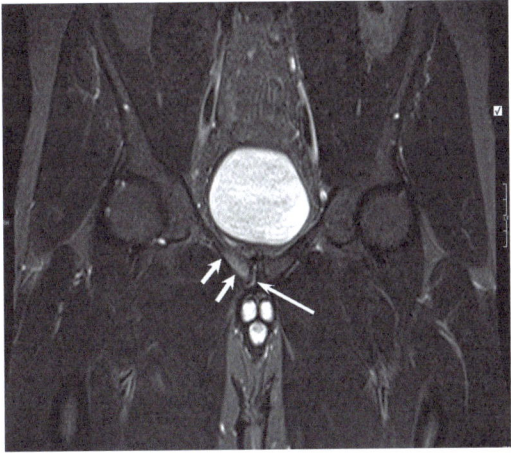

Fig. 17.5 Pelvis MRI that shows right-sided pubis edema (*short arrows*) and a secondary cleft (*longer arrow*). R rectus, P pubis. The secondary cleft is a curvilinear fluid cleft extending from the inferior aspect of the pubis

Surgical Treatment

The majority of sports-related groin injuries resolve with rest, ice, nonsteroidal anti-inflammatory drugs, and physical therapy. Deep tissue massage, or active tissue release, may also be effective in the appropriate setting. Injections with local anesthetic and steroids may be both diagnostic and therapeutic in the treatment algorithm if the pain is well-localized on the abdominal wall. Some centers have used platelet-rich plasma (PRP) injections at the site of injury, but reports have been limited to isolated case reports [15–17] and use of PRP for treatment of other sports-related injuries [18]. Anecdotally, PRP has been associated with heterotopic calcification and should be avoided in the area of the adductor tendon or insertion.

Abdominal Wall Repair

Surgery is indicated in athletes who fail 2–3 months of conservative management and who have the appropriate clinical features and supportive imaging findings. In some cases, earlier intervention may be warranted in high-level athletes who have an acute rectus insertional injury that is seen on MRI. There have been two randomized clinical trials that compared operative treatment to non-operative treatment for sports-hernia-type groin pain [19–20]. In both series, athletes who underwent surgical management had significantly reduced pain at 3–6 months and returned to sports sooner than those who received non-operative management. In addition, there was significant crossover from the non-operative arms to the operative arm in each study (51% [19] and 23% [20]) due to persistent pain. In both studies, participants who crossed over experienced significant improvement in their pain after surgery. These trials support the use of surgical intervention to treat athletes who have failed conservative management and have the appropriate exam and imaging findings.

The first key to choosing the proper surgical intervention is accurate diagnosis of the problem.

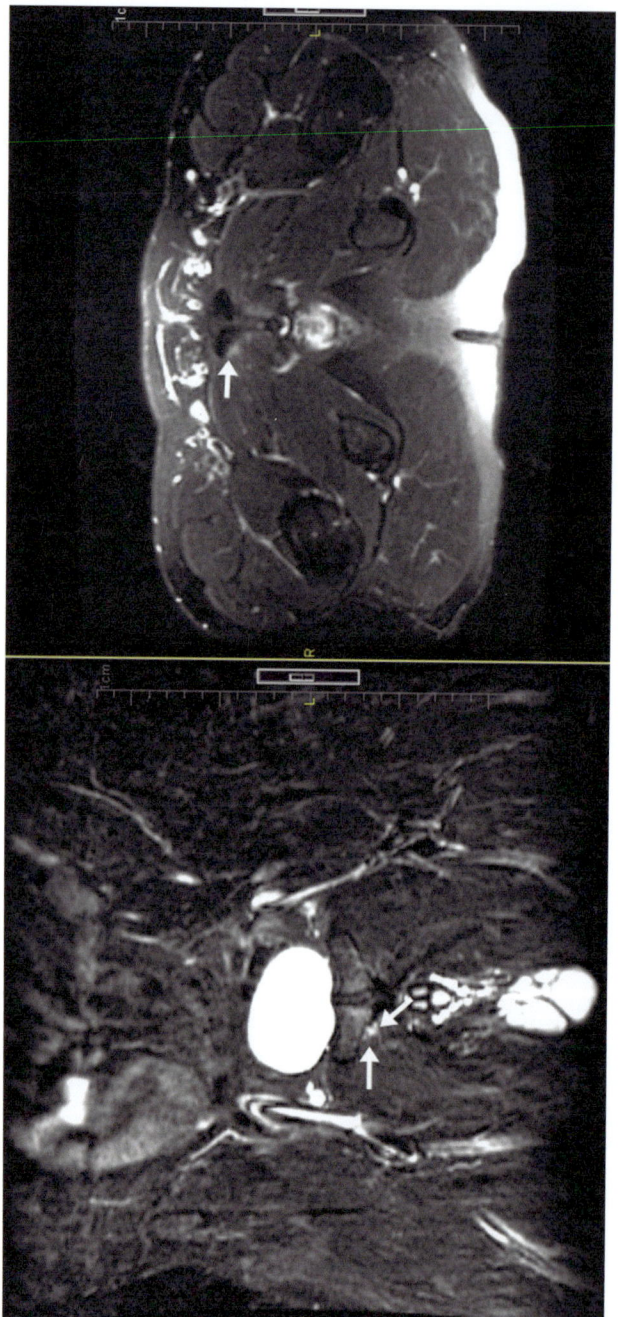

Fig. 17.6 Pelvic MRI that shows an adductor tear (*arrows*). Left panel, coronal *view*; right panel, axial image

A variety of operative approaches have been utilized by various groups to treat the abdominal/inguinal floor pathology of athletic pubalgia. Broadly, these consist of (1) open primary suture repairs, (2) open tension-free mesh repairs, and (3) laparoscopic mesh repairs. Regardless of the approach, the goal of surgery is to provide support and stability to the posterior inguinal floor and rectus insertion at the pubis, thereby strengthening the latter.

Primary Repairs

Two principal types of primary suture repairs have been described. Meyers, who has the world's largest experience with surgical treatment of athletic pubalgia injuries, sutures the inferolateral edge of the rectus fascia to the pubis and adjacent anterior ligaments [21]. This approach differs from a standard Bassini inguinal hernia repair in that the sutures are oriented in a near vertical line and the internal ring is not tightened since it is usually normal caliber. Muschawek and colleagues carry out a "minimal" repair technique in which only the weakened posterior inguinal floor is opened [22] The repair then consists of running two imbricating monofilament sutures up and down the inguinal floor between the transversalis/internal oblique layers and the iliopubic tract and inguinal ligament. This repair is analogous somewhat to a Shouldice repair except only the weakened section of the floor is repaired with the goal to lateralize the rectus. In selected cases, a genital neurectomy is also performed.

Tension-Free Mesh Repairs

The rationale for a tension-free mesh repair is that these repairs have largely replaced primary suture repairs over the last 20 years, and, for athletes who exert tremendous forces around the pubic region, this should result in a durable long-term repair. For open mesh repairs, the mesh is placed similar to a Lichtenstein repair with two exceptions: (1) the mesh is anchored medially to the rectus sheath and (Fig. 17.7), when possible, (2) the internal oblique is brought over the mesh and sutured to the inguinal ligament to insinuate native tissue between the mesh and the spermatic cord (Fig. 17.7c). Splitting the mesh and bringing

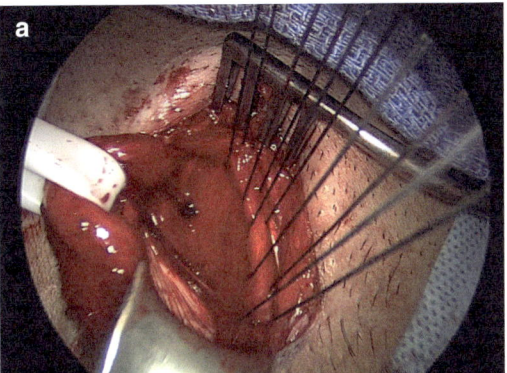

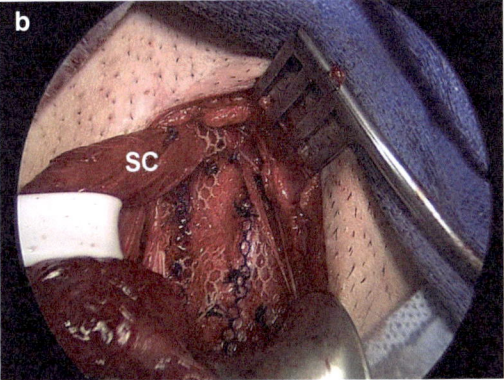

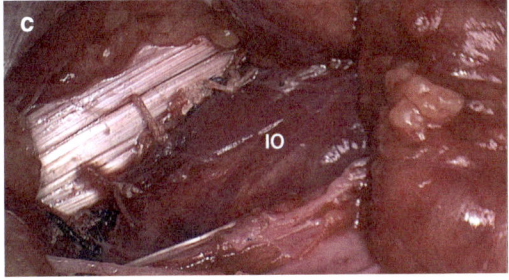

Fig. 17.7 Open repair of inguinal floor. (**a**) Sutures anchored to healthy transversalis fascia and rectus sheath. (**b**) Completed tension-free mesh repair of floor. SC = spermatic cord. (**c**) Internal oblique (IO) covering the mesh floor repair by suturing it to the inguinal ligament

the two tails around the spermatic cord is done not because the internal ring is abnormal but so that the mesh lies flat and evenly along the floor. An additional advantage of the open approach is that it allows repair of the external oblique which is often markedly attenuated in these athletes.

Some groups [20, 23] have advocated a laparoscopic approach to this problem. Paajanen et al. describe a total extraperitoneal (TEP) approach with dissection of the preperitoneal plane in the same fashion as one would do for an inguinal hernia repair [20]. The preperitoneal space is initially developed with a balloon dilator and then is dissected bluntly from the pubic symphysis to the inferior epigastric vessels bilaterally as well as caudally behind the pubic symphysis. A lightweight polypropylene mesh is fixed to the rectus abdominis, conjoined tendon, and Cooper's ligament (Fig. 17.8). This procedure may also be carried out using a transabdominal preperitoneal (TAPP) approach. Some groups advocate bilateral floor repair laparoscopically even when patients have unilateral injuries or symptoms, although repair of an asymptomatic groin is controversial. Lloyd et al. release the inguinal ligament by detaching the medial insertion of the inguinal ligament at the pubis based on the concept that the pain is primarily related to tension at the inguinal ligament [23]. This approach is

followed by placement of a large polypropylene mesh in the preperitoneal plane to buttress the entire inguinal floor on the side of the injury.

The senior author's practice is to perform an open tension-free mesh repair in most cases for the reasons given above. For young athletes who are still in their growth phase or women athletes, a primary suture repair is preferred analogous to that described above in which the lateral rectus is sutured to the pubis and inguinal ligament with interrupted nonabsorbable sutures [21]. In a series of 257 cases treated at our institution over the past 12 years, 83% underwent open mesh repair, 5% were treated with primary tissue repairs, and 13% underwent laparoscopic TEP repair with an overall success rate of return to sports of 90%. The laparoscopic approach was used primarily in athletes who had prior open inguinal surgery and demonstrable rectus aponeurosis tears on imaging.

No comparative trials have been done to assess outcomes of the different surgical approaches for the treatment of sports-hernia-related inguinal pain, although a trial is currently underway in Finland to compare laparoscopic vs. open minimal suture repair in athletes who have failed conservative management (NCT01876342). Reported series have also not shown differences in outcomes between open or laparoscopic approaches [24], but this issue remains controversial. Athletes are in most cases able to return to competitive sports within 5–8 weeks of surgery [4, 13, 23].

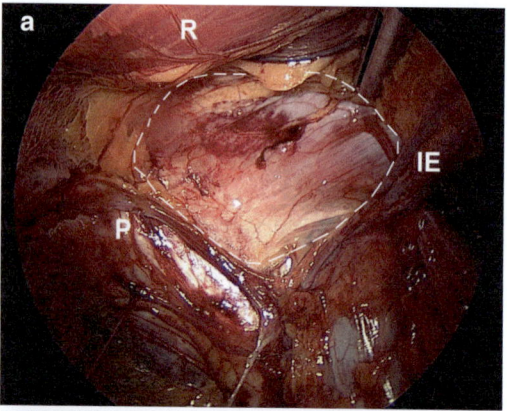
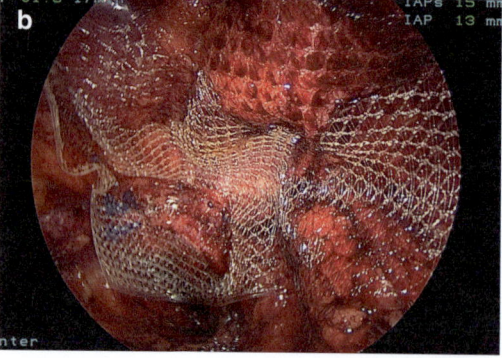

Fig. 17.8 Laparoscopic view of right inguinal floor. (**a**) The dotted circle shows a defect in the medial posterior inguinal floor similar to that on the anterior view seen in Fig. 17.7. (P = pubis, R = rectus, IE = inferior epigastrics). (**b**) Mesh repair of inguinal floor, laparoscopic approach

Adductor Tenotomy

If the symptoms, exam, and imaging findings are primarily related to adductor tendon pathology, an adductor tenotomy can be performed, either as an isolated procedure or in conjunction with inguinal floor repair. In these cases, patients have pain inferior to the inguinal ligament near the attachment of the adductor longus tendon to the pubis and have discomfort with resisted adduction on that side. MRI typically shows adductor tendon thickening, chronic tendinopathy, or a tear at the insertion site. A small incision is made 2–3 cm below the adductor insertion on the pubis.

Several incisions are made into the tendon sheath to stimulate neovascularity and to release tension in the adductor compartment. Occasionally, calcifications in the tendon are found and should be debrided (Fig.17.9). Percutaneous approaches to adductor tenotomy have also been described [25]. Return to sports with these approaches has been reported at 4–14 weeks postoperatively [25–27].

The role of primary surgical repair vs. conservative management of adductor tendon tears is unclear. In one study of National Football League players, the mean time to return to play was 6.1 ± 3.1 weeks in 12 conservatively treated athletes compared to 12.0 ± 2.5 weeks in 5 surgically managed patients [28]. In a second study of 15 elite athletes, adductor repair was performed between 5 and 34 days from injury using bone anchors to reattach the tendon at the pubis. These

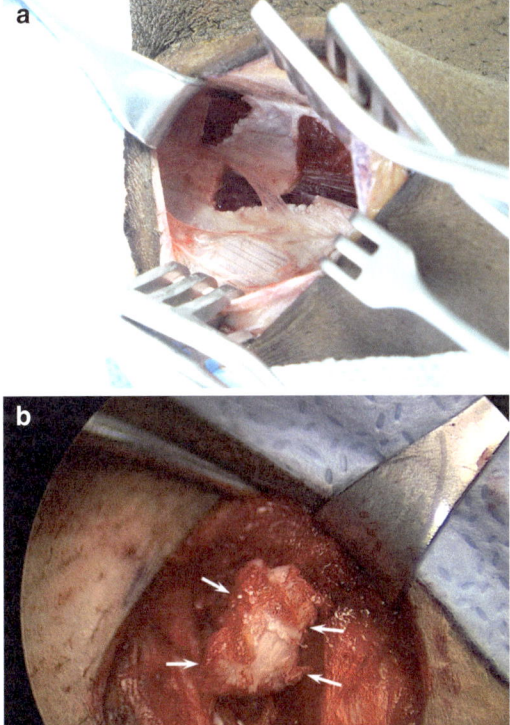

Fig. 17.9 (**a**) Operative view of partial adductor longus release. (**b**) Calcified adductor tendon (*arrows*) that is undergoing debridement

athletes were able to return to sports at a mean of 13 weeks after repair (range 10–21 weeks). Seven of these athletes also underwent simultaneous mesh repair of an injury on the abdominal side. No recurrences were observed over 1 year of follow-up [4].

Postoperative Care

Rehabilitation after surgery for a sports-related groin injury should entail a structured approach with gradually increasing activity levels. Ellsworth et al. have published a detailed, well-defined regimen [29]. Regardless of the type of surgery performed, patients in the senior author's practice are instructed to resume light activities and stretching from the day of surgery. Within 5 days they should begin a program of structured walking progressing to light running within 2 weeks. Cycling for conditioning and light resistance exercises may begin as soon as is comfortable for the athlete. Light sports-specific activities (e.g., dribbling a soccer ball, light skating, or football drills) may also be resumed within 2–3 weeks according to comfort level with gradual progression to higher-level drills. Functional strengthening and core stabilization exercises should be included in the rehabilitation along with scar mobilization with deep tissue massage. Finally, progression to team practices, scrimmage, and simulated game conditions should precede return to play. It is important to note that progression of recovery should be based on function and symptoms and not a rigid time-based approach. Recovery will vary according to the athlete, sports, and extent of injury. Most athletes can return to competitive sports within 5–8 weeks, though longer may be required for more complex injuries and those with adductor involvement.

Summary

Sports-related groin injuries are common and can be difficult to diagnose and manage. Surgical treatment is indicated for athletes who fail conservative therapy and who have the appropriate exam and radiographic features. Hernia surgeons who become involved in the evaluation of these athletes should understand the diverse conditions that cause athletic groin pain, be familiar with the special exam and imaging components necessary to make the diagnosis, and have a well-constructed surgical approach to management. A multidisciplinary approach with the sports medicine or orthopedist specialist, musculoskeletal radiologist, and athletic trainer/physical therapist with experience in managing these athletes is also essential to successful outcomes.

References

1. Minnich JM, Hanks JB, Muschaweck U, Brunt LM, Diduch DR. Sports hernia: diagnosis and treatment highlighting a minimal repair surgical technique. Am J Sports Med. 2011;39:1341–9.
2. Nicholas SJ, Tyler TF. Adductor muscle strains in sport. Sports Med. 2002;32:339–44.
3. Harris NH, Murray RO. Lesions of the symphysis in athletes. BMJ. 1974;4:211–4.
4. Tansey RJ, Benjamin-Laing H, Jassim S, Liekens K, Shankar A, Haddad FS. Successful return to high-level sports following early surgical repair of combined adductor complex and rectus abdominis avulsion. Bone Joint J. 2015;97-b:1488–92.
5. Holmich P, Thorborg K, Dehlendorff C, Krogsgaard K, Gluud C. Br J Sports Med. 2014;48:1245–50.
6. Sheen AJ, Stephenson BM, Lloyd DM, et al. 'Treatment of the sportsman's groin' British hernia Society's 2014 position statement based on the Manchester consensus conference. Br J Sports Med. 2013;0:1–9.
7. Weir A, Brukner P, Delahunt E, Ekstrand J, Griffin D, Khan KM, et al. Doha agreement meeting on terminology and definitions in groin pain athletes. Br J Sports Med. 2015;49:768–74.
8. Meyers WC, Yoo E, Devon ON, Jain N, Horner M. Understanding "sports hernia" (athletic pubalgia): the anatomic and pathophysiologic basis for abdominal and groin pain in athletes. Oper Tech Sports Med. 2007;15:165–77.
9. Meyers WC, Greenleaf R, Saad A. Anatomic basis for evaluation of abdominal and groin pain in athletes. Oper Tech Sports Med. 2005;13:55–61.
10. Steele P, Annear P, Grove JR. Surgery for posterior inguinal wall deficiency in athletes. J Sci Med Sport. 2004;7(4):415–21.
11. Ziprin P, Williams P, Foster ME. External oblique aponeurosis nerve entrapment as a cause of groin pain in the athlete. Br J Surg. 1999;86:566–8.

12. de Sa D, Holmich P, Phillips M, Heaven S, Simunovic N, Philippon MJ, et al. Athletic groin pain: a systematic review of surgical diagnoses, investigations, and treatment. Br J Sports Med. 2016;50:1181–6.
13. Hammoud S, Bedi A, Magennis E, Meyers WC, Kelly BT. High incidence of athletic pubalgia symptoms in professional athletes with symptomatic femoracetabular impingement. Arthroscopy: J Arthr Rel Surg. 2012;28:1388–95.
14. Mei-Dan O, Lopez V, Carmont MR, McConkey MO, Steinbacher G, Alvarez PD, et al. Adductor tenotomy as a treatment for groin pain in professional soccer players. Orthopedics. 2013;36(9):e1189-e1197.
15. Scholten PM, Massimi S, Dahmen N, Diamond J, Wyss J. Successful treatment of athletic pubalgia in a lacrosse player with ultrasound-guided needle tenotomy and platelet-rich plasma injection: a case report. PM&R. 2015;7(1):79–83.
16. Singh JR, Roza R, Bartolozzi AR. Platelet rich plasma therapy in an athlete with adductor longus tendon tear. U Penn Ortho J. 2010;20:42–3.
17. St-Onge E, Macintyre IG, Galea AM. Multidisciplinary approach to non-surgical management of inguinal disruption in a professional hockey player treated with platelet-rich plasma, manual therapy and exercise: a case report. J Can Chiropr Assoc. 2015;59(4):390–7.
18. Fader RR, Mitchell JJ, Traub S, et al. Platelet-rich plasma treatment improves outcomes for chronic proximal hamstring injuries in an athletic population. Muscles Ligaments Tendons J. 2014;4(4):461–6.
19. Ekstrand J, Ringborg S. Surgery versus conservative treatment in soccer players with chronic groin pain: a prospective randomized study in soccer players. Eur J Sports Traumatol Rel Res. 2001;23:141–5.
20. Paajanen H, Brinck T, Hermunen H, Airo I. Laparoscopic surgery for chronic groin pain in athletes is more effective than nonoperative treatment: a randomized clinical trial with magnetic resonance imaging of 60 patients with sportsman's hernia (athletic pubalgia). Surg. 2011;150:99–107.
21. Meyers WC, McKechnie A, Philippon MJ, Horner MA, Zoga AC, Devon ON. Experience with "sports hernia" spanning two decades. Ann Surg. 2008;248:656–65.
22. Muschaweck U, Berger L. Minimal repair technique of sportsmen's groin: an innovative open-suture repair to treat chronic inguinal pain. Hernia. 2010;14:27–33.
23. Lloyd Dm SCD, Altafa A, Fareed K, Bloxham L, Spencer L, et al. Laparoscopic inguinal ligament tenotomy and mesh reinforcement of the anterior abdominal wall: a new approach for the management of chronic groin pain. Surg Laparosc Endosc Percutan Tech. 2008;18:363–8.
24. Ingoldby CJ. Laparoscopic and conventional repair of groin disruption in sportsmen. Br J Surg. 1997;84(2):213–5.
25. Atkinson HD, Johal P, Falworth MS, Ranawat VS, Dala-Ali B, Martin DK. Adductor tenotomy: its role in the management of sports-related groin pain. Arch Orthop Trauma Surg. 2010;130:965–70.

26. Schilders E, Dimitrakopoulou A, Cooke M, Bismil Q, Cooke C. Effectiveness of a selective partial adductor release for chronic adductor-related groin pain in professional athletes. Am J Sports Med. 2013;41:603–7.

27. Vezeridis P, Gill TJ. Adductor injuries and the role of adductor tenotomy for groin pain in athletes. In: Diduch D, Brunt LM, editors. Sports hernia and athletic pubalgia: diagnosis and treatment. New York: Spring; 2014. p. 173–81.

28. Schlegel TF, Bushnell BD, Godfrey J, Boublik M. Success of nonoperative management of adductor longus tendon ruptures in National Football League athletes. Am J Sports Med. 2009;37:1394–9.

29. Ellsworth AA, Zoland MP, Tyler TF. Athletic pubalgia and associated rehabilitation. Int J Sports Phys Ther. 2014;9:774–84.

Inguinal Hernia Repair in Children

18

Domenic R. Craner, Ian C. Glenn,
and Todd A. Ponsky

Epidemiology

Inguinal hernia repair is one of the most common procedures performed by pediatric surgeons across the world. The incidence of inguinal hernia in male children is higher than that in females, by almost a 10:1 ratio [1]. The overall incidence in children worldwide is often quoted as being 0.8–4% and decreasing as age increases, with 85% of hernias presenting as unilateral [1, 2]. Studies have hypothesized that the incidence of patent processus vaginalis without hernia, however, is much higher. Weaver and colleagues identified 20% of their patients who underwent any type of laparoscopic procedure to have an asymptomatic patent processus vaginalis, while only 6% of patients identified with a patent processus vaginalis ever returned to their clinic with inguinal hernia symptoms [3].

In children, inguinal hernias are generally a congenital disease, with the indirect type being the more commonly occurring defect. A direct hernia in the pediatric population is a rare finding, with the incidence often being estimated as less than 1% of all inguinal hernias in children. Some risk factors for inguinal hernia in children and infants include prematurity and low birth weight.

In patients under 18 years of age, incarceration occurs in 6–18% of inguinal hernias and commonly involving the bowel or omentum, as well as ovaries in females. The highest risk of incarceration is during infancy, occurring at a rate of 30% [4].

Pathophysiology

The pathophysiology of indirect inguinal hernia in children is related to defects in the development of the gonads and abdominal wall, occurring well before the birth of the child. The gonads begin to form around the 5th week of gestation and start their descent around 7 months gestation. The descent occurs along the gubernaculum, inside a peritoneal diverticulum referred to as the processus vaginalis, in the direction of the internal ring.

In normal development, the processus vaginalis should obliterate between 36 and 40 weeks gestation, with complete closure occurring in 60% of children within the first 2 years of life [5, 6]. Failure of closure of the processus vaginalis creates a communication between the scrotum and the peritoneal cavity which allows for abdominal contents to descend. In females, it is the canal of Nuck which undergoes closure, analogous to the processus vaginalis. Persistence of the canal of Nuck allows for inguinal hernias in females.

D. R. Craner · I. C. Glenn · T. A. Ponsky (✉)
Akron Children's Hospital, Department of Pediatric
Surgery, Akron, OH, USA

© Springer International Publishing AG, part of Springer Nature 2018
M. P. LaPinska, J. A. Blatnik (eds.), *Surgical Principles in Inguinal Hernia Repair*,
https://doi.org/10.1007/978-3-319-92892-0_18

Diagnosis

The diagnosis of inguinal hernia is typically made clinically. Most inguinal hernias are asymptomatic. Physical exam is the most reliable method for diagnosis, especially when paired with history of an inguinal or scrotal bulge [6]. However, patients may present with signs of obstruction, localized erythema, and nausea/vomiting which can be indicative of a more acute and emergent problem. More commonly, inguinal hernias will present as right-sided defect.

Imaging is not required for the diagnosis of inguinal hernia. However, ultrasound has occasionally been used to identify structures contained within the hernia. It should be noted that negative ultrasound findings do not necessarily rule out the presence of inguinal hernia [6].

Management

Expectant versus surgical management of pediatric inguinal hernias is controversial. There is great debate over the appropriate timing for repair. In children, there is a much higher rate of incarceration of inguinal hernia than in adults. Thus, pediatric repairs should be performed in a more expeditious manner. There are a variety of techniques currently employed by pediatric surgeons for repair, both open and laparoscopic.

Open Repair

Even with the advancing technology of laparoscopic repair, open herniorrhaphy is still considered the gold standard for repair of inguinal hernias in the pediatric population. The open repair technique involves an inguinal crease incision, followed by sharp and blunt dissection through Scarpa's fascia to the external oblique aponeurosis. The external oblique aponeurosis is sharply incised to exposed the internal inguinal ring and allow for a view of the inguinal canal. The ilioinguinal nerve, vas deferens, and gonadal vessels are identified and moved away from the sac for protection. Next, the hernia sac is clamped

and divided, with any sac contents reduced as needed, followed by ligation of the patent processus vaginalis with 3-0 or 4-0 braided absorbable sutures [7]. There is no indication for the use of mesh in the pediatric population.

Laparoscopic Repair

Initially performed only in females due to fear of injury to the vas deferens, the laparoscopic hernia repair technique was first described in 1997 by El-Gohary [8]. In 2000, Schier described laparoscopic technique for hernioplasty in both sexes [9]. Now, there are multiple techniques for laparoscopic herniorrhaphy, ranging from single-port techniques to multiple-port technique as well as intra- and extraperitoneal ligation of the patent processus vaginalis. While there are multiple laparoscopic approaches, there is little evidence supporting one single technique [10]. Choice of laparoscopic approach is largely surgeon preference. Here we will discuss various methods of both techniques, paying extra attention to the extraperitoneal repairs.

Intraperitoneal Repair

Intraperitoneal repair methods involve accessing the abdomen laparoscopically and then ligating the patent processus vaginalis completely intraperitoneally. These options often involve a minimum of two laparoscopic ports and can consist of excision of the hernia sac by itself, suture ligation, or even a combination [10]. The first of these approaches to be described was Schier's in 1998 where he used two or three Z-stitches to bring the edges of the ring together creating a closure. This was initially only conducted in females; it has been successfully performed in males as well [9, 11]. Of note, this technique was later shown to have very high recurrence rate [10].

In 2004, Yip and colleagues [12] described a "laparoscopic flip-flap hernioplasty." This technique involves dividing the anterolateral border of the hernia sac at the level of the internal ring and then bringing it medially. The lateral edge is then sewn to the medial edge of the internal ring which closes the patent processus vaginalis while also moving the closing site away from the opening in the muscle. Also in 2004, Becmeur described a technique consisting of incision of the peritoneum on the external portion of the internal inguinal ring, dividing the processus vaginalis, and subsequent stitching of the edges of the peritoneum with 3-0 Vicryl suture [13].

Zallen and Glick [14] described a technique referred to as the laparoscopic inversion ligation used solely for hernia repair in females, which involves inserting graspers through abdominal wall stab incisions made bilaterally at the level of the anterior iliac crest. Contralateral to the defect, an Endoloop with absorbable monofilament suture is placed around the opening to the patent processus vaginalis. The ipsilateral grasper is placed through the Endoloop and into the processus vaginalis. The sac is grasped and then inverted (into the peritoneal cavity) allowing for dissection to be performed to free the contents of the sac. Following this, a second Endoloop is placed around the processus vaginalis, which is twisted until high ligation is completed.

Another intraperitoneal technique of note is the laparoscopic sac excision described by Riquelme, which involves resection of the peritoneal sac associated with the processus vaginalis with no ligation [15]. In this technique, blunt and sharp dissection of hernia sac is followed by eversion of the sac into the peritoneal cavity. A small cut is made in the parietal peritoneum above the internal inguinal ring. Following dissection of the hernia sac away from the gonadal vasculature and vas deferens, a small portion of peritoneum is taken, leaving a small, circular area of deperitonealized surface around the internal ring. The hernia sac is then completely resected allowing the peritoneal scar tissue to close around the ring and obliterate the patent processus vaginalis.

Extraperitoneal Repair

Our preferred method of repair involves using a percutaneous inguinal ring suturing (PIRS) technique, which is a modification of the technique described by Patkowski et al. [10, 16]:

- Prior to beginning the procedure, two 18G spinal needles are bent into a gentle curve and threaded with a looped 3-0 monofilament suture, with the loop coming out of the tip of the needle. The loop is pulled just inside the tip of the needle.
- Local anesthesia is injected and an umbilical incision is made. A Veress needle is used for insufflation of the abdomen to 8–10 mmHg (Fig. 18.1).
- A 3-mm port is placed, a 3-mm 70° scope inserted, and the internal ring is identified. The contralateral side is also inspected for a patent processus vaginalis or undiagnosed hernia, although there is controversy regarding the need for repair of asymptomatic patent processus vaginalis without hernia.
- Another 3-mm stab incision is made in the ipsilateral lower abdominal quadrant and a 3-mm Maryland dissector is placed through the incision. This is used to assist in passing the peritoneum over the needle and to cauterize the peritoneum for scar formation.
- The peritoneum is then cauterized from the 8 o'clock to 5 o'clock position of the internal ring (opposite the cord structures), with care taken to spare the area overlying the cord structures as shown in Fig. 18.2.

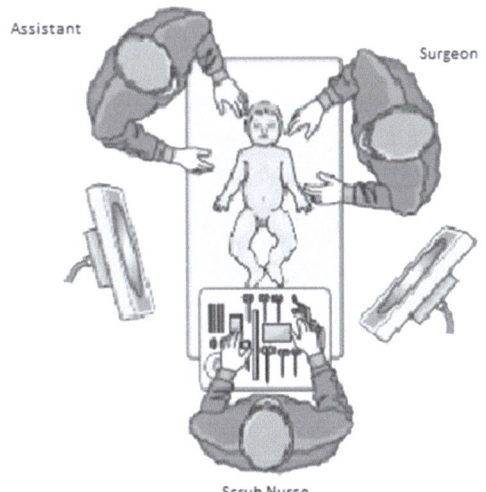

Fig. 18.1 Patient positioning and proper preparation of operative field [17]

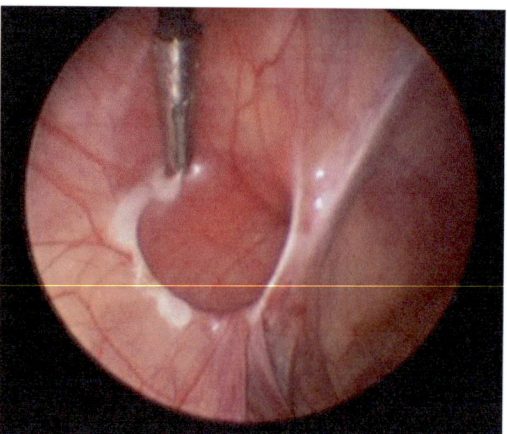

Fig. 18.2 Peritoneum is cauterized from the 8 o'clock to 5 o'clock position of the internal ring

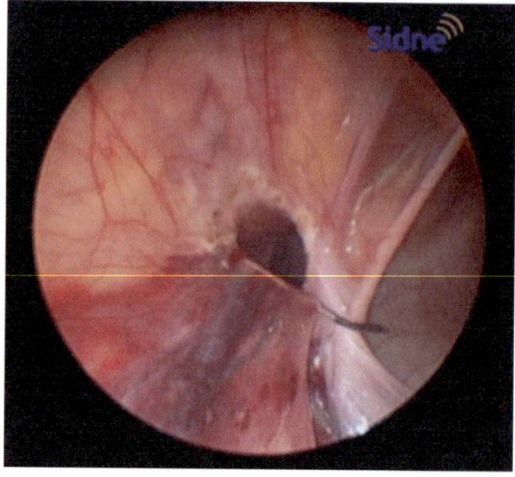

Fig. 18.3 18G spinal needle is passed *laterally* around the internal ring between the abdominal wall and peritoneum, where previously hydrodissected

- A 25-gauge finder needle is then used to identify the 12 o'clock position of the internal ring at the level of the patent processus vaginalis, and a 1-mm skin incision is made at this point.
- Hydrodissection beneath the peritoneum is performed, using local anesthetic, to elevate the peritoneum away from the abdominal wall and cord structures.
- The previously prepared 18G spinal needle is passed through the 1-mm skin incision until seen beneath the peritoneum at 12 o'clock position. It is then passed *laterally* around the internal ring between the abdominal wall and peritoneum, where previously hydrodissected (Fig. 18.3).
- The needle is passed beneath the peritoneum, over the vessels and vas deferens. The Maryland grasper may be used to assist with lifting the peritoneum away from the cord structures.
- The spinal needle is pushed through the peritoneum into the peritoneal cavity once the vessels have been traversed. The loop of suture is pushed out of the needle.
- The needle is then removed, leaving the looped suture in place with tails exiting the skin incision.
- Repeat the previous step with 18G needle passing from the 12 o'clock position *medially* around the ring.

- The needle is passed through the initially placed suture loop, and the laterally placed loop is pulled snug against the needle. The threaded suture contained in the needle is pushed out into the peritoneal cavity.
- The needle is removed, resulting in the lateral loop snuggly securing the medial loop, thereby functioning as a snare.
- The lateral suture is pulled out of the peritoneal cavity pulling the medial loop circumferentially around the ring and out through the skin.
- A braided, nonabsorbable suture is passed through the monofilament loop currently around the hernia sac, and the free ends of monofilament are pulled retrograde, in order to pull the braided suture through the same space around the internal ring and out through the skin incision.
- The looped, braided suture is then cut at the apex of loop allowing for a double ligation of the ring.
- The suture is then tied, obliterating the hernia sac. The knot is positioned in the subcutaneous tissue.
- The umbilical incision is closed with absorbable 3-0 suture. The skin at the umbilicus and the inguinal puncture sites are closed with surgical glue.

While the PIRS technique is our preferred method for inguinal hernia repair, it is important that we also discuss the other laparoscopic techniques that are successfully employed for herniorrhaphy in pediatric populations.

Another technique, the subcutaneous endoscopically assisted ligation, was described by Michael Harrison [18]:

- A 2.7-mm 30° scope is passed through a 3-mm umbilical port so that both sides can be visualized allowing for diagnosis of an occult contralateral defect.
- The internal ring is visualized and identified with the use of the endoscope.
- At the point of the abdominal wall superficial to the internal ring, a suture on a large needle (T12 or T20) is passed from one side through the extraperitoneal space surrounding the internal ring and out of the skin, avoiding the cord structures.
- The needle is then "backed" through the subcutaneous tissue anterior to the internal ring, and the butt end is brought through the original stab wound.
- The suture is then tied, obliterating the internal ring with the vas and vessels remaining outside the obliterated ring.
- There are many variations to this technique.

Yeung [19] has described his own technique involving extraperitoneal ligation of the processus vaginalis:

- Infraumbilical incision is made and a 3- or 5-mm cannula is inserted.
- A 2- to 3-mm stab incision made at a point midway between umbilicus and pubic.
- A 3-mm laparoscopic grasper, which will be used to provide countertraction of the peritoneum during dissection of the hernia sac, is passed through the stab incision under laparoscopic guidance.
- Herniotomy hook is prepared by threading a looped 3-0 polydioxanone suture through the tip to form two loops.
- An additional 2-mm stab incision is made at the 12 o'clock position superficial to the internal inguinal orifice so that the tip of the blade is just visible underneath, but not penetrating, the peritoneum.
- The loaded herniotomy hook is passed through the second stab incision until the tip is seen stretching the peritoneum at the level of inguinal ring.
- The hook is manipulated in the extraperitoneal plane to dissect the peritoneum circumferentially around the ring, and off surrounding structures, while using the grasper to provide countertraction intraperitoneally.
- Dissection is carried out from anterior to posterior and lateral to medial on right-sided hernias, vice versa on the left side.
- Once the hook is passed over the vas deferens and spermatic vessels, the tip is rotated toward the peritoneal cavity to pierce through the peritoneum into the abdominal cavity.
- The grasper is used to take the double suture loop from the hook and bring it into abdominal cavity.
- The hook is withdrawn through its original tract with the suture withdrawn to the previous 12 o'clock position and then passed around the other half of the circumference of the internal orifice just beneath the peritoneum until the point where the suture exits into the peritoneal cavity.
- Dissection is completed, and the herniotomy hook is manipulated through the opening that the suture loop exits into the peritoneal cavity.
- Now the double suture loop should completely encircle the neck of the hernia sac.
- The abdomen is desufflated and the sutures tied securely, enclosing only the peritoneal layer, while excluding other intervening tissues.

Controversy in Repair

There continues to be controversy as to the most appropriate surgical approach for repair of inguinal hernia in children. With the advancement of laparoscopic technique, the argument for laparoscopic over open repair has grown stronger. Studies have demonstrated that laparoscopic repair has a diminished risk for complications when compared with open technique [20]. Furthermore, in unilateral and recurrent hernia, laparoscopic repair has shown decreased operative times in the pediatric population. Previous authors have concluded that laparoscopic repair is also technically easier than open repair. This is due to the ability of the laparoscopic surgeon to identify the important anatomic structures in a way not capable in open techniques [21]. Due to these findings, there have been many evidence-based proposals to make laparoscopic repair the standard for hernia repair in children. However, these recommendations have not been widely adopted.

Special Considerations

While most of the techniques discussed above are used for uncomplicated repairs, there are many circumstances that can change the management of inguinal hernias in children.

Incarcerated Hernias

The greatest risk of an unrepaired inguinal hernia is incarceration/strangulation. In fact, this is the most frequent complication of not surgically repairing an inguinal hernia. While the repair of the actual, anatomic defect resembles that of the unincarcerated hernia, there are measures that must be taken in terms of reduction of the incarcerated hernia.

Presentation

Incarcerated hernias in children can present in a multitude of ways. Most commonly, incarcerated hernias contain ovaries, omentum, small bowel, and appendix [22]. Children can often appear with signs of obstruction such as abdominal pain and nausea/vomiting. As well, they can appear tachycardic and toxic when the incarceration has progressed to contain strangulated and dead tissue.

Manual Reduction of Incarcerated Hernia

In many patients presenting with incarcerated inguinal hernia, it is safe to proceed with manual reduction, as the patient is not exhibiting signs or symptoms of ischemic or necrotic bowel. Manual reduction has been shown to be successful in 70–95% of cases of incarcerated inguinal hernia [6]. Due to the anatomic nature of incarceration and the likelihood of edematous bowel, it is often difficult to manually push the hernia contents back through the external ring by applying direct pressure to the hernia contents alone. Consequently, we recommend applying pressure with one hand above the external ring to keep the hernia contents fixed in place. A second hand is simultaneously used to push the hernia contents slowly back through the defect. By using two hands and applying pressure to both the contents and above the external ring, the tendency for bowel to slide superior to (instead of into) the external ring is often inhibited. The continuous, direct pressure applied to the bowel also allows for some of the bowel edema to be pushed out. This technique should be performed slowly and can often take 5–10 min to complete [6].

Surgical Management

The standard management of incarcerated hernia is an attempt at manual reduction of the hernia contents upon initial presentation, unless there is concern for bowel perforation or strangulation. If the hernia can be manually reduced, then repair is frequently delayed for 1–2 days to allow resolution of inflammation of tissues [23]. Inability to manually reduce the hernia is an indication for urgent surgical management [6].

Once the decision to treat surgically has been made, one should determine the appropriate technique. Many of the open and laparoscopic techniques described previously have been employed for surgical treatment of incarcerated hernia, with variations to account for the incarcerated contents. Following closure of the processus vaginalis, and repair of the hernia, abdominal contents should be thoroughly examined for viability and injury. Repair and resection should take place as needed.

Controversies in Management of Incarceration

As laparoscopic technique has advanced, the argument over open versus laparoscopic management has shifted to include incarcerated hernias as well. While open repair is more commonly used, laparoscopic repair has been shown to have similar outcomes [24]. As well, there are many benefits to the laparoscopic repair that open techniques do not provide. The insufflation of the abdominal compartment with carbon dioxide allows for widening of the internal inguinal ring, providing for easier reduction of incarcerated contents if manual reduction is unsuccessful. Additionally, the incarcerated bowel can be visualized after it is reduced to assess viability which may not be fully examined during open repair [23]. However, neither technique is without complication.

Most agree that when a patient presents with an incarcerated hernia, it is best to attempt manual reduction of hernia, and if successful, then plan on hernia repair in 24 h to 5 days of presentation [25, 26]. Delaying repair allows for the tissue to become less inflamed, thus allowing for a safer repair. However, there is an increased risk for re-incarceration if repair is delayed [26]. Studies have reported an incidence of re-incarceration to be above 50% [27].

Recurrence Rates

The most common complication in inguinal hernia repair is recurrence. However, it is difficult to compare recurrence rates among techniques due to variation in patient follow-up between studies.

It has been estimated that the recurrence rate of the open is 1–2%, with 96% of those recurrences occurring within 5 years of repair [28]. Recurrence rates for laparoscopic repair have been found to be between 0 and 5.5% [4, 21, 29]. When comparing open and laparoscopic technique, some studies have shown a trend toward higher rates of recurrence for the laparoscopic technique. In a meta-analysis in 2011, Alzahem and colleagues showed a 2% versus 4% difference between open and laparoscopic technique,

respectively. However, this was not statistically significant [30].

Most of the comparative studies in pediatric hernia repair are between open and laparoscopic repairs. However, Shalaby et al. [31] analyzed intraperitoneal and extraperitoneal repairs. They found a statistically significant difference between the two techniques in terms of recurrence, with 4% of the intraperitoneal group experiencing a recurrence, while only 1.3% of the extraperitoneal group experienced a recurrence within 24 months postoperatively. There could certainly be benefit to further comparison between the various laparoscopic techniques for management of inguinal hernia.

The Role of Scar Tissue

Multiple studies, in both the adult [32–34] and pediatric populations [35, 36], have described open, indirect inguinal herniorrhaphy with excision of the hernia sac, but without suture ligation. This is predicated upon the belief that the key to closure is not the ligation of the sac but scarring of the sac from the injury from dividing it.

The authors tested the role of injury in the laparoscopic repair [37] by simulating a pediatric laparoscopic inguinal hernia showed in rabbits and found that intentional sharp trauma to the internal inguinal ring plus suture repair was superior to suture repair alone.

The best evidence to date for the significance of scar formation comes from Riquelme et al. [15]. Patients with internal rings of 10-mm diameter or less were successfully treated with laparoscopic resection of the patent processus vaginalis and associated peritoneum without suture. In addition to potentially shorter operative times, the primary advantage of this technique is reducing the risk of damage to the spermatic cord structures.

Conclusions

In conclusion, inguinal hernia repair is one of the most commonly performed procedures for the pediatric surgeon. Understanding the anatomy and pathophysiology of the childhood hernia can help a surgeon to choose the best possible method of repair. Here we have presented multiple repair techniques which are employed throughout the world. It is important to continue to develop these techniques to minimize complications and the need for future repeat repairs.

References

1. Chang SJ, Chen JY, Hsu CK, Chuang FC, Yang SS. The incidence of inguinal hernia and associated risk factors of incarceration in pediatric inguinal hernia: a nation-wide longitudinal population-based study. Hernia. 2016;20(4):559–63. Epub 2015/11/30, PubMed PMID: 26621139. https://doi.org/10.1007/s10029-015-1450-x.

2. Esposito C, Escolino M, Turrà F, Roberti A, Cerulo M, Farina A, et al. Current concepts in the management of inguinal hernia and hydrocele in pediatric patients in laparoscopic era. Semin Pediatr Surg. 2016;25(4):232–40. Epub 2016/05/11, PubMed PMID: 27521714. https://doi.org/10.1053/j.sempedsurg.2016.05.006.

3. Weaver KL, Poola AS, Gould JL, Sharp SW, St Peter SD, Holcomb GW. The risk of developing a symptomatic inguinal hernia in children with an asymptomatic patent processus vaginalis. J Pediatr Surg. 2017;52(1):60–4. Epub 2016/10/28, PubMed PMID: 27842956. https://doi.org/10.1016/j.jpedsurg.2016.10.018.

4. Esposito C, Escolino M, Cortese G, Aprea G, Turrà F, Farina A, et al. Twenty-year experience with laparoscopic inguinal hernia repair in infants and children: considerations and results on 1833 hernia repairs. Surg Endosc. 2016. Epub 2016/08/05, PubMed PMID: 27495342;31:1461. https://doi.org/10.1007/s00464-016-5139-8.

5. Rowe MI, Copelson LW, Clatworthy HW. The patent processus vaginalis and the inguinal hernia. J Pediatr Surg. 1969;4(1):102–7. PubMed PMID: 5779274

6. Abdulhai S, Glenn I, Ponsky T. Incarcerated pediatric hernias. Surg Clin N Am. 2017;97:129–45.

7. Fraser J, Inguinal Hernias SC. Hydroceles. In: Holcomb G, Murphy P, Ostlie D, editors. Ashcraft's pediatric surgery. 6th ed. New York: Elsevier; 2014. p. 679–88.

8. El-Gohary M. Laparoscopic ligation of inguinal hernia in girls. Pediatr Endosurg Innov Techn. 1997;1:185–8.

9. Schier F. Laparoscopic surgery of inguinal hernias in children--initial experience. J Pediatr Surg. 2000;35(9):1331–5. https://doi.org/10.1053/jpsu.2000.9326. PubMed PMID: 10999691

10. Ostlie DJ, Ponsky TA. Technical options of the laparoscopic pediatric inguinal hernia repair. J Laparoendosc Adv Surg Tech A. 2014;24(3):194–8.

https://doi.org/10.1089/lap.2014.0081. PubMed PMID: 24625350

11. Schier F. Laparoscopic herniorrhaphy in girls. J Pediatr Surg. 1998;33(10):1495–7. PubMed PMID: 9802799

12. Yip KF, Tam PK, Li MK. Laparoscopic flip-flap hernioplasty: an innovative technique for pediatric hernia surgery. Surg Endosc. 2004;18(7):1126–9. Epub 2004. PubMed PMID: 15162239.

13. Becmeur F, Philippe P, Lemandat-Schultz A, Moog R, Grandadam S, Lieber A, et al. A continuous series of 96 laparoscopic inguinal hernia repairs in children by a new technique. Surg Endosc. 2004;18(12):1738–41. Epub 2004/10/26, PubMed PMID: 15809780. https://doi.org/10.1007/s00464-004-9008-5.

14. Zallen G, Glick PL. Laparoscopic inversion and ligation inguinal hernia repair in girls. J Laparoendosc Adv Surg Tech A. 2007;17(1):143–5. https://doi.org/10.1089/lap.2006.0553. PubMed PMID: 17362194

15. Riquelme M, Aranda A, Riquelme-Q M. Laparoscopic pediatric inguinal hernia repair: no ligation, just resection. J Laparoendosc Adv Surg Tech A. 2010;20(1):77–80. https://doi.org/10.1089/lap.2008.0329. PubMed PMID: 19489678

16. Patkowski D, Czernik J, Chrzan R, Jaworski W, Apoznański W. Percutaneous internal ring suturing: a simple minimally invasive technique for inguinal hernia repair in children. J Laparoendosc Adv Surg Tech A. 2006;16(5):513–7. https://doi.org/10.1089/lap.2006.16.513. PubMed PMID:17004880

17. Schier F. Laparoscopic herniorraphy. In: Bax KMA, Georgeson KE, Rothenberg SS, Valla JS, Yeung CK, editors. Endoscopic surgery in infants and children. 1st ed. New York: Springer; 2008. p. 575–84.

18. Harrison MR, Lee H, Albanese CT, Farmer DL. Subcutaneous endoscopically assisted ligation (SEAL) of the internal ring for repair of inguinal hernias in children: a novel technique. J Pediatr Surg. 2005;40(7):1177–80. https://doi.org/10.1016/j.jpedsurg.2005.03.075. PubMed PMID: 16034766

19. Yeung C, Lee K. Inguinal herniotomy: laparoscopic-assisted extraperitoneal technique. In: Bax K, Georgeson K, Rothenberg S, Valla J, Yeung C, editors. Endoscopic surgery in infants and children. Berlin/Heidleberg: Springer; 2008. p. 591–6.

20. Feng S, Zhao L, Liao Z, Chen X. Open versus laparoscopic inguinal Herniotomy in children: a systematic review and meta-analysis focusing on postoperative complications. Surg Laparosc Endosc Percutan Tech. 2015;25(4):275–80. https://doi.org/10.1097/SLE.0000000000000161. PubMed PMID: 26018053

21. Parelkar SV, Oak S, Gupta R, Sanghvi B, Shimoga PH, Kaltari D, et al. Laparoscopic inguinal hernia repair in the pediatric age group--experience with 437 children. J Pediatr Surg. 2010;45(4):789–92. https://doi.org/10.1016/j.jpedsurg.2009.08.007. PubMed PMID: 20385288

22. Esposito C, Turial S, Alicchio F, Enders J, Castagnetti M, Krause K, et al. Laparoscopic repair of incarcer-

ated inguinal hernia. A safe and effective procedure to adopt in children. Hernia. 2013;17(2):235–9. Epub 2012/07/08, PubMed PMID: 22772871. https://doi.org/10.1007/s10029-012-0948-8.

23. Kaya M, Hückstedt T, Schier F. Laparoscopic approach to incarcerated inguinal hernia in children. J Pediatr Surg. 2006;41(3):567–9. https://doi.org/10.1016/j.jpedsurg.2005.11.066. PubMed PMID: 16516636

24. Mishra PK, Burnand K, Minocha A, Mathur AB, Kulkarni MS, Tsang T. Incarcerated inguinal hernia management in children: 'a comparison of the open and laparoscopic approach'. Pediatr Surg Int. 2014;30(6):621–4. Epub 2014/05/08, PubMed PMID: 24805115. https://doi.org/10.1007/s00383-014-3507-9.

25. Vaos G, Gardikis S, Kambouri K, Sigalas I, Kourakis G, Petoussis G. Optimal timing for repair of an inguinal hernia in premature infants. Pediatr Surg Int. 2010;26(4):379–85. Epub 2010/02/19, PubMed PMID: 20169441. https://doi.org/10.1007/s00383-010-2573-x.

26. Gahukamble DB, Khamage AS. Early versus delayed repair of reduced incarcerated inguinal hernias in the pediatric population. J Pediatr Surg. 1996;31(9):1218–20. PubMed PMID: 8887087

27. Niedzielski J, Kr 1 R, Gawłowska A. Could incarceration of inguinal hernia in children be prevented? Med Sci Monit. 2003;9(1):CR16–8. PubMed PMID: 12552244

28. Ein SH, Njere I, Ein A. Six thousand three hundred sixty-one pediatric inguinal hernias: a 35-year review. J Pediatr Surg. 2006;41(5):980–6. https://doi.org/10.1016/j.jpedsurg.2006.01.020. PubMed PMID: 16677897

29. Schier F. Laparoscopic inguinal hernia repair-a prospective personal series of 542 children. J Pediatr Surg. 2006;41(6):1081–4. https://doi.org/10.1016/j.jpedsurg.2006.02.028. PubMed PMID: 16769338

30. Alzahem A. Laparoscopic versus open inguinal herniotomy in infants and children: a meta-analysis. Pediatr Surg Int. 2011;27(6):605–12. https://doi.org/10.1007/s00383-010-2840-x. PubMed PMID: 21290136

31. Shalaby R, Ismail M, Dorgham A, Hefny K, Alsaied G, Gabr K, et al. Laparoscopic hernia repair in infancy and childhood: evaluation of 2 different techniques. J Pediatr Surg. 2010;45(11):2210–6. https://doi.org/10.1016/j.jpedsurg.2010.07.004. PubMed PMID: 21034946

32. Jiang ZP, Yang B, Wen LQ, Zhang YC, Lai DM, Li YR, et al. The etiology of indirect inguinal hernia in adults: congenital or acquired? Hernia. 2015;19(5):697–701. Epub 2014/11/28, PubMed PMID: 25431254. https://doi.org/10.1007/s10029-014-1326-5.

33. Othman I, Hady HA. Hernia sac of indirect inguinal hernia: invagination, excision, or ligation? Hernia. 2014;18(2):199–204. Epub 2013/04/02, PubMed PMID: 23546863. https://doi.org/10.1007/s10029-013-1081-z.

34. Gharaibeh KI, Matani YY. To ligate or not to ligate the hernial sac in adults? Saudi Med J. 2000;21(11):1068–70. PubMed PMID: 11360071

35. Ali K, Kamran H, Khattak IU, Latif H, Non-ligation of Indirect Hernial sac in children. J Ayub Med Coll Abbottabad. 2015;27(1):180–2. PubMed PMID: 26182771

36. Mohta A, Jain N, Irniraya KP, Saluja SS, Sharma S, Gupta A. Non-ligation of the hernial sac during herniotomy: a prospective study. Pediatr Surg Int. 2003;19(6):451–2. Epub 2003/05/28, PubMed PMID: 12774253. https://doi.org/10.1007/s00383-002-0940-y.

37. Blatnik JA, Harth KC, Krpata DM, Kelly KB, Schomisch SJ, Ponsky TA. Stitch versus scar--evaluation of laparoscopic pediatric inguinal hernia repair: a pilot study in a rabbit model. J Laparoendosc Adv Surg Tech A. 2012;22(8):848–51. Epub 2012/09/18, PubMed PMID: 22989037. https://doi.org/10.1089/lap.2012.0137.

Inguinal Hernia Repair in the Setting of Bowel Injury/Resection

19

Garth R. Jacobsen and Jessica L. Reynolds

The use of permanent synthetic mesh in the repair of inguinal hernias is considered standard of care regardless of whether a laparoscopic or open approach is used. The use of mesh has been shown to reduce the recurrence rate tenfold to less than 1% compared to primary repair with no significant mesh-related complications [1, 2]. However, when repair of the inguinal hernia involves resection of the bowel or injury to the bowel, the use of mesh becomes more controversial due to concerns with seeding the mesh with enteric bacteria. This can be a devastating complication resulting in chronic mesh infection requiring mesh explantation. This question also arises when considering repair of an inguinal hernia during an unrelated abdominal procedure such as cholecystectomy or small bowel obstructions from adhesive disease or malignancy.

Inguinal hernia repair can involve a spectrum of contaminated wound classifications ranging from a clean-contaminated case that involves resection of a dusky loop of the bowel with minor spillage to contaminated cases involving injury to the bowel with gross spillage and dirty cases with perforation and necrosis. Our repair options depend on the level of contamination of the wound. It is important to keep in mind that there is no permanent synthetic mesh that is approved for use in contaminated fields, though it is becoming increasingly popular to use macroporous meshes in these situations. There is however abundant data related to the safe use of biologic or some absorbable synthetic meshes. Of course, the option is open to do a primary tissue repair in the acute setting a good one, with the option to perform a definitive laparoscopic or open repair should the patient develop a recurrence.

Clean Contaminated

The CDC defines a clean-contaminated wound in this case as one in which the alimentary tract was entered under controlled conditions and without unusual contamination. Current evidence would suggest that using appropriate synthetic mesh in clean-contaminated settings is safe with wound morbidity rates not significantly different from non-mesh repairs [3–8]. It is our practice to use lightweight, macroporous polypropylene mesh in these cases. It is also acceptable to use an absorbable mesh or biologic mesh.

Typically, a clean-contaminated case involves a strangulated hernia that requires resection of the reduced small bowel due to questionable viability, but there is no perforation. We prefer to approach incarcerated and strangulated hernias laparoscopically using a transabdominal

G. R. Jacobsen (✉) · J. L. Reynolds
University of California San Diego,
San Diego, CA, USA
e-mail: gjacobsen@ucsd.edu

© Springer International Publishing AG, part of Springer Nature 2018
M. P. LaPinska, J. A. Blatnik (eds.), *Surgical Principles in Inguinal Hernia Repair*,
https://doi.org/10.1007/978-3-319-92892-0_19

approach. After induction of anesthesia, the bowel usually can be reduced with a combination of gentle traction and external pressure and sometimes relaxing incisions. Once the bowel is reduced, it can be determined if it is not viable and will need resection. We proceed with repair of the hernia and mesh placement prior to resecting the bowel to allow the mesh to be placed in the preperitoneal space prior to contaminating the peritoneal space. We prefer the transabdominal approach as this offers the best access to the peritoneal cavity to further assess for bowel viability. After raising the peritoneal flap, reducing the hernia sack completely, and ensuring there is an adequate pocket for the mesh with good inferior and medial coverage of the myopectineal orifice, the mesh is tacked in place at Cooper's ligament and then superior on either side of the epigastric vessels. The peritoneal flap is then sutured closed with a running stich. In a clean-contaminated case, we recommend using a lightweight macroporous synthetic meshes as these have been shown to be more resistant to infection than other types of synthetic mesh while still being very durable. The bowel resection can then be completed either intracorporeally or extracorporeally by extending the umbilical incision.

If the bowel cannot be reduced laparoscopically as described above, it may be necessary to perform a relaxing incision. This is most typically utilized during incarcerated femoral hernias. The inguinal ligament can be incised using hook electrocautery anteriorly and medially. If reduction still cannot be achieved, a groin incision can be performed. The bowel resection can be done at this point if necessary allowing for reduction and subsequent anastomosis. The anastomosis can be done through the groin. If this is unsuccessful, then we would complete the bowel resection through the inguinal incision and repair the hernia using a Lichtenstein approach with lightweight macroporous polypropylene mesh.

Contaminated

The CDC defines a contaminated wound in this case as hernia-related bowel pathology in which gross spillage occurred. If the bowel injury and contamination occur during a laparoscopic procedure and the soilage is limited to the peritoneal cavity, then the best option is to convert to an open repair of the inguinal hernia, after repairing or resecting the injured bowel as described above. This avoids placing permanent mesh in the contaminated field and reduces the risk of mesh infection. If, however, there is gross spillage within the inguinal canal that would mandate exposure of the repair to the gross contamination, more care should be exercised. This is often the case in the late presenting patient with evidence of sepsis and some degree of ischemia in a large inguinal hernia but has not yet perforated. Though laparoscopy may be useful, anterior approach is often needed. Should resection be needed and spillage occur consideration for primary tissue-based repair should be had. One may also consider utilizing a biologic or absorbable synthetic mesh such as Gore Bio-A in the manner of Lichtenstein. Current data does not support the use of permanent synthetic mesh in this setting.

Dirty

Dirty wounds are those in which there is retained devitalized tissue and those that involve existing clinical infection or perforated viscera. The patient presentation is similar to the above but more extreme as the patient has now perforated the viscus. Patients who have a strangulated hernia with perforation and gross contamination in our practice are no longer considered a "hernia" case. The primary concern is to resect the bowel, wash out the contaminated space, and prevent intra-abdominal sepsis. This can be done through either an inguinal or abdominal incision. If the patient does not have peritonitis, we prefer an inguinal approach to limit the intra-abdominal contamination. The bowel usually can be pulled into the wound to perform the resection and anastomosis and then returned to the abdomen. If adequate length to do the resection cannot be achieved, the operation can be hybridized utilizing either a laparoscopic approach or a midline laparotomy. Again, the primary consideration in this case is a gastrointestinal one, and control of the bowel injury is the most important. Depending on the size of the hernia defect, it can then either be repaired primarily or repair can be staged. We do not routinely place any mesh, including absorbable or biologic, in a dirty wound, and prefer to stage the repair. If the patient is unstable, then the wound should just be washed out and closed over the drain with plans to return for repair of the hernia when the patient is stable and the wound is clean.

Patients who have peritonitis require a laparotomy with exploration and washout of the abdominal cavity in addition to bowel resection. We prefer a staged approach to hernia repair in these patients, first treating the bowel perforation and sepsis and returning to the OR for hernia repair when the infection has resolved.

<hr>

Conclusion

The repair of hernias in the face of concomitant bowel injury and resection should be addressed in a systematic fashion which is most easily approached by addressing the degree of wound contamination. We struggle as hernia surgeons to define the best repair for a clean groin hernia. Should we do open or laparoscopic? TEPP or TAPP? Mesh or no mesh? These questions are just as relevant in the approach to the inguinal hernia in the face of various degrees of contamination. However, we believe the systematic approach laid out above helps to prioritize the nature of the problem. Is the problem mostly hernia (clean contaminated) or mostly visceral (contaminated)? Once that determination has been made, the treatment options become clearer. The utilization of prosthetic meshes (particularly macroporous and certain absorbable synthetics) in these situations is becoming increasingly prevalent and in fact is likely safe for clean-contaminated wounds but more controversial in higher wound classification. Finally, as evidenced by the discussion above, the surgeon approaching inguinal hernia repair in this complex setting is best served by having knowledge and skill in a variety of laparoscopic and open techniques so as to best serve their patient.

<hr>

References

1. Amid PK, Shulman AG, Lichtenstein IL. Critical scrutiny of the open "tension-free" hernioplasty. Am J Surg. 1993;165:369–71.
2. Shulman AG, Amid PK, Lichtenstein IL. The safety of mesh repair for primary inguinal hernias: results of 3,019 operations from five diverse surgical sources. Am Surg. 1992;58:255–7.
3. Carbonell AM, Cobb WS. Safety of prosthetic mesh hernia repair in contaminated fields. Surg Clin N Am. 2013;93:1227–39.
4. Carbonell AM, Criss CN, Cobb WS, Novitsky YW, Rosen MJ. Outcomes of synthetic mesh in contaminated ventral hernia repairs. J Am Coll Surg. 2013;217:991–8.
5. Kelly ME, Behrman SW. The safety and efficacy of prosthetic hernia repair in clean-contaminated and contaminated wounds. Am Surg. 2002;68:524–8; discussion 528-529
6. Souza JM, Dumanian GA. Routine use of bioprosthetic mesh is not necessary: a retrospective review of 100 consecutive cases of intra-abdominal midweight polypropylene mesh for ventral hernia repair. Surgery. 2013;153:393–9.
7. Hentati H, Dougaz W, Dziri C. Mesh repair versus non-mesh repair for strangulated inguinal hernia: systematic review with meta-analysis. World J Surg. 2014;38:2784–90.
8. Bessa SS, Abdel-fattah MR, Al-Sayes IA, Korayem IT. Results of prosthetic mesh repair in the emergency management of the acutely incarcerated and/or strangulated groin hernias: a 10-year study. Hernia: J Hernias Abdominal Wall Surg. 2015;19:909–14.

Inguinal Hernia Repair Around Prostatectomy

20

Stephen Masnyj and Matthew I. Goldblatt

Introduction

Inguinal hernias and prostate cancer are two of the most common medical conditions affecting males in the United States today. The annual incidence of inguinal hernias is 0.5–1%, with a 25% lifetime risk in males [1]. The lifetime risk of developing prostate cancer is about 1 in 7, or 14% [2]. Inguinal hernia repair and radical prostatectomy are among the most frequently performed procedures in males. Given the demographic overlap between inguinal hernia and prostate cancer patients, there are a large number of patients undergoing radical prostatectomy who have had previous mesh inguinal hernia repair and vice versa. Today a majority of prostatectomies are performed using minimally invasive techniques, with either laparoscopic or robotic assistance. There has been a similar rise in minimally invasive surgery for inguinal herniorrhaphy. The aim of this chapter is to investigate this crossroads between radical prostatectomy (RP) and laparoscopic inguinal hernia repair (LIHR). We will investigate three distinct groups: those who undergo LIHR prior to prostatectomy, those who undergo concurrent LIHR and RP, and finally those who undergo LIHR following RP. The majority of the chapter will focus on the first group, with brief reviews of the data pertaining to the other two groups.

Anatomy

Minimally invasive techniques for LIHR and RP both share a common preperitoneal dissection plane. Dissection within the anatomical spaces of Retzius and Bogros is integral to proper performance of both procedures. Prior dissection within these spaces may compromise the future performance of RP after LIHR and vice versa. Understanding the anatomy of these shared spaces is integral to understanding why LIHR may interfere with RP.

The preperitoneal space is situated between the peritoneum posteriorly and the transversalis fascia anteriorly. Bogros described the homonymous space of Bogros in his 1823 thesis [3]. This triangular space lies between the iliac fascia, transversalis fascia, and parietal peritoneum. In 1858 Retzius went on to describe the prevesical space named for him. The space of Retzius lies anterior and lateral to the urinary bladder and posterior to the pubic symphysis. The space of Bogros is a lateral extension of the space of Retzius. With increased anatomic understanding of these two spaces, there has come an advancement of laparoscopic preperitoneal approaches to both inguinal hernia repair and prostatectomy. The preperitoneal space dissection was first

S. Masnyj · M. I. Goldblatt (✉)
Medical College of Wisconsin, Milwaukee, WI, USA
e-mail: mgoldbla@mcw.edu

utilized for ligation of inferior epigastric or exter-nal iliac artery aneurysms in the late 1800s. The first preperitoneal approach to herniorrhaphy was likely utilized by Annandale in 1876 [3]. In 1921 Cheatle described a preperitoneal approach to inguinal hernia repair using a paramedian incision to dissect within the space of Bogros. McKernon and Laws described the first total extraperitoneal approach to hernia repair in 1993 [4]. Since that time, LIHR has become a frequently performed procedure by general surgeons. Radical prosta-tectomy has undergone a similar revolution with the advancement of laparoscopic equipment and skills. More recently, robotic-assisted radical prostatectomy has become the favored procedure.

Laparoscopic Inguinal Hernia Repair Before Radical Retropubic Prostatectomy

With the increase in laparoscopic inguinal her-nia repairs, more men with prostate cancer are presenting with previous preperitoneal dissec-tion and mesh placement within the preperito-neal space. Radical retropubic prostatectomy requires development of this same preperitoneal space, which can be rendered inaccessible by prior mesh placement. In order to prevent hernia recurrence during repairs, the mesh must cover a large portion of the preperitoneal space. This mesh induces a local inflammatory response that leads to scar formation and distortion of the anatomical planes [5]. Subsequent development of Retzius' space during prostatectomy requires meticulous dissection through often-dense adhe-sions. This adds time to the procedure and may lead to increased complications.

In the early 2000s, case reports described aborted open radical prostatectomies in patients with prior LIHR. They blamed dense adhesions and an obliterated preperitoneal space secondary to the mesh placed at the time of inguinal hernia repair [6]. These papers called into question the safety and feasibility of radical prostatectomy following LIHR. Some went so far as to urge against performing LIHR in all males, because, they argued, it would make future prostatectomy

impossible. They argued that the preperitoneal space could not be created safely and that there was too high risk of injury to nerves and sur-rounding structures. In 2002 Katz et al. reported two of the first cases of aborted open retropubic prostatectomy following LIHR. In their first case, Retzius' space was completely obliterated by a large polypropylene mesh that took up the entire width of the pelvis and covered bilateral inguinal hernias. They encountered significant scarring and inflammation, the procedure was aborted, and the patient was treated with hormonal and radiation therapy. In a second case, the mesh was densely adherent to the endopelvic fascia, but they were able to remove it. In the process of removing the mesh, the anterior bladder wall was stripped, thus making subsequent urethrovesical anastomosis challenging. From their analysis of these two case reports, the authors concluded that laparoscopic inguinal hernia repair complicated and in some cases made it impossible to perform open retropubic radical prostatectomy. They urged general surgeons to counsel their patients prior to LIHR on the potential limitations the sur-gery could have on future prostatectomy.

Subsequent research has shown that despite the added difficulty, minimally invasive radical pros-tatectomy is both feasible and safe following lapa-roscopic inguinal hernia repair. A recent review by Haifler et al. attempted to synthesize the current data concerning LIHR before open, laparoscopic, or robotic-assisted RP (RARP) [7]. In their review, any of the three approaches to RP were found to be feasible and safe following LIHR. They also acknowledged the significant added technical difficulty imposed by the mesh and subsequent inflammatory response to the mesh.

Saint-Elie et al. reported on 21 cases of open prostatectomy after LIHR, wherein none of the operations had to be aborted. Operative time and blood loss were slightly increased, but they recorded no intraoperative complications. In six of the patients, complete pelvic lymph node dis-section was not possible due to prior LIHR [8].

Do and colleagues [9] investigated the feasibil-ity and safety of laparoscopic prostatectomy fol-lowing LIHR. Their larger cohort of 92 patients with prior LIHR had a higher complication rate at 12% vs 5.85% in those without prior LIHR; however this result was not statistically significant ($P = 0.06$). They noted no increase in operative time, transfusion rate, blood loss, or ability to perform a nerve sparing operation. In addition, they examined functional and oncological outcomes and found that their rate of positive margins was unaffected by prior preperitoneal mesh hernia repair. This is likely due to the fact that once the extraperitoneal space is developed, resection of the prostate can proceed in usual fashion. They reiterated that open RP seems to be more difficult to perform than laparoscopic RP following LIHR. They advocated for minimally invasive prostatectomy over open prostatectomy in cases that follow LIHR.

Another criticism of prior LIHR is that it complicates pelvic lymph node dissection at the time of prostatectomy. There is controversy over whether or not PLND affects overall prognosis of prostate cancer [10]. Extended lymphadenectomy may affect the clinical stage, but not the overall survival. The decision to perform PLND is based upon the T stage, serum PSA level, and Gleason score. Low-risk patients do not require extensive PLND. This includes patients with disease in one lobe of the prostate (T1–T2a), a serum PSA < 10 ng/mL, and a Gleason score ≤ 6. In addition nomograms exist that predict the probability of lymph node metastasis; and if the probability of lymph node spread is <2%, no PLND is recommended [11]. Adequate staging involves excision of four to ten lymph nodes according to Joslyn and Konety [12].

Pelvic lymphadenectomy involves clearance of nodes in the obturator fossa as well as along the external and internal iliac vessels up to where they bifurcate. Mesh placed at the time of LIHR often covers the external iliac and obturator fossa nodes, and may make their removal difficult, if not impossible. In the study by Do et al., 51 of their 92 patients required PLND. Of those 51 patients, 39 could only undergo unilateral PLND since the contralateral side had mesh [9]. Additionally, five patients with bilateral LIHR could not undergo PLND. Postoperative surveillance with PSA showed that at 6 and 12 months, there was no difference between those who had undergone previous LIHR and those who had not.

Over the last decade, robot-assisted radical prostatectomy (RARP) has taken over as the preferred operation for prostate cancer. The added maneuverability and visualization of RARP are especially beneficial for difficult dissections complicated by prior mesh LIHR. Siddiqui et al. [13] reported on a population of 3950 patients who underwent RARP, 166 of whom had previous inguinal hernia repair with mesh. Those with prior IHR had more extensive adhesions and required increased operative times. They noted no increase in blood loss or intraoperative complications and concluded that inguinal surgery was not a contraindication to performing RARP.

In a meta-analysis and systematic review, Picozzi et al. investigated the feasibility and outcomes of open, laparoscopic, and robotic-assisted radical prostatectomy following mesh herniorrhaphy [14]. They identified 7497 patients, 462 of which had undergone prior mesh IHR. In the open prostatectomy group, 159 of 1699 patients had undergone prior mesh IHR. There was no significant difference between groups in terms of blood loss and operative times. The number of lymph nodes removed and the length of hospital stay with catheterization were, however, statistically significant. The number of lymph nodes removed was three to four vs six to eight for patients without prior IHR. In the laparoscopic RP group, 116 study patients were compared to 2020 controls. They found no statistically significant difference between mesh and control groups in terms of blood loss, operative time, or catheterization time. Their data sets did not have enough information to make any assessment of lymph nodes removed or hospital stay. Finally, the authors investigated robotic prostatectomy after IHR, and 187 study patients were compared to 3475 controls. Due to lack of data comparison of blood loss, operative time, hospital stay, catheterization time, and number of lymph nodes could not be performed. The lack of data indicates a need for more research in patients with RARP after LIHR.

Spernat and colleagues performed a retrospective analysis of 57 patients who underwent RP after LIHR [15]. Of the 57 patients, 19 underwent open RP, 33 laparoscopic RP, and 5 robot-assisted RP. All cases were completed successfully. In terms of PLND, only 10 of 18 PLND were completed in the open, 4 of 22 in the laparoscopic, and 5 of 5 in the robot-assisted groups. In total, PLND was attempted in 44 patients; however it was unsuccessful in 25 of 44 patients. In other words, over 50% of the time, PLND was not possible in patients with prior LIHR. On the other hand, 100% of patients who underwent robot-assisted RP had a successful PLND, although this cohort was small. This study again demonstrates the possible superiority of robot assistance when it comes to performing the PLND, but more data is needed to draw any conclusions. The added visualization and maneuverability may make the dissection easier.

Regardless of the approach, RP after LIHR is both safe and feasible. The technical demands of the procedure are increased by prior mesh placement within the preperitoneal space. Despite the added difficulty, the number of intraoperative complications is not increased. Additionally, the oncological outcomes are similar. The biggest criticism of LIHR before RP is that PLND may be compromised. Completion of PLND has been described as the "Achilles heel" of RP after LIHR by several studies. This is particularly true during open and laparoscopic cases following LIHR. Robot-assisted surgery, on the other hand, claims to offer superior visualization and maneuverability, which make PLND feasible for most patients with previous LIHR. More data, however, is needed to further support RARP as the superior approach to prostate cancer patients with prior LIHR. RARP may in fact make the lymphadenectomy argument a mute point. Additional newer research is now calling into question the utility and added benefit of PLND for prostate cancer. Newer surveillance with PSA levels may also make PLND unnecessary.

The general surgeon should keep in mind the future implications of mesh LIHR on radical prostatectomy. Prior to operation, they must counsel their male patients on the potential complications the mesh can create at the time of prostatectomy. Men over 50 should be screened for prostate cancer with PSA testing prior to undergoing LIHR. At the time of LIHR, there are several steps the general surgeon can take to make future dissection of the preperitoneal space more amenable for the urologist. This includes not placing the mesh too far inferior to Cooper's ligament and the pubic ramus. In the case of bilateral inguinal hernia repair, two separate meshes should be placed with sparing of the midline [16]. When counseling patients with prior LIHR for prostatectomy, urologists must discuss the possibility of hernia recurrence, mesh infection, need for mesh explantation, and possibility that mesh may compromise completion of pelvic lymphadenectomy.

LIHR at the Same Time as Prostatectomy

Inguinal hernias are a common complication following radical prostatectomy. The rate of IH following radical prostatectomy was reported to be 11.9% by Regan and his group [17]. Zhu et al. reported a 15.9% inguinal hernia rate following open RP and a rate of 6.7% following laparoscopic RP [18]. Stranne et al. tracked inguinal hernia rates at 4 years following open radical prostatectomy compared to robot-assisted radical prostatectomy and found the rate to be 12.2% vs 5.8% [19]. In most cases, the hernias were apparent within 2 years of operation. The factors that contributed to hernias included a low BMI, advanced age, previous IH repair, and postoperative anastomotic stricture. Factors that did not contribute to IH rate included prostate-specific antigen level, hypertension, diabetes, and operative time. Nielsen evaluated the incidental inguinal hernia rate at the time of prostatectomy and noted a 33% hernia detection rate [20]. There is uncertainty as to whether the high inguinal hernia rate is from the dissection or rather a failure to detect and treat subclinical hernias at time of prostatectomy. Given the high incidence of postoperative as well as the high lifetime incidence of inguinal hernias in males, there is interest in treating subclinical inguinal hernias prophylactically at the time of prostatectomy. The question is whether this can be done safely and without risk of mesh complications.

Do et al. [21] reported on 93 cases of concurrent LIHR and laparoscopic preperitoneal radical prostatectomy. Repair was performed for all reducible hernias identified from 2125 consecutive prostatectomies. Most of the exposure and early dissection required for completion of LIHR was performed during their standard prostatectomy procedure. They noted no increase in postoperative complications such as lymphoceles, bladder neck stenosis, hernia recurrence, or mesh infection. Oncologic outcomes were unaffected as well. Celik report similarly low complication rates and no mesh-related infections without compromising either the cancer operation or the hernia repair [22]. They conclude that LIHR can be combined with prostatectomy without any adverse effects.

There are prophylactic procedures described in the urology literature that aid in preventing future occurrences of inguinal hernias. Extensive description of these procedures is beyond the scope of this text, but they do warrant some consideration. Some of these techniques included transection of the processus vaginalis during RP [23] or release of the spermatic cord from the peritoneum [24]. Both methods work by obliterating an easy pathway for a hernia sac to travel along the cord structures.

LIHR After Prostatectomy

Many surgeons consider previous radical prostatectomy a contraindication to laparoscopic inguinal hernia repair. The shared preperitoneal space used for dissection during both procedures becomes scarred down following prostatectomy. Additionally, any lower abdominal surgery complicates dissection within this plane. Dulucq et al. investigated the feasibility of totally extraperitoneal (TEP) hernia repair following prostatectomy or lower abdominal surgery [25]. They identified 202 patients undergoing TEP hernia repair, 10 who had prior prostatectomy and 15 who had prior lower abdominal surgery. They

noted increased difficulty of the dissection and three episodes of inferior epigastric artery bleeding that were all controlled laparoscopically. There were no hernia recurrences in any of the patients, regardless of prior surgical history. The authors conclude that TEP repair is both feasible and safe following prostatectomy or lower abdominal surgery. This study, like others that look at TEP after radical prostatectomy, is limited by small sample size and short follow-up. Most general surgeons, when faced with a post-prostatectomy inguinal hernia, would elect to use an open approach in order to avoid dissecting in a plane with a large amount of scar tissue. Laparoscopic approaches to post-prostatectomy hernias are best left up to those with experience working in the scarred down preperitoneal plane following prostatectomy.

References

1. Stranne J, Lodding P. Inguinal hernia after radical retropubic prostatectomy: risk factors and prevention. Nat Rev Urol. 2011;8:267.
2. Howlader N, Noone AM, Krapcho M, Miller D, Bishop K, Altekruse SF, Kosary CL, Yu M, Ruhl J, Tatalovich Z, Mariotto A, Lewis DR, Chen HS, Feuer EJ, Cronin KA (eds). SEER Cancer Statistics Review, 1975–2013, National Cancer Institute. Bethesda, http://seer.cancer.gov/csr/1975_2013/, based on November 2015 SEER data submission, posted to the SEER web site, April 2016.
3. Mirilas P, Colborn GL, McClusky DA III, et al. The history of anatomy and surgery of the preperitoneal space. Arch Surg. 2005;140(1):90–4.
4. JB MK, Laws HL. Laparoscopic repair of inguinal hernias using a totally extraperitoneal prosthetic approach. Surg Endosc. 1993;7:26–8.
5. LeBlanc KA, Booth WV, Whitaker JM, Baker D. In vivo study of meshes implanted over the inguinal ring and external iliac vessels of uncastrated pigs. Surg Endosc. 1998;12:247–51.
6. Katz EE, Patel RV, Sokoloff MH, et al. Bilateral inguinal hernia repair can complicate subsequent radical retropubic prostatectomy. J Urol. 2002;167:637–8.
7. Haifler M, Benjamin B, Ghinea R, Avital S. The impact of previous laparoscopic inguinal hernia repair on radical prostatectomy. J Endourol. 2012;26(11):1458–62. https://doi.org/10.1089/end.2012.0285. Epub 2012 Sep 13
8. Saint-Elie DT, Marshall FF. Impact of laparoscopic inguinal hernia repair mesh on open radical retropubic prostatectomy. Urology. 2010;76:1078–82.

9. Do HM, Turner K, Dietel A, et al. Previous laparoscopic inguinal hernia repair does not adversely affect the functional or oncological outcomes of endoscopic extraperitoneal radical prostatectomy. Urology. 2011;77:963–7.

10. DiMarco DS, Zincke H, Sebo TJ, et al. The extent of lymphadenectomy for pTXNO prostate cancer does not affect prostate cancer outcome in the prostate specific antigen era. J Urol. 2005;173:1121–5.

11. National Comprehensive Cancer Network (NCCN). NCCN Clinical practice guidelines in oncology. http://www.nccn.org/professionals/physician_gls/f_guidelines.asp.

12. Joslyn SA, Konety BR. Impact of extent of lymphadenectomy on survival after radical prostatectomy for prostate cancer. Urology. 2006;68:121–5.

13. Siddiqui SA, Krane LS, Bhandari A, et al. The impact of previous inguinal or abdominal surgery on outcomes after robotic radical prostatectomy. Urology. 2010;75:1079–82.

14. Picozzi SCM, Ricci C, Bonavina L, et al. Feasibility and outcomes regarding open and laparoscopic radical prostatectomy in patients with previous synthetic mesh inguinal hernia repair: meta-analysis and systematic review of 7,497 patients. World J Urol. 2015;33:59.

15. Spernat D, Sofield D, Moon D, Louie-Johnsun M, Woo H. Implications of laparoscopic inguinal hernia repair on open, laparoscopic, and robotic radical prostatectomy. Prostate Int. 2014;2:8–11.

16. Cooperberg MR, Downs TM, Carroll PR. Radical retropubic prostatectomy frustrated by prior laparoscopic mesh herniorrhaphy. Surgery. 2004;135:452–4.

17. Regan TC, Mordkin RM, Constantinople NL, et al. Incidence of inguinal hernias following radical retropubic prostatectomy. Urology. 1996;47:536.

18. Zhu S, Zhang H, Xie L, Chen J, Niu Y. Risk factors and prevention of inguinal hernia after radical prostatectomy: a systematic review and meta-analysis. J Urol. March 2013;189(3):884–90.

19. Stranne J, Johansson E, Nilsson A, Bill-Axelson A, Carlsson S, Holmberg L, et al. Inguinal hernia after radical prostatectomy for prostate cancer: results from a randomized setting and a nonrandomized setting. Eur Urol. 2010;58:719–26.

20. Nielsen ME, Walsh PC. Systematic detection and repair of subclinical inguinal hernias at radical retropubic prostatectomy. Urology. 2005;66:1034–7.

21. Do M, Liatsikos EN, Kallidonis P, Wedderburn AW, Dietel A, Turner KJ, et al. Hernia repair during endoscopic Extraperitoneal radical prostatectomy: outcome after 93 cases. J Endourol. April 2011;25(4):625–9.

22. Celik O, Akand M, Ekin G, Duman I, Ilbey YO, Erdogru T. Laparoscopic radical prostatectomy alone or with laparoscopic Herniorrhaphy. JSLS: J Soc Laparoendoscopic Surgeons. 2015;19(4):e2015.00090.

23. Fujii Y, Yamamoto S, Yonese J, Kawakami S, Okubo Y, Suyama T, et al. A novel technique to prevent post-radical retropubic prostatectomy inguinal hernia: the processus vaginalis transection method. Urology. 2010;75:713–7.

24. Stranne J, Aus G, Bergdahl S, Damber JE, Hugosson J, Khatami A, et al. Post-radical prostatectomy inguinal hernia: a simple surgical intervention can substantially reduce the incidence – results from a prospective randomized trial. J Urol. 2010;184:984–9.

25. Dulucq JL, Wintringer P, Mahajna A. Totally extraperitoneal hernia repair after radical prostatectomy or previous lower abdominal surgery. Surg Endosc. 2006;20:473.

Recurrent Inguinal Hernia Repair

Jared McAllister and Jeffrey A. Blatnik

Introduction

Inguinal hernia repair is one of the most common operations performed by general surgeons in the USA, with about 800,000 operations performed annually [1]. Recurrence rates vary significantly with the type of repair performed, hernia characteristics, and clinical context. The percentage of inguinal hernia repair done for recurrence has decreased over time, from 16% in 1992 to 9% in 2008, according to the Swedish hernia database [2, 3]. This change is also reflected in data from Olmsted County, Minnesota, showing the incidence of recurrent inguinal hernia repair (IHR) decreasing from 66 to 26 per 100,000 person-years over the 19-year period from 1989 to 2008 [3]. This trend has been accompanied by increasing prevalence of modern techniques, including the use of mesh to obtain a tension-free repair and new minimally invasive methods, with tissue repair falling out of favor. Meta-analysis from the Cochrane database shows that mesh repairs decrease the relative risk of recurrence by 50–75% in comparison to tissue repairs [4, 5],

J. McAllister
Section of Minimally Invasive Surgery, Department of Surgery, Washington University School of Medicine, St. Louis, MO, USA

J. A. Blatnik (✉)
Section of Minimally Invasive Surgery, Department of Surgery, Washington University Medical Center Department of Surgery, St. Louis, MO, USA

leaving traditional tissue repairs for contaminated settings where mesh is contraindicated. The optimal method of repair in the setting of recurrence is still debated and depends on the method of primary repair and clinical setting.

Current Techniques for Repair

The major inguinal hernia repair techniques in use today all utilize mesh and can be categorized as open or laparoscopic and anterior or posterior. The Lichtenstein repair is the classic open approach and is a form of anterior repair, where mesh is placed anterior to the transversalis fascia, covering only the inguinal space. One popular variation of this repair adds a mesh plug placed in the indirect space after the hernia sac is reduced. The Nyhus or open preperitoneal mesh repair (OPMR) is a form of open posterior repair, where mesh is placed deep to transversalis muscle in the preperitoneal plane, allowing coverage of the femoral as well as inguinal spaces. A third open technique utilizes a connected bilayer polypropylene mesh device (BPMD) to place mesh in both the anterior and posterior planes, combining aspects of the Lichtenstein and OPMR repairs.

The two major laparoscopic repair techniques are the transabdominal preperitoneal (TAPP) approach and the totally extraperitoneal (TEP) approach. Both place mesh in the posterior preperitoneal position and cover the femoral and

© Springer International Publishing AG, part of Springer Nature 2018
M. P. LaPinska, J. A. Blatnik (eds.), *Surgical Principles in Inguinal Hernia Repair*,
https://doi.org/10.1007/978-3-319-92892-0_21

inguinal spaces. The TEP technique allows the surgeon to stay totally extraperitoneal and completely avoid violation of the peritoneal cavity, but has a somewhat harder learning curve and can be difficult in the setting of previous lower abdominal surgery, including Pfannenstiel incisions and prior posterior hernia repair. Both approaches have also been described utilizing robotic surgical technology with increasing prevalence.

Recurrence

Location of Recurrence

Hernia recurrence can be described as occurring in either the direct or indirect space. The data after Lichtenstein repair is mixed, with earlier series showing the direct space as the most common location of recurrence [6]. However, recent studies including a Swedish database study of over 700 patients found that recurrences after Lichtenstein repair most commonly occur in the same space as the original hernia, with 81% of recurrences after primary indirect hernia occurring in the indirect space on subsequent laparoscopy [7, 8]. Evidence regarding recurrence after laparoscopic repair is also somewhat mixed, with several small series showing most recurrences in the indirect space, thought to be caused by inadequate lateral fixation, small mesh size, or inadequate dissection of the cord structures [9, 10]. A larger series looking at 53 recurrences after previous TAPP repair, however, found that two thirds of recurrences were located caudally or medially from the previously placed mesh [11].

Risk Factors for Recurrence

Numerous risk factors have been suggested to predispose patients to recurrence after primary inguinal hernia repair. Large studies have found that female sex, direct hernia type at primary repair, reoperation for recurrent hernia, and smoking were significant risk factors for inguinal hernia recurrence. Of these, smoking is the only modifiable risk factor, and smoking cessation should be strongly encouraged in all patients

undergoing repair [7, 12]. Sliding hernia type, where one wall of the hernia is formed from an organ such as the colon or bladder, is also an independent risk factor for recurrence [13]. In addition, postoperative complications and specific operative techniques have been shown to increase risk of recurrence, with tissue repairs having the highest rates of recurrence [14]. Recent evidence also suggests that recurrence rates depend on hospital type and volume, with specialized hernia centers and centers reporting greater than 50 procedures per year having significantly lower recurrence rates [15, 16].

Multiple repairs are another clear risk factor, and each failed hernia repair increases the subsequent rate of recurrence [12, 17]. One 8-year study found recurrence and reoperation rates after primary inguinal hernia repair of 3.1%. After having a first recurrence requiring reoperation, the risk of a subsequent recurrence requiring reoperation increased to 8% [18]. A growing body of literature now points to systemic connective tissue disease as a cause of hernia creation and recurrence. There is a clear association with abdominal aortic aneurysm (AAA) and abdominal wall defects. The vascular literature shows that patients undergoing AAA treatment are 2.3-fold more likely to have an inguinal hernia than those undergoing treatment for aortoiliac occlusive disease ($p < 0.0001$), with the mechanism likely related to connective tissue defects in both disease states [19]. This data points to two important ideas: (1) the first inguinal hernia repair provides the best chance to obtain a durable repair; and (2) some patients have an increased propensity for hernia development due to systemic connective tissue disease and thus may be more resistant to definitive repair.

Of note, heavy lifting and return to normal physical activity soon after inguinal hernia repair have not been shown to increase the risk of recurrence [20]. One large study compared three groups of postoperative hernia repair patients: group 1 was instructed to resume usual work and daily activities the day after surgery ($n = 1059$), group 2 was a cohort of patients presenting in similar clinics with no specific instructions given ($n = 1306$), and group 3 consisted of patients in the Danish Hernia Database ($n = 8297$) and were given no specific instructions. At a median time of 16 months postoperatively, the patients instructed to resume activity the day after surgery (group 1) had reoperation rates of 0.7%, compared to 1.6% and 1.4% for groups 2 and 3 (p = NS). Despite these instructions, a significant portion of patients in group 1 had not returned to full activity at 7 days, and pain was cited as the most common reason for delay in full activity. Regardless, the study demonstrates that instructions for next-day return to full activity do not increase rates of short-term recurrence [21]. Similarly, evidence has not shown increased rates of recurrence related to the use of lightweight mesh or use of alternative fixation such as fibrin glue or self-adhering mesh [22–24].

Approach to the Recurrent Hernia

Symptomatology in recurrent inguinal hernia is like that of primary hernia and includes inguinal swelling, pain, and history of obstructive symptoms. Signs of mesh infection should be noted on history and physical exam and may include skin changes, warmth, erythema, and draining sinus tracts. An infected mesh will significantly affect operative planning and may require multiple future procedures beginning with excision of the affected mesh and pathogen clearance. Additional imaging is not generally required to make a diagnosis of recurrent hernia but should be utilized if the diagnosis is unclear due to atypical symptomatology or exam findings. Ultrasound (US), CT scan, and magnetic resonance imaging (MRI) have all been found to have adequate sensitivity and specificity for detection of inguinal hernia. Ultrasound is the appropriate initial study if expertise in this modality is available [25, 26].

Indications for repair of recurrent inguinal hernia are primarily guided by symptomatology. As in primary hernia, signs of strangulation, obstruction, or bowel perforation require urgent operative repair. Watchful waiting is considered safe with low rates of serious complication when the recurrent hernia is asymptomatic or minimally symptomatic, but repair is generally recommended for symptomatic patients who are fit to undergo surgery [27].

Evaluation of patients with recurrent inguinal hernia should always seek to identify the technique and mesh location used in the primary repair. In the case of prior mesh repair, the surgeon will want to know whether the mesh was placed in an anterior or posterior position and whether mesh plugs or other novel devices were used, as this may alter the anatomy and approach of subsequent repair.

The Optimal Repair Type

Attempts to identify an optimal method for repairing the recurrent hernia have yielded somewhat mixed results. A meta-analysis of 12 randomized prospective trials comparing Lichtenstein with laparoscopic techniques in recurrent inguinal repair showed that laparoscopic repair was associated with significantly less chronic pain (9.2% vs. 21.5%, p = 0.003) and shorter return to daily activities (13.9 vs. 18.4 days), but with significantly longer operative time (62.9 vs 54.2 min). This analysis also found a nonsignificant trend toward lower rates of re-recurrence among the laparoscopic group (8.3% vs. 11.6%, p = 0.16) [28].

Current guidelines from the European and international hernia societies suggest that the optimal type of repair in the setting of recurrence depends on the primary repair type and surgical expertise available. In general, when the primary repair is an open anterior repair (i.e., Lichtenstein type), recurrent repair should utilize a laparoscopic posterior approach. When the primary hernia is repaired with a posterior approach, the open anterior approach should be used for recurrent repair [26, 29]. With this strategy in mind, previously placed inguinal mesh is not routinely removed and often not encountered on reoperation. Exceptions to this occur when the mesh is a suspected source of chronic pain and in the case of mesh infection, where mesh removal is usually warranted. In the setting of a prior tissue-based repair, both anterior and posterior mesh-based repairs are acceptable options for reoperation, though evidence points to decreased pain and shorter return to activity with laparoscopic approaches [28, 30, 31].

Posterior mesh repair for recurrent hernia after open anterior mesh repair may lead to decreased recurrences and improved patient-reported outcomes. The Danish Hernia Database, which captures >98% of all inguinal hernia repairs done in Denmark, looked retrospectively at all inguinal hernias that underwent Lichtenstein repair and found that reoperation with laparoscopic repair (TEP or TAPP) resulted in significantly lower rates of subsequent recurrence than if the reoperation was performed with open techniques (Fig. 21.1). As a retrospective database study, these results are limited by lack of randomization, selection bias, and tendency to miss smaller recurrences that do not require reoperation [18]. Other studies have not shown decreased recurrence rates with laparoscopic repair after previous open repair, but have shown that this method results in decreased postoperative pain, decreased chronic pain, shorter convalescence time, and lower rates of wound infection [29, 32, 33].

These results are not surprising given that reentry into the groin with the same approach has the potential to be significantly more difficult and require dissection through significant scar tissue that obscures planes and makes important structures more vulnerable to injury. In contrast, the laparoscopic approach to the groin after previous open anterior repair (Fig. 21.1) completely avoids the anterior mesh and scar, allowing the surgeon to dissect through clean tissue planes and place mesh well away from the prior repair, covering both the inguinal and femoral spaces. The choice of TAPP versus TEP in the reoperative groin is dependent on surgeon experience and comfort level with each procedure, and data is not convincing that one technique is superior [34]. However, patients with a previous plug-and-patch repair represent a special case in which TAPP is preferred over TEP [35] (Fig. 21.2). Mesh plugs cause peritoneal adhesions that can lead to large tears in the peritoneum during initial TEP balloon dissection. These plugs also often need to be removed during the reoperation due to chronic pain issues and to create a flat plane for mesh placement.

Similarly, reports of open preperitoneal mesh repair after previous anterior mesh repair have shown favorable results, with one trial of 107 patients showing a 2.8% recurrence rate after a minimum of 3 years of follow-up and no instances of chronic pain [36].

Conversely, in cases of recurrence after previous laparoscopic repair, the open anterior approach is often recommended as it avoids a repeat preperitoneal dissection. Evidence is not as strong in this setting, and some surgeons prefer to use a laparoscopic approach for reoperation. In that case, the TAPP procedure is generally preferred over the TEP, as the latter requires mostly blind preperitoneal dissection and is prone to large peritoneal tears when significant preperitoneal scar tissue is present [11, 35].

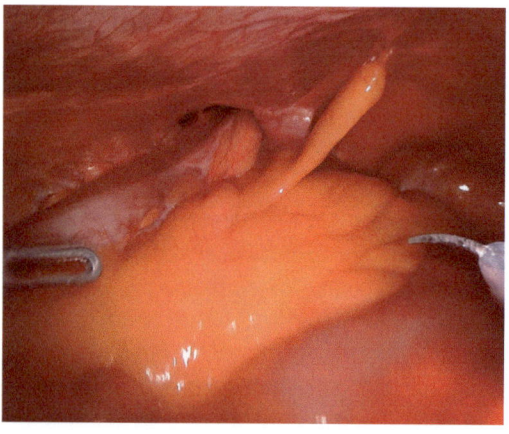

Fig. 21.1 A minimally invasive view of a recurrent inguinal right inguinal hernia with sigmoid colon involvement

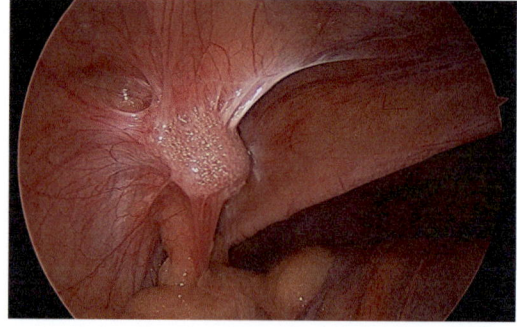

Fig. 21.2 A minimally invasive view of a previously placed open groin plug used for hernia repair. The plug can be visualized protruding into the peritoneal cavity with associated adhesions

With TAPP, the surgeon separates the peritoneum from the abdominal wall under direct visualization and thus can avoid larger peritoneal rents.

Summary

Recurrent inguinal hernia repair is a source of morbidity for patients and difficulty for surgeons. Types of mesh repair can be classified as anterior or posterior based on the location of the resultant mesh. Several factors can increase the risk of recurrence, including smoking, recurrent hernia, prior tissue repair, postoperative complications, and low hospital hernia volume. In addition, evidence suggests that hernia formation is linked to systemic connective tissue disease, and thus patient biology may play a role in recurrence. Type of mesh fixation and postoperative activity restriction do not appear to affect hernia recurrence.

When approaching the recurrent hernia, the patient's symptomatology, functional status, and prior repair type should be considered. Where the diagnosis is unclear, ultrasound is a good initial test, and the surgeon should keep the possibility of femoral hernia in mind. The optimal surgical approach for repair is a matter of some debate. Generally, laparoscopic repair for recurrent hernia results in less pain and shorter return to full activity. However, evidence suggests that anterior repair is preferred after prior laparoscopic repair, and laparoscopic repair is preferred after prior open anterior repair. This recommendation allows the surgeon to avoid prior scar tissue and avoid complications. Nonetheless, these conventions continue to be challenged by surgeons experienced in certain techniques, and case series show good results with many different methods of repair.

References

1. Rutkow IM. Demographic and socioeconomic aspects of hernia repair in the United States in 2003. Surg Clin North Am. 2003;83(5):1045–51–v–vi. https://doi.org/10.1016/S0039-6109(03)00132-4.

2. Sevonius D, Gunnarsson U, Nordin P, Nilsson E, Sandblom G. Recurrent groin hernia surgery. Br J Surg. 2011;98(10):1489–94. https://doi.org/10.1002/bjs.7559.

3. Zendejas B, Ramirez T, Jones T, et al. Incidence of inguinal hernia repairs in Olmsted County, MN: a population-based study. Ann Surg. 2013;257(3):520–6. https://doi.org/10.1097/SLA.0b013e31826d41c6.

4. Scott NW, McCormack K, Graham P, Go PM, Ross SJ, Grant AM. Open mesh versus non-mesh for repair of femoral and inguinal hernia Scott N, ed. Cochrane Database Syst Rev. 2002;(4):CD002197. https://doi.org/10.1002/14651858.CD002197.

5. Bay-Nielsen M, Kehlet H, Strand L, et al. Quality assessment of 26,304 herniorrhaphies in Denmark: a prospective nationwide study. Lancet. 2001;358(9288):1124–8. https://doi.org/10.1016/S0140-6736(01)06251-1.

6. Bay-Nielsen M, Nordin P, Nilsson E, Kehlet H. Danish Hernia Data Base and the Swedish Hernia Data Base. Operative findings in recurrent hernia after a Lichtenstein procedure. Am J Surg. 2001;182(2):134–6.

7. Burcharth J, Andresen K, Pommergaard H-C, Bisgaard T, Rosenberg J. Recurrence patterns of direct and indirect inguinal hernias in a nationwide population in Denmark. Surgery. 2014;155(1):173–7. https://doi.org/10.1016/j.surg.2013.06.006.

8. Bringman S, Holmberg H, Österberg J. Location of recurrent groin hernias at TEP after Lichtenstein repair: a study based on the Swedish Hernia Register. Hernia. 2016;20(3):387–91. https://doi.org/10.1007/s10029-016-1490-x.

9. Lamb ADG, Robson AJ, Nixon SJ. Recurrence after totally extraperitoneal laparoscopic repair: implications for operative technique and surgical training. Surgeon. 2006;4(5):299–307.

10. Felix E, Scott S, Crafton B, et al. Causes of recurrence after laparoscopic hernioplasty. A multicenter study. Surg Endosc. 1998;12(3):226–31.

11. van den Heuvel B, Dwars BJ. Repeated laparoscopic treatment of recurrent inguinal hernias after previous posterior repair. Surg Endosc. 2013;27(3):795–800. https://doi.org/10.1007/s00464-012-2514-y.

12. Burcharth J, Pommergaard H-C, Bisgaard T, Rosenberg J. Patient-related risk factors for recurrence after inguinal hernia repair: a systematic review and meta-analysis of observational studies. Surg Innov. 2015;22(3):303–17. https://doi.org/10.1177/1553350614552731.

13. Andresen K, Bisgaard T, Rosenberg J. Sliding inguinal hernia is a risk factor for recurrence. Langenbeck's Arch Surg. 2015;400(1):101–6. https://doi.org/10.1007/s00423-014-1262-y.

14. Magnusson N, Nordin P, Hedberg M, Gunnarsson U, Sandblom G. The time profile of groin hernia recurrences. Hernia. 2010;14(4):341–4. https://doi.org/10.1007/s10029-010-0648-1.

15. Andresen K, Friis-Andersen H, Rosenberg J. Laparoscopic repair of primary inguinal hernia

performed in public hospitals or low-volume centers have increased risk of reoperation for recurrence. Surg Innov. 2016;23(2):142–7. https://doi.org/10.1177/1553350615596636.

16. Malik A, Bell CM, Stukel TA, Urbach DR. Recurrence of inguinal hernias repaired in a large hernia surgical specialty hospital and general hospitals in Ontario, Canada. Can J Surg. 2016;59(1):19–25. https://doi.org/10.1503/cjs.003915.

17. Søndenaa K, Nesvik I, Breivik K, Kørner H. Long-term follow-up of 1059 consecutive primary and recurrent inguinal hernias in a teaching hospital. Eur J Surg. 2001;167(2):125–9. https://doi.org/10.1080/110241501750070583.

18. Bisgaard T, Bay-Nielsen M, Kehlet H. Re-recurrence after operation for recurrent inguinal hernia. A nationwide 8-year follow-up study on the role of type of repair. Ann Surg. 2008;247(4):707–11. https://doi.org/10.1097/SLA.0b013e31816b18e3.

19. Antoniou GA, Georgiadis GS, Antoniou SA, Granderath FA, Giannoukas AD, Lazarides MK. Abdominal aortic aneurysm and abdominal wall hernia as manifestations of a connective tissue disorder. J Vasc Surg. 2011;54(4):1175–81. https://doi.org/10.1016/j.jvs.2011.02.065.

20. Bittner R, Montgomery MA, Arregui E, et al. Update of guidelines on laparoscopic (TAPP) and endoscopic (TEP) treatment of inguinal hernia (International Endohernia Society). Surg Endosc. 2015;29(2):289–321. https://doi.org/10.1007/s00464-014-3917-8.

21. Bay-Nielsen M, Thomsen H, Andersen FH, et al. Convalescence after inguinal herniorrhaphy. Br J Surg. 2004;91(3):362–7. https://doi.org/10.1002/bjs.4437.

22. Tabbara M, Genser L, Bossi M, et al. Inguinal hernia repair using self-adhering sutureless mesh: Adhesix™: a 3-year follow-up with low chronic pain and recurrence rate. Am Surg. 2016;82(2):112–6.

23. Sun P, Cheng X, Deng S, Hu Q, Sun Y, Zheng Q. Mesh fixation with glue versus suture for chronic pain and recurrence in Lichtenstein inguinal hernioplasty. Zheng Q, ed. Cochrane Database Syst Rev. 2017;2:CD010814. https://doi.org/10.1002/14651858.CD010814.pub2.

24. Ozmen J, Choi V, Hepburn K, Hawkins W, Loi K. Laparoscopic totally extraperitoneal groin hernia repair using a self-gripping mesh: clinical results of 235 primary and recurrent groin hernias. J Laparoendosc Adv Surg Tech A. 2015;25(11):915–9. https://doi.org/10.1089/lap.2015.0056.

25. Robinson A, Light D, Kasim A, Nice C. A systematic review and meta-analysis of the role of radiology in the diagnosis of occult inguinal hernia. Surg Endosc. 2013;27(1):11–8. https://doi.org/10.1007/s00464-012-2412-3.

26. Simons MP, Aufenacker T, Bay-Nielsen M, et al. European Hernia Society guidelines on the treatment of inguinal hernia in adult patients. Hernia. 2009;13(4):343–403. https://doi.org/10.1007/s10029-009-0529-7.

27. Fitzgibbons RJ, Giobbie-Hurder A, Gibbs JO, et al. Watchful waiting vs repair of inguinal hernia in minimally symptomatic men: a randomized clinical trial. JAMA. 2006;295(3):285–92. https://doi.org/10.1001/jama.295.3.285.

28. Pisanu A, Podda M, Saba A, Porceddu G, Uccheddu A. Meta-analysis and review of prospective randomized trials comparing laparoscopic and Lichtenstein techniques in recurrent inguinal hernia repair. Hernia. 2015;19(3):355–66. https://doi.org/10.1007/s10029-014-1281-1.

29. Miserez M, Peeters E, Aufenacker T, et al. Update with level 1 studies of the European Hernia Society guidelines on the treatment of inguinal hernia in adult patients. Hernia. 2014;18(2):151–63. https://doi.org/10.1007/s10029-014-1236-6.

30. Erdas E, Medas F, Gordini L, et al. Tailored anterior tension-free repair for the treatment of recurrent inguinal hernia previously repaired by anterior approach. Hernia. 2016;20(3):393–8. https://doi.org/10.1007/s10029-016-1475-9.

31. Li J, Ji Z, Li Y. Comparison of laparoscopic versus open procedure in the treatment of recurrent inguinal hernia: a meta-analysis of the results. Am J Surg. 2014;207(4):602–12. https://doi.org/10.1016/j.amjsurg.2013.05.008.

32. Yang J, Tong DN, Yao J, Chen W. Laparoscopic or Lichtenstein repair for recurrent inguinal hernia: a meta-analysis of randomized controlled trials. ANZ J Surg. 2013;83(5):312–8. https://doi.org/10.1111/ans.12010.

33. Sevonius D, Montgomery A, Smedberg S, Sandblom G. Chronic groin pain, discomfort and physical disability after recurrent groin hernia repair: impact of anterior and posterior mesh repair. Hernia. 2016;20(1):43–53. https://doi.org/10.1007/s10029-015-1439-5.

34. Köckerling F, Bittner R, Kuthe A, et al. TEP or TAPP for recurrent inguinal hernia repair-register-based comparison of the outcome. Surg Endosc. 2017:1–11. https://doi.org/10.1007/s00464-017-5416-1.

35. Chen X, Li J-W, Zhang Y, Sun J, Zheng M-H, Dong F. The surgical strategy for laparoscopic approach in recurrent inguinal hernia repair: 213 cases report. Zhonghua Wai Ke Za Zhi. 2013;51(9):792–5.

36. Yang B, Jiang Z-P, Li Y-R, Zong Z, Chen S. Long-term outcome for open preperitoneal mesh repair of recurrent inguinal hernia. Int J Surg. 2015;19:134–6. https://doi.org/10.1016/j.ijsu.2015.05.029.

Training General Surgery Residents in Inguinal Hernia Repair

Nicole Kissane Lee, Vandana Botta, and Mariah Alexander Beasley

Introduction

In the United States, inguinal hernia repairs are the most commonly performed surgical procedures with over 700,000 cases per year in 2003 [17]. Due to the high prevalence of inguinal hernias, general surgery residents across the country often have early and extensive experience in performing inguinal herniorrhaphies. Despite this early exposure, variations in operative training, clinical curriculum, case loads, and expertise of teaching staff in combination with the lack of a unanimous teaching protocol inherently lead to differences in resident training between surgical residency programs.

The volume of inguinal hernia cases has likely remained constant over time; however the variety of surgical intervention has broadened such that the same number of cases is now being performed via three different modalities: open, laparoscopic, and robotic [13]. Increasing favor of laparoscopic and minimally invasive surgical [MIS] operations has consequently led to decreased resident exposure to open hernia repair [13]. As such, we feel that residents need further teaching and learning opportunities in open hernia repair. In the paragraphs to follow, we will discuss our institution's successful and well-received open hernia lab. Of note, in this lab we teach non-mesh repairs, specifically the Bassini and McVay techniques, as they are of historical significance, rarely performed in current times, and frequently seen on national exams. In addition, we have found benefit in teaching these open repair techniques to our residents who may necessitate this specific skill while in operative settings where no mesh or advanced resources are available for hernia repair.

Training Modalities

Surgical training has traditionally established its foundations in the Halstedian model of "See one, do one, teach one" in which residents earn graduated clinical responsibilities and operative autonomy as they progress through their training [15]. Although hands-on instruction in the operating room remains a vital component of surgical training, rapidly emerging innovations in the field of surgery have necessitated a simultaneous expansion of surgical training modalities [2-4, 7 and 8].

Duty hour restrictions and increasingly stringent standards for patient safety may also contribute to decreased resident autonomy and

N. K. Lee (✉)
Indiana University School of Medicine, Department of Surgery, Indianapolis, IN, USA

V. Botta
University of Tennessee School of Medicine, Memphis, TN, USA

M. A. Beasley
University of Tennessee School of Medicine, Department of Surgery, Knoxville, TN, USA

operative time, forcing residency programs to implement training strategies in addition to the Halsted model [1].

Most surgical training programs adhere to Ericsson et al.'s emphasis on the importance of teaching and assessing both cognitive and technical skills [6, 9]. This may be achieved through a combination of teaching tools. Visual presentations whether in the form of brief videos or slides can provide didactic information such as relevant anatomy, indications and contraindications, potential intraoperative and postoperative complications, and details of surgical technique prior to learning the technique itself. Baseline assessment of knowledge may be evaluated with pretests or oral discussion. Live video adjuncts and post-video assessment with immediate feedback on a trainee's technical strengths and weaknesses have also been proven as effective modalities of surgical training [1]. Dry labs with simulators, models, or mannequins may serve as effective adjuncts prior to transitioning to ex vivo wet labs in which animal or cadaveric models. In a study by Sharma et al. [18], resident operative competency and confidence were significantly improved by simply participating in a brief, 8-week, procedurally oriented cadaver anatomy review course.

Training Residents at Our Institution

The primary modalities utilized for training our residents are visual adjuncts and cadaveric wet labs. Prior to the procedure, residents are provided an overview of relevant inguinal anatomy and surgical techniques through slides and are required to complete a pretest on these concepts. The pretest serves as an objective analysis of knowledge and preparation for this lab and consists of basic hernia repair techniques and surgical considerations. Residents are encouraged to review hernia repair techniques prior to the lab by accessing online modules. In our program, we recommend the SCORE curriculum [5].

The cadaveric wet lab is facilitated by general surgery attendings with extensive experience in

inguinal hernia repair as well as experience in formal teaching of proper surgical technique. The ratio of instructor to student is 1:2. The learning objectives for this lab include:

1. Understand and describe relevant anatomy for inguinal hernia repair.
2. Create a surgical plan for repair utilizing open repair, without mesh.
3. Identify elements of successful hernia repair including anatomic considerations, suture composition, instrumentation, and tissue handling.
4. Determine the most appropriate hernia repair technique for patient care and long-term outcomes, and describe indications and potential intraoperative and postoperative complications.
5. Develop a comprehensive management plan for hernias repaired by open technique, without the use of mesh. Contrast this management plan with respective plans for open repair with mesh, laparoscopic repair, and robotic repair.

The lab begins with an overall review of anatomy led by faculty and adjunct faculty expertise provided by Chief Residents in general surgery. A short 10-min didactic lecture reviews basic inguinal anatomy and various types of hernias. The focus then turns to the cadaveric models.

The cadaver is marked to identify important anatomical landmarks including the anterior superior iliac spine, pubic tubercle, anticipated locations of the deep and superficial inguinal rings and inguinal canal, and the ilioinguinal and iliohypogastric nerves. Discussion then ensues regarding placement of the ilioinguinal nerve block and adequate administration of local anesthetic (Fig. 22.1).

After all pertinent surface anatomy is marked and reviewed by faculty for accuracy, the residents begin dissection and identify anatomic layers, including but not limited to Camper's, Scarpa's, and external oblique fasciae (Fig. 22.2). In the usual fashion, the students are directed to open the external oblique aponeurotic fibers

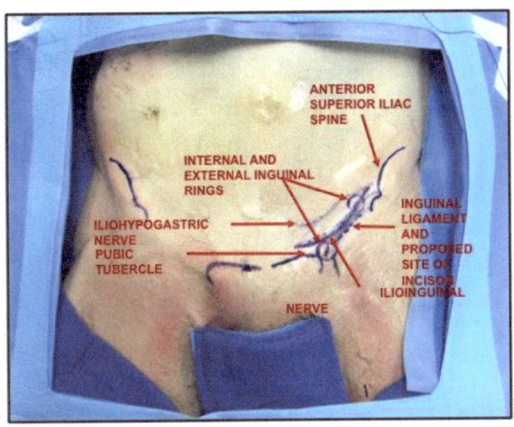

Fig. 22.1 Surface anatomy and pertinent anatomical landmarks

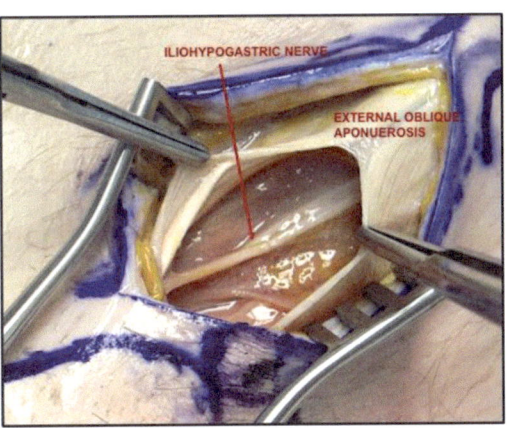

Fig. 22.3 Division of external oblique aponeurosis and identification of iliohypogastric nerve

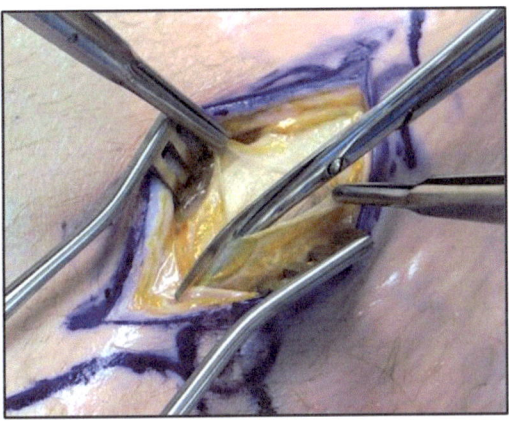

Fig. 22.2 Incisions through Camper's and Scarpa's fasciae

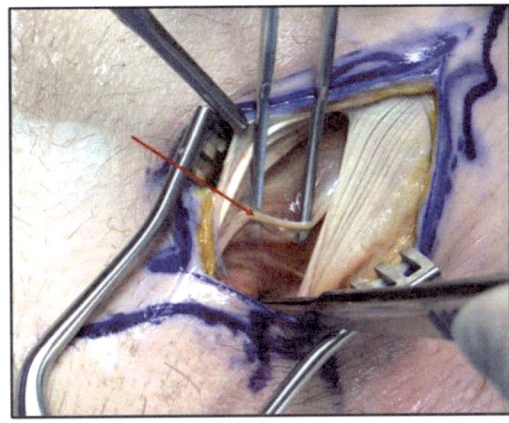

Fig. 22.4 Care is taken to dissect the ileohypogastric nerve and prevent inadvertent injury

along their length and identify and protect cord structures, specifically the overlying nerve tissue (Figs. 22.3 and 22.4).

The cord is then navigated circumferentially, again reinforcing discussion of relevant anatomical considerations (Fig. 22.5). Teaching faculty are encouraged to discuss nearby vessels, specifically the femoral vessels, and illustrate them for the learners if possible (Fig. 22.6). The inguinal region is then examined for direct, indirect, or femoral hernia defects, and any cord lipomas are removed as necessary (Fig. 22.7). The content of the cord itself is examined, identified, and preserved (Fig. 22.8).

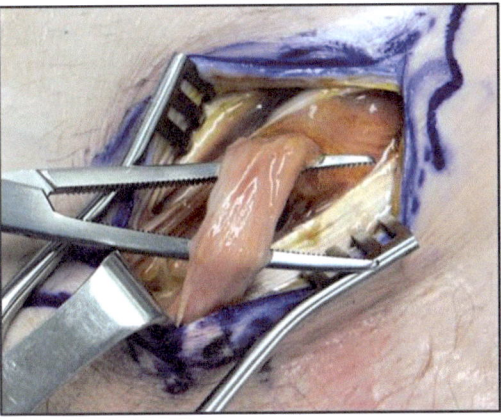

Fig. 22.5 Identification of spermatic cord

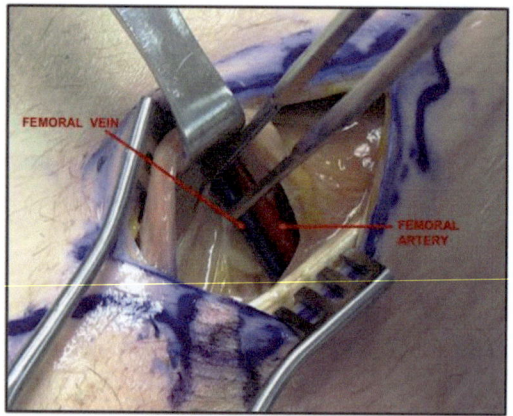

Fig. 22.6 Identification of femoral vessels

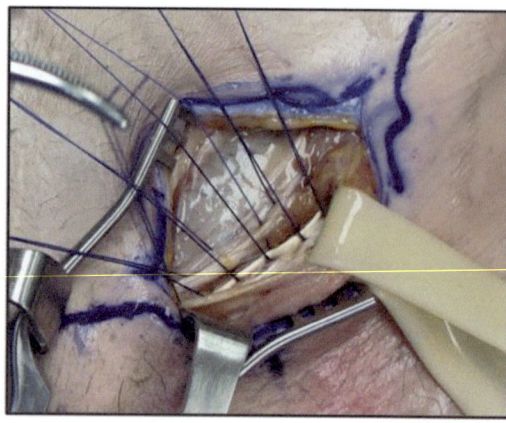

Fig. 22.9 Bassini repair: triple layer approximated to inguinal ligament (Poupart's ligament)

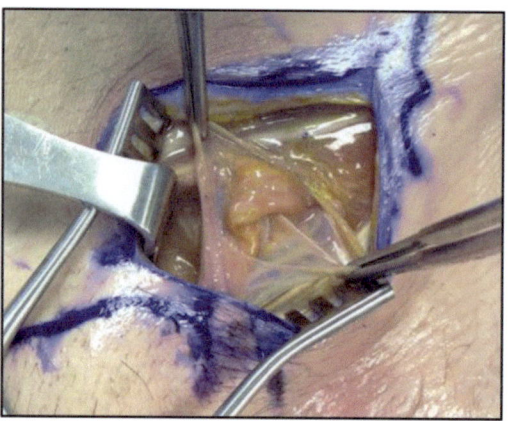

Fig. 22.7 Dissection of cord

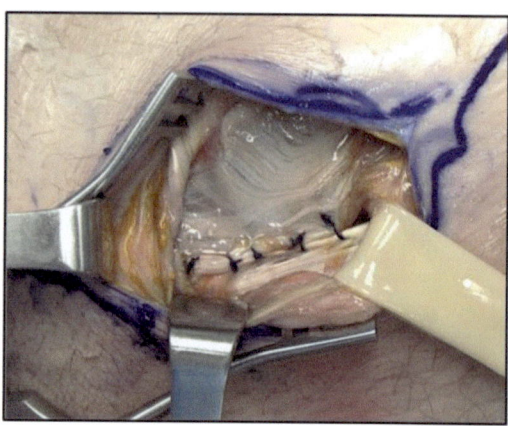

Fig. 22.10 Closure of internal ring with non-absorbable, interrupted sutures in Bassini repair

We then proceed with non-mesh Bassini repair, suturing the transversalis fascia and conjoint tendon to the inguinal ligament (Figs. 22.9 and 22.10).

Upon completion of the Bassini repair, faculty guide students through the McVay repair, again discussing relevant anatomical considerations. The McVay repair reapproximates the transversus abdominis aponeurosis and transversalis fascia to Cooper's ligament and the iliopubic tract (Fig. 22.11). Finally, a relaxing incision is performed and discussed given the high-tension nature of this repair (Fig. 22.12). The hernia defect is then closed in layers in the

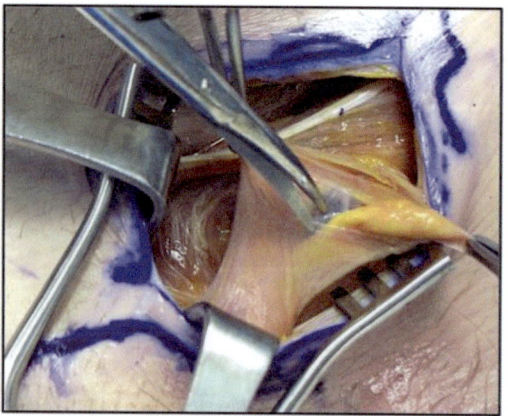

Fig. 22.8 Exploration of cord contents and identification and dissection of hernia sac

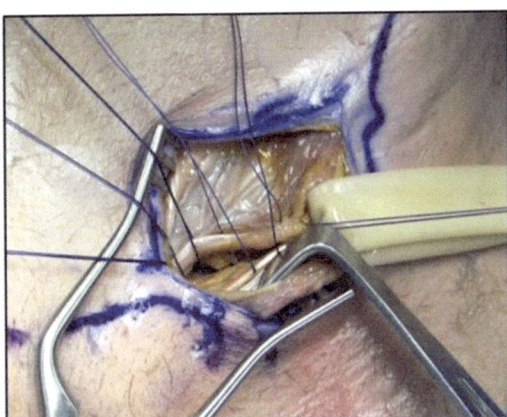

Fig. 22.11 McVay repair: triple layer approximated to Cooper's ligament with lateral transition stitch

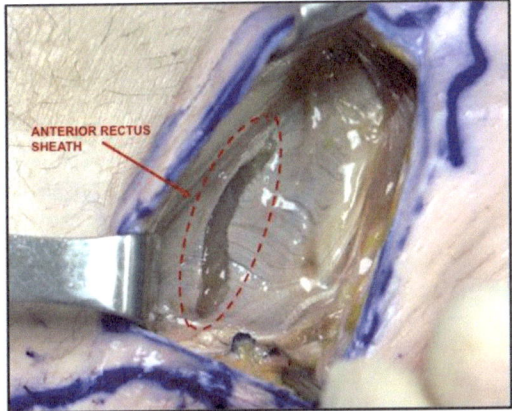

Fig. 22.12 Relaxing incision through anterior rectus sheath

usual fashion, beginning with the external oblique fibers and concluding with the epidermis.

As each cadaver has two inguinal regions, students are provided with additional lab time to perform herniorrhaphy on the contralateral side. We encourage junior residents to guide one another through the case to experience learning and dissection from a faculty perspective. Faculty remain available to mentor and coach this repair as necessary.

Upon completion of the lab, residents and faculty are assessed for performance and learning. The objectives noted previously are highlighted in this assessment, as are performance benchmarks appropriate to student level. Using an assessment module based upon the Objective Structured Assessment of Technical Skills [OSATS] criteria, we evaluate each resident for critical deficiencies and level of competency as seen in Fig. 22.13 [11, 12 14]. This assessment module is used during the lab by observing faculty to evaluate residents as they progress through procedure. The assessment focuses on tissue handling, dexterity, effort, and efficiency. The participating residents complete a posttest as an adjunct, objective assessment module; this test specifically highlights open, non-mesh herniorrhaphy and the relevant anatomy and surgical considerations.

Future Directions

With the rapidly expanding body of knowledge in surgery, surgical training, and biomedical innovation, many novel training modalities are emerging. Several studies have supported the efficacy of medical simulation and virtual reality [VR] simulators in not only improving residents' technical skills and proficiency but also patient outcomes [9, 16, 21]. VR simulation could potentially serve as a high-fidelity, cost-effective surgical training modality [10]. With growing enthusiasm for robotic hernia repair, particularly inguinal and ventral hernia repair, surgery residents stand to benefit from the development of standardized robotic simulator modules for such repairs on currently available robotic training simulators [19]. Lastly, the development of a universal education on core hernia techniques would standardize residency education internationally and provide a better basis for both patient care and future exam preparation [20].

OPEN, NON-MESH, INGUINAL HERNIA REPAIR

PRACTICE DOMAIN	COMPETENCY	CRITICAL DEFICIENCIES	LEVEL 1	LEVEL 2	LEVEL 3	LEVEL 4
SELF-DIRECTED LEARNING (SDL)	PRACTICE-BASED LEARNING AND IMPROVEMENT (PBLI2)	• Unable to meet minimum benchmarks. • The resident dose not complete simulation assignments. The resident is frequently absent for scheduled simulation exercises without a valid excuse. • The trainee is not motivated or focused and makes little progress. • The trainee is not open to suggestion for improvement.	• Knowledge of inguinal anatomy & pathology. • Basic operative skills. • Identifies the basic anatomy and pathology of the inguinal canal. • Knows the steps of inguinal dissection. • The trainee struggles to use both hands equally or uses only one instrument at a time. • The trainee requires more practice and needs to focus on skills development.	• The trainee uses two hands but not equally. • The trainee becomes frustrated and rushed or is easily distracted. • Knowledge of the different types of inguinal repairs and complications and indications of each.	• The trainee uses both hands but tends to use a large volume of space to work. • The trainee is putting in the effort but is slow to implement changes that will improve efficiency when critiqued.	• The trainee smoothly uses bimanual dexterity with optimum economy of motion. • The trainee is focused on the task, not easily distracted, and finds unique ways to increase efficiency.
			1	1.5	2	2.5	3	3.5	4

(Score scale below LEVEL columns: 1 | 1.5 | 2 | 2.5 | 3 | 3.5 | 4)

COMMENTS:

Trainee: _____   Date: _____   Final Score: _____

Assessor: _____

UT Center for Advanced Medical Simulation   Department of Surgery

Fig. 22.13 Objective Structured Assessment of Technical Skills [OSATS] assessment for general surgery residents participating in cadaveric open inguinal herniorrhaphy lab

Acknowledgments The authors would like to thank Hobart Akin, MD, FACS, Sperry Nelson, MD, FACS, and the staff at the University of Tennessee Center for Advanced Medical Simulation for their invaluable contributions to this hernia curriculum.

References

1. Abdelsattar JM, Pandian TK, Finnesgard EJ, El Khatib MM, Rowse PG, Buckarma EN, et al. Do you see what I see? How we use video as an adjunct to general surgery resident education. J Surg Educ. 2015;72(6):e145–50.

2. Andresen K, Laursen J, Rosenberg J. Teaching the Onstep technique for inguinal hernia repair, results from a focus group interview. Surg Res Pract. 2016;2016:4787648.

3. Balayla J, Bergman S, Ghitulescu G, Feldman LS, Fraser SA. Knowing the operative game plan: a novel tool for the assessment of surgical procedural knowledge. Can J Surg. 2012;55(4):S158–62.

4. Cauraugh JH, Martin M, Martin KK. Modeling surgical expertise for motor skill acquisition. Am J Surg. 1999;177(4):331–6.

5. Colonna AL. Inguinal and femoral hernia repair. The Surgical Council on Resident Education [SCORE] Portal. http://www.surgicalcore.org. Published March 16, 2017.

6. Ericsson KA, Krampe RT, Tesch-Römer C. The role of deliberate practice in the acquisition of expert performance. Psychol Rev. 1993;100(3):363–406.

7. Ericsson KA. Deliberate practice and the acquisition and maintenance of expert performance in medicine and related domains. Acad Med. 2004;79(10 Suppl):S70–81.

8. Hall JC. Imagery practice and the development of surgical skills. Am J Surg. 2002;184(5):465–70.

9. Hamilton EC, Scott DJ, Kapoor A, Nwariaku F, Bergen PC, Rege RV, et al. Improving operative performance using a laparoscopic hernia simulator. Am J Surg. 2001;182(6):725–8.

10. Hernández-Irizarry R, Zendejas B, Ali SM, Farley DR. Optimizing training cost-effectiveness of simulation-based laparoscopic inguinal hernia repairs. Am J Surg. 2016;211(2):326–35.

11. Martin JA, Regehr G, Reznick R. Objective structured assessment of technical skill (OSATS) for surgical residents. Br J Surg. 1997;84(2):273–8.

12. Masters RS, Lo CY, Maxwell JP, Patil NG. Implicit motor learning in surgery: implications for multitasking. Surgery. 2008;143(1):140–5.

13. McCoy AC, Gasevic E, Szlabick RE, Sahmoun AE, Sticca RP. Are open abdominal procedures a thing of the past? An analysis of graduating general surgery residents' case logs from 2000 to 2011. J Surg Educ. 2013;70(6):683–9.

14. Niitsu H, Hirabayashi N, Yoshimitsu M, et al. Using the Objective Structured Assessment of Technical Skills (OSATS) global rating scale to evaluate the skills of surgical trainees in the operating room. Surg Today. 2013;43:271–5.

15. Polavarapu HV, Kulaylat AN, Sun S, Hamed OH. 100 years of surgical education: the past, present, and future. Bull Am Coll Surg. 2013;98(7):22–7.

16. Rochlen LR, et al. First-person point-of-view-augmented reality for central line insertion training. Simul Healthc. 2017;12(1):57–61.

17. Rutkow IM. Demographic and socioeconomic aspects of hernia repair in the United States in 2003. Surg Clin North Am. 2003;83(5):1045–51, v–vi.

18. Sharma G, Aycart MA, Najjar PA, van Houten T, Smink DS, Askari R, et al. A cadaveric procedural anatomy course enhances operative competence. J Surg Res. 2016;201(1):22–8.

19. Waite KE, Herman MA, Doyle PJ. Comparison of robotic versus laparoscopic transabdominal preperitoneal (TAPP) inguinal hernia repair. J Robot Surg. 2016;10(3):239–44.

20. Wilkiemeyer M, Pappas TN, Giobbie-Hurder A, Itani KM, Jonasson O, Neumayer LA. Does resident post graduate year influence the outcomes of inguinal hernia repair? Ann Surg. 2005;241(6):879–82; discussion 882–4.

21. Zendejas B, Cook DA, Bingener J, Huebner M, Dunn WF, Sarr MG, et al. Simulation-based mastery learning improves patient outcomes in laparoscopic inguinal hernia repair: a randomized controlled trial. Ann Surg. 2011;254(3):502–9.

Index

© Springer International Publishing AG, part of Springer Nature 2018
M. P. LaPinska, J. A. Blatnik (eds.), *Surgical Principles in Inguinal Hernia Repair*,
https://doi.org/10.1007/978-3-319-92892-0

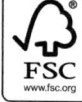

MIX
Papier aus verantwortungsvollen Quellen
Paper from responsible sources
FSC® C105338

If you have any concerns about our products,
you can contact us on
ProductSafety@springernature.com

In case Publisher is established outside the EU,
the EU authorized representative is:
Springer Nature Customer Service Center GmbH
Europaplatz 3, 69115 Heidelberg, Germany

Printed by Libri Plureos GmbH
in Hamburg, Germany